EAI/Springer Innovations in Communication and Computing

Series Editor

Editor's Note

The impact of information technologies is creating a new world yet not fully understood. The extent and speed of economic, life style and social changes already perceived in everyday life is hard to estimate without understanding the technological driving forces behind it. This series presents contributed volumes featuring the latest research and development in the various information engineering technologies that play a key role in this process.

The range of topics, focusing primarily on communications and computing engineering include, but are not limited to, wireless networks; mobile communication; design and learning; gaming; interaction; e-health and pervasive healthcare; energy management; smart grids; internet of things; cognitive radio networks; computation; cloud computing; ubiquitous connectivity, and in mode general smart living, smart cities, Internet of Things and more. The series publishes a combination of expanded papers selected from hosted and sponsored European Alliance for Innovation (EAI) conferences that present cutting edge, global research as well as provide new perspectives on traditional related engineering fields. This content, complemented with open calls for contribution of book titles and individual chapters, together maintain Springer's and EAI's high standards of academic excellence. The audience for the books consists of researchers, industry professionals, advanced level students as well as practitioners in related fields of activity include information and communication specialists, security experts, economists, urban planners, doctors, and in general representatives in all those walks of life affected ad contributing to the information revolution.

Indexing: This series is indexed in Scopus, Ei Compendex, and zbMATH.

About EAI

EAI is a grassroots member organization initiated through cooperation between businesses, public, private and government organizations to address the global challenges of Europe's future competitiveness and link the European Research community with its counterparts around the globe. EAI reaches out to hundreds of thousands of individual subscribers on all continents and collaborates with an institutional member base including Fortune 500 companies, government organizations, and educational institutions, provide a free research and innovation platform.

Through its open free membership model EAI promotes a new research and innovation culture based on collaboration, connectivity and recognition of excellence by community.

More information about this series at http://www.springer.com/series/15427

Lalit Garg • Chinmay Chakraborty • Saïd Mahmoudi
Victor S. Sohmen
Editors

Healthcare Informatics for Fighting COVID-19 and Future Epidemics

Springer

EAI
RESEARCH MEETS INNOVATION

Editors
Lalit Garg
Information and Communication Technology
University of Malta
Msida, Malta

Saïd Mahmoudi
University of Mons
Mons, Belgium

Chinmay Chakraborty
Electronics & Communication Engineering
Birla Institute of Technology
Jharkhand, India

Victor S. Sohmen
Harrisburg University of Science and Tec
Harrisburg, PA, USA

ISSN 2522-8595 ISSN 2522-8609 (electronic)
EAI/Springer Innovations in Communication and Computing
ISBN 978-3-030-72751-2 ISBN 978-3-030-72752-9 (eBook)
https://doi.org/10.1007/978-3-030-72752-9

This Springer imprint is published by the registered company Springer Nature Switzerland AG
The registered company address is: Gewerbestrasse 11, 6330 Cham, Switzerland

Preface

The COVID-19 outbreak is among the most significant tragedies the world has ever faced. It has already killed millions of people; hundreds of millions of people are infected, billions of people faced lockdown and costing trillions of USDs to the world economy. Intelligent healthcare informatics can play a vital role in this challenging time. This book titled "Healthcare Informatics for Fighting COVID-19 and Future Epidemics" within the *EAI/Springer Innovations in Communication and Computing* series is a set of 21 chapters selected after peer-review from total 40 chapters received as the response to a closed call for chapters attracting submissions from contacts including eminent researchers, academicians and practitioners worldwide. We take this opportunity to profoundly appreciate the reviewers for their work reviewing the chapters for this book.

The book's objective is to present innovative solutions utilising informatics to deal with various issues related to the COVID-19 outbreak. The book will focus on health data analytics, information exchange, knowledge sharing, Internet of Things (IoT)-based solutions, healthcare informatics solutions' applications, management, implementation, assessment and adoption. The chapters present innovative approaches utilising various healthcare informatics to analyse COVID-19 data to characterise the COVID-19 infection spread in the population, its impact, tools available to diagnose and manage the infection, and forecasting its progression. These chapters survey the state-of-the-art developments in the literature and propose novel intelligent methods to address COVID-19 pandemic. This book primarily covers COVID-19 research needs to be urgently available to researchers, academicians, practitioners and policymakers. This research can also be helpful in better preparing for better controlling and managing future epidemics.

The first chapter titled "Novel COVID-19 Recognition Framework based on Conic Functions Classifier" by Ahmad M. Karim from Ankara Yildirim Beyazit University (AYBU), Ankara, Turkey and Alok Mishra from Molde University College-Specialized University in Logistics, Norway and Atilim University, Ankara, Turkey. The authors proposed a solution aiming to diagnose COVID-19 by using local binary patterns (LBP) and factor analysis, based on the conic functions classifier. The conic functions classifier presents remarkable results compared with the popular classifiers and state-of-the-art studies presented in the literature. The aim of using LBP is to analyse the input COVID-19 image and extract salient features.

The second chapter titled "A Real-Time Review of Social Health Protection and Health Informatics Support for COVID-19 Outbreak" is authored by Chokri Arfa from National Institute of Labour and Social Studies, University of Carthagee, Ariana, Tunisia, Ilker Dastan from the World Health Organization's Regional Office for Eastern Mediterranean, Cairo, Egypt, Kamel Barkaoui from Conservatoire National des Arts et Metiers, Paris, France and Borgi Taoufik from the Computer Center of the Ministry of Health, Tunis, Le Belvedere, Tunisia. The authors present a review of decision support systems and electronic health record management as tools for data analysis and data sharing and their integration in real time into health supply chains and social health protection, making health policies more efficient, particularly those targeting patients infected with coronaviruses in need of health assistance.

The third chapter is titled "Active Learning Based Estimation of COVID-19 Pandemic: A Synergetic Case Study in Selective Regions Population" and authored by Arijit Chakraborty from The Heritage Academy, Kolkata, India, Sajal Mitra and Dipankar Das from Heritage Institute of Technology, Kolkata, India, Debnath Battacharyya from K L Deemed to be University, KLEF, Guntur, India, Debashis De and Sankar Prasad Mondal from the Maulana Abul Kalam Azad University of Technology, Kolkata, India and Anindya J. Pal from the University of Burdwan, Burdwan, India. This chapter used the support vector machine-based regression (SVR) method in predicting the adversities induced by this global pandemic in China and India and achieved a reasonably small root mean square error (RMSE). In contrast, conventional regression better estimated the outbreak pattern in Italy.

The fourth chapter title is "Management of Future Outbreaks Risks (Prevention, Control, and Treatment)". The authors are Abhinay Thakur and Ashish Kumar from Lovely Professional University, Phagwara, Punjab, India. The authors summarised the existing state of awareness of COVID-19 infection spread by addressing prevention steps, monitoring and treatment protocols to help manage current and future outbreak risks. Further, strongly support the fastest strategy to vaccinate the population that may make them immune to any new mutations that this virus could trigger in the future.

The fifth chapter is titled "Statistical Analysis of Novel COVID-19 Based on Real-Time Data and Future Epidemics" and authored by C. H. Sekhar and M. Srinivasa Rao from Vignan's Institute of Information Technology, Visakhapatnam, India, Debnath Battacharyya from K L Deemed to be University, KLEF, Guntur, India. The chapter carried out statistical analysis of COVID-19 death and recovered cases among India's various states using the dataset prepared based on the real-time data provided by the Indian Council of Medical Research (ICMR).

The sixth chapter is titled "A Real-Time Approach with Deep Learning for Pandemic Management" authored by Raghavendra Rao A. and Debabrata Samanta from CHRIST (Deemed to be University), Bangalore, India. In the chapter, an attempt was made to put together some Artificial Intelligence (AI) thoughts and healthcare to relate them to pandemic management's frequent subject. Caution is drawn towards some crucial aspects, such as security and transparency, that cannot be compromised. Some of the prominent approaches are looked at from a pandemic management point of view, which can start a more in-depth discussion on AI and healthcare going hand in hand in managing this pandemic situation. Important areas of pandemic management, such as building on the knowledge gathered over a period, plugging in the real-time data from the society, building efficient data management systems and building transparent and interpretable solutions are the focus areas of exploration in this chapter.

The seventh chapter titled, "Personal Protective Equipment for COVID-19: A Comprehensive Review" is authored by Debangana Das, Shreya Nag, Hemanta Naskar, Srikanta Acharya, Sourav Bakchi, Sheikh Saharuk Ali, Runu Banerjee Roy and Bipan Tudu from Jadavpur University, Kolkata, India and Dr. Rajib Bandyopadhyay from ITMO University, Saint Petersburg, Russia. This chapter reviews personal protective equipment (PPE) for COVID-19, medical devices (including PPE) standards, infection transmission and prevention advice.

The eighth chapter "Extensive Statistical Analysis on Novel Corona Virus, Towards Worldwide Health Using Apache Spark" is authored by Eali Stephen Neal Joshua, Bhanu Prakash Doppala and Midhun Chakkravarthy from Lincoln University College, Malaysia and Debnath Battacharyya from K L Deemed to be University, KLEF, Guntur, India. This chapter determines and compares the total case sufferer death price (CFR) for Italy, South Korea and China. Further, the chapter discusses an epidemiological effort using the ideal mathematical versions to design the results of these steps and examine the various arrangements used by scientists to anticipate precisely how the instance infection price boosts.

The ninth chapter titled "Visual Exploratory Data Analysis Technique for Epidemiological Outbreak of COVID-19 Pandemic" is authored by Joseph Bamidele Awotunde from the University of Ilorin, Ilorin, Nigeria, Roseline Oluwaseun Ogundokun and Emmanuel Abidemi Adeniyi from Landmark University, Omu-Aran, Nigeria and Sanjay Misra from Covenant University Ota, Nigeria. The chapter describes and analyses the exploration of coronavirus data reported worldwide from January to August 2020 to monitor the total number of confirmed, discharged active and death cases. For the primary analysis of the dataset, linear regression was used. It was discovered that the virus is contagious but less deadly as the total number of deaths recorded for the four months is lower compared to the recovery cases. The analysis shows that the early test of COVID-19 will eliminate the critical/severe cases and reduce the death case. The real time, generation of comprehensive and vigorous data for evolving sickness outbursts could help engender strong indication and significant support and inform public health workers and government to make a strategic decision for the citizens' wellbeing.

The tenth chapter titled, "Machine Learning Approach Using KPCA-SVMs for Predicting COVID-19" authored by Micheal Olaolu Arowolo and Roseline Oluwaseun Ogundokun from Department of Computer Science, Landmark University, Omu-Aran, Nigeria, Sanjay Misra from Covenant University, Ota, Nigeria and Akeem Femi Kadri and Tahir Olanrewaju Aduragba from Kwara State University, Malete, Nigeria. The chapter identifies relevant prognostic factors for

COVID-19 that is required to regulate the difficulties in apprehending the disease's increase. The algorithms used for the prediction are kernel principal component analysis (KPCA) and support vector machines (SVM) implemented in MATLAB. The results are evaluated using matrices like accuracy, sensitivity, specificity, *F*-score, Matthews correlation coefficient, precision and negative predictive value. A machine learning approach is proposed for COVID-19 predicting health status concerning actions and symptoms observed to help healthcare persons recognise and record incidence to verify qualified healthcare across nations.

The 11th chapter "COVID-19 Epidemic Impact on Various Society Sectors" is authored by Mohandas V. Pawar, Asha M. Pawar, Sudarshan Sanap, Rajneesh Kaur Sachdeo, Kishore Ravande, Jyoti Malhotra, H. R. Bhapkar from MIT School of Engineering, MIT ADT University, Pune, India, J. Anuradha from VIT University, Vellore, India and Pranav Pawar from Barllan University, Israel. The chapter is a detailed literature review on the various sectors of society and COVID-19 pandemic impact, providing multiple solutions using Big Data and AI measures.

The 12th chapter is titled "A New Collaborative Platform for COVID-19 Benchmark Datasets" and authored by Olivier Debauche, Saïd Mahmoudi, Sidi Ahmed Mahmoudi, and Pierre Manneback from the University of Mons, Belgium. This chapter presents a new collaborative platform allowing exchange and sharing both medical benchmark datasets and developed applications rapidly and securely between research teams. This platform aims to facilitate and encourage the exploration of new fields of research. This platform implements proven data security techniques that guarantee confidentiality, mainly Argon2id password hashing algorithm, anonymisation, expiration of forms, and datasets double encryption and decryption with AES 256-GCM XChaCha20Poly1305 algorithms.

The 13th chapter is titled "Artificial Intelligence Approaches for the COVID-19 Pandemic" and authored by Pilla Srinivas from Dadi Institute of Engineering & Technology, Anakapalle, India and Debnath Battacharyya from K L Deemed to be University, KLEF, Guntur, India. The chapter is mainly focused on digital technologies like artificial intelligence, virtual reality/augmented reality, 3D-printing, robotics, nanotechnology and their vital role for faster and effective solutions to many diseases.

The 14th chapter is titled "Towards the Development of Triboelectricity-Based Virus Killer Face Mask for COVID-19: Role of Different Inputs" and authored by Sanjay Banerjee and Sk. Babar Ali from Future Institute of Engineering and Management, Kolkata, India, Barnali Ghatak, Bipan Tudu, Krittish Roy and Kuntal Maity from Jadavpur University, Kolkata, India, Nityananda Das from Jagannath Kishore College, Purulia, West Bengal, India, Rajib Bandyopadhyay from ITMO University, Saint Petersburg, Russia and Dipankar Mandal from Habitat Centre, Mohali, India. The chapter proposes a self-powered (no external power source) face mask that does not require to be sterilised, comprising two differently charged Tribo-series materials with the outer electrocution layer.

The 15th chapter is titled "SmartCovSens: A Multimodal Approach for Detection of COVID-19" and authored by Sanjoy Banerjee and Sk. Babar Ali from Future Institute of Engineering and Management, Kolkata, India, Debangana Das,

Nilava Debabhuti, Prolay Sharma, Barnali Ghatak and Rajib Bandyopadhyay from Jadavpur University, Kolkata, India and Anwesha Sengupta from National Institute of Technology Rourkela, Rourkela, India, Saurabh Pal from the University of Calcutta, Kolkata, India, Nityananda Das from Jagannath Kishore College, Purulia, West Bengal, India, Prabal Patra and Chitresh Kundu from Tata Steel Jamshedpur, India and Arunangshu Ghosh from National Institute of Technology Patna, Patna, Bihar, India. The chapter describes a multimodal approach for rapid screening of potential COVID-19 carriers based on symptomatic sensing using a combination of sensors, followed by generation of a metric to indicate the severity of symptoms. The proposed system is likely to be a significant addition to scan COVID-19 carriers.

The 16th chapter is "Explainable Deep Learning for COVID-19 Detection Using Chest X-Ray and CT-Scan Images" authored by Sidi Ahmed Mahmoudi, Sédrick Stassin, Xavier Lessage and Saïd Mahmoudi from the University of Mons, Mons, Belgium and Mostafa El Habib Daho from the University of Tlemcen, Algeria. The chapter proposes an explainable DL model for COVID-19 images classification and segmentation with two modalities: X-ray images and CT scans. The provided explanations were evaluated by doctors and physicians that confirmed that accuracy of our results.

The 17th chapter is "Innovative Solutions to the Clinical Challenges of COVID-19" authored by S. M. Kadri and Samir Mattoo from the Directorate of Health Services, Kashmir, India, Ailbhe H. Brady from Warrington and Halton Teaching Hospitals NHS Foundation Trust, Warrington, United Kingdom and Marija Petkovic from the University of Medicine, Belgrade, Serbia. This chapter reviews the literature addressing COVID-19 clinical challenges retrospectively through the lens of informatics and detailing examples of how these challenges have been tackled.

The 18th chapter is "Being Resilient to Deal with Attrition of Nurses in Private COVID-19 Hospitals: Critical Analysis with Respect to the Crisis in Kolkata, India" authored by Soumik Gangopadhyay from the Institute of Engineering and Management, Kolkata, India and Amitava Ukil from the Eminent College of Management and Technology, Barbaria, Barasat, Kolkata, India. This chapter is a case study critically analysing the issue of nurses attrition in private COVID-19 hospitals and proposes its solutions especially focusing on 3I approach (Information, Integration and Innovation).

The 19th chapter is "Healthcare Technology for Reducing the Risk and the Spread of COVID-19 Pandemic and Other Epidemics" authored by Suchandra Dutta and Dhrubasish Sarkar from Amity Institute of Information Technology, Amity University, Kolkata, India, Premananda Jana from Netaji Subhas Open University, Kalyani, West Bengal, India and Dipak K. Kole from Jalpaiguri Government Engineering College, Jalpaiguri, West Bengal, India. This chapter addresses the outbreak of coronavirus and how digital healthcare technologies can help navigate and resolve COVID-19 and future epidemics.

The 20th chapter is "Real-Time Alert System for Delivery Operators Through Artificial Intelligence in Last-Mile Delivery" authored by Vinod Kumar Shukla and Leena Wanganoo from Amity University, Dubai, UAE and Nibhrita Tiwari from Radicon Institute of Radiology, Dubai, UAE. This chapter proposes an algorithm to predict operator's behaviour and an AI-based real-time alert system to provide a smart solution incorporating the delivery operator's behaviour such as driving pattern, fatigue check, eye blink, braking and curved angles and other road conditions alert notification on a real-time basis to avoid accidents, streamline the processes and ultimately improve the customer experience for the timely delivery of the product based in UAE.

Finally, the last chapter is "Chest X-Ray Images Analysis with Deep Convolutional Neural Networks (CNN) for COVID-19 Detection" authored by Xavier Lessage, Saïd Mahmoudi, Sidi Ahmed Mahmoudi, Sohaib Laraba, Olivier Debauche, Mohammed Amin Belarbi from the University of Mons, Mons, Belgium. This chapter proposes an approach H. R. Bhapkar of transfer learning and fine-tuning from pre-trained CNN models (InceptionV3, VGG16, MobileNet, EfficientNet, etc.) to detect COVID-19 from chest X-ray images.

The book reviews the state-of-the-art development and deals with informatics applications in COVID-19 outbreak management, including disease diagnosis, understanding and characterising infection spread, its prediction, tools to manage the spread and patient management. The book chapters are authored by 88 authors affiliated to 43 Universities, institutes, government and private organisations including WHO and national ministries. The research presented in the book will also boost our understanding of COVID-19 pandemic and its spread, trends and prepare us with novel means to manage the pandemic better.

Msida, Malta Lalit Garg

Jharkhand, India Chinmay Chakraborty

Mons, Belgium Saiïd Mahmudi

Harrisburg, PA, USA Victor S. Sohmen

Contents

Contributors

Srikanta Acharya Department of Instrumentation and Electronics Engineering, Jadavpur University, Kolkata, West Bengal, India

Emmanuel Abidemi Adeniyi Department of Computer Science, Landmark University, Omu-Aran, Nigeria

Tahir Olanrewaju Aduragba Department of Computer Science, Kwara State University, Malete, Nigeria

Sheikh Saharuk Ali Department of Instrumentation and Electronics Engineering, Jadavpur University, Kolkata, West Bengal, India

Sk. Babar Ali Department of Electronics and Communication Engineering, Future Institute of Engineering and Management, Kolkata, West Bengal, India

J. Anuradha School of Computer Science and Engineering, VIT University, Vellore, India

Chokri Arfa The National Institute of Labour and Social Studies, University of Carthage, Ariana, Tunisia

Micheal Olaolu Arowolo Department of Computer Science, Landmark University, Omu-Aran, Nigeria

Joseph Bamidele Awotunde Department of Computer Science, University of Ilorin, Ilorin, Nigeria

Sourav Bakchi Department of Instrumentation and Electronics Engineering, Jadavpur University, Kolkata, West Bengal, India

Rajib Bandyopadhyay Department of Instrumentation and Electronics Engineering, Jadavpur University, Kolkata, West Bengal, India

Sanjay Banerjee Department of Applied Electronics and Instrumentation Engineering, Future Institute of Engineering and Management, Kolkata, India

Sanjoy Banerjee Department of Applied Electronics and Instrumentation Engineering, Future Institute of Engineering and Management, Kolkata, India

Runu Banerjee Roy Department of Instrumentation and Electronics Engineering, Jadavpur University, Kolkata, West Bengal, India

Kamel Barkaoui Conservatoire National des Arts et Metiers, Computer Science Department, Lab. Cedric, Paris, France

H. R. Bhapkar MIT School of Engineering, MIT ADT University, Pune, India

Mohammed Amin Belarbi University of Mons, Mons, Belgium

Debnath Battacharyya Department of Computer Science and Engineering, K L Deemed to be University, KLEF, Guntur, India

Ailbhe H. Brady National Health Service, Manchester, United Kingdom

Divya Midhun Chakkravarthy Department of Computer Science and Multimedia, Lincoln University College, Petaling Jaya, Malaysia

Midhun Chakkravarthy Department of Computer Science and Multimedia, Lincoln University College, Petaling Jaya, Malaysia

Arijit Chakraborty Bachelor of Computer Application Department, The Heritage Academy, Kolkata, India

Mostafa El Habib Daho University of Tlemcen, Chetouane, Algeria

Debangana Das Department of Instrumentation and Electronics Engineering, Jadavpur University, Kolkata, West Bengal, India

Dipankar Das Bachelor of Computer Application Department, The Heritage Academy, Kolkata, India

Nityananda Das Department of Physics, Jagannath Kishore College, Purulia, West Bengal, India

Ilker Dastan The World Health Organization, Regional Office for Eastern Mediterranean, Cairo, Egypt

Olivier Debauche University of Mons, Mons, Belgium

Debashis De Department of Computer Science and Engineering, Maulana Abul Kalam Azad University of Technology, Kolkata, India

Nilava Debabhuti Department of Instrumentation and Electronics Engineering, Jadavpur University, Kolkata, West Bengal, India

Bhanu Prakash Doppala Department of Computer Science and Multimedia, Lincoln University College, Petaling Jaya, Malaysia

Suchandra Dutta Amity Institute of Information Technology, Amity University, Kolkata, West Bengal, India

Soumik Gangopadhyay Business Administration Institute of Engineering and Management, Kolkata, India

Barnali Ghatak Department of Instrumentation and Electronics Engineering, Jadavpur University, Kolkata, West Bengal, India

Arunangshu Ghosh Department of Electrical Engineering, National Institute of Technology Patna, Patna, Bihar, India

Premananda Jana Netaji Subhas Open University, Kalyani, West Bengal, India

Eali Stephen Neal Joshua Department of Computer Science and Multimedia, Lincoln University College, Petaling Jaya, Malaysia

Akeem Femi Kadri Department of Computer Science, Kwara State University, Malete, Nigeria

S. M. Kadri Disease Control, Directorate of Health Services, Kashmir, UT of Jammu and Kashmir, India

Ahmad M. Karim Computer Engineering Department, AYBU, Ankara, Turkey

Dipak K. Kole Department of CSE, Jalpaiguri Government Engineering College, Jalpaiguri, West Bengal, India

Ashish Kumar Department of Chemistry, Faculty of Technology and Sciences, Lovely Professional University, Phagwara, Punjab, India

Chitresh Kundu Automation Division, Tata Steel Jamshedpur, Jamshedpur, Jharkhand, India

Sohaib Laraba University of Mons, Mons, Belgium

Xavier Lessage University of Mons, Mons, Belgium

Saïd Mahmoudi University of Mons, Mons, Belgium

Sidi Ahmed Mahmoudi University of Mons, Mons, Belgium

Kuntal Maity Department of Physics, Jadavpur University, Kolkata, India

Jyoti Malhotra MIT School of Engineering, MIT ADT University, Pune, India

Dipankar Mandal Institute of Nano Science and Technology (INST), Habitat Centre, Mohali, India

Pierre Manneback University of Mons, Mons, Belgium

Samir Mattoo Directorate of Health Services, Kashmir, UT of Jammu and Kashmir, India

Alok Mishra Molde University College-Specialized University in Logistics, Molde, Norway

Sanjay Misra Department of Electrical and Information Engineering, Covenant University, Ota, Nigeria

Sajal Mitra Department of Computer Science and Engineering, Heritage Institute of Technology, Kolkata, India

Sankar Prasad Mondal Department of Applied Science, Maulana Abul Kalam Azad University of Technology, Kolkata, India

Shreya Nag Department of Instrumentation and Electronics Engineering, Jadavpur University, Kolkata, West Bengal, India

Hemanta Naskar Department of Instrumentation and Electronics Engineering, Jadavpur University, Kolkata, West Bengal, India

Roseline Oluwaseun Ogundokun Department of Computer Science, Landmark University, Omu-Aran, Nigeria

Anindya J. Pal University of Burdwan, Burdwan, India

Saurabh Pal Department of Applied Physics, University of Calcutta, Kolkata, West Bengal, India

Prabal Patra Automation Division, Tata Steel Jamshedpur, Jamshedpur, Jharkhand, India

Asha M. Pawar MIT School of Engineering, MIT ADT University, Pune, India

Mohandas V. Pawar MIT School of Engineering, MIT ADT University, Pune, India

Pranav Pawar Bar-Ilan University, Tel Aviv, Israel

Marija Petkovic University of Medicine, Belgrade, Serbia

A. Raghavendra Rao Data Science Department, CHRIST (Deemed to be) University and Specialist-QMS, First American India Private Ltd., Bengaluru, India

Kishore Ravande MIT School of Engineering, MIT ADT University, Pune, India

Krittish Roy Department of Physics, Jadavpur University, Kolkata, India

Rajneesh Kaur Sachdeo MIT School of Engineering, MIT ADT University, Pune, India

Debabrata Samanta Department of Computer Science, CHRIST (Deemed to be University), Bangalore, India

Sudarshan Sanap MIT School of Engineering, MIT ADT University, Pune, India

Dhrubasish Sarkar Amity Institute of Information Technology, Amity University, Kolkata, West Bengal, India

C. H. Sekhar Department of Computer Science and Engineering, Vignan's Institute of Information Technology, Visakhapatnam, India

Anwesha Sengupta Department of Electrical Engineering, National Institute of Technology Rourkela, Rourkela, Odisha, India

Prolay Sharma Department of Instrumentation and Electronics Engineering, Jadavpur University, Kolkata, West Bengal, India

Vinod Kumar Shukla Department of Engineering and Architecture, Amity University, Dubai, UAE

Pilla Srinivas Department of Computer Science and Engineering, Dadi Institute of Engineering & Technology, Anakapalle, India

M. Srinivasa Rao Department of Computer Science and Engineering, Vignan's Institute of Information Technology, Visakhapatnam, India

Sédrick Stassin University of Mons, Mons, Belgium

Borgi Taoufik Computer Center of the Ministry of Health, Tunis, Tunisia

Abhinay Thakur Department of Chemistry, Faculty of Technology and Sciences, Lovely Professional University, Phagwara, Punjab, India

Nibhrita Tiwari Radicon Institute of Radiology, Dubai, UAE

Bipan Tudu Department of Instrumentation and Electronics Engineering, Jadavpur University, Kolkata, West Bengal, India

Amitava Ukil Department of Business Administration, Eminent College of Management & Technology, Kolkata, India

Leena Wanganoo Department of Management and Commerce, Amity University, Dubai, UAE

Chapter 1
Novel COVID-19 Recognition Framework Based on Conic Functions Classifier

Ahmad M. Karim and Alok Mishra

1.1 Introduction

Many infectious illnesses have affected many human lives in the history and lead to severe cases, causing scientists to spend a long time researching for a cure for such illnesses. An illness that arises within a definite period is known as an epidemic or a pandemic [1–3]. An epidemic arises when infectious illness spread rapidly to many people in countries or several countries. For instance, the SARS epidemic affected 26 nations with 8000 confirmed cases in 2003. The transmission of SARS-CoV is mainly from human to human. Symptoms of the disease generally appear 1–2 weeks after the infection. In contrast, a pandemic is a kind of epidemic which has spread across a wider geographic range and which has affected the whole country or the entire world.

COVID-19 began as an epidemic and within a few weeks' time became a pandemic that spread to most countries in the world. According to the last statistics dated 11 September 2020, there are 29 million confirmed, 19.6 million recovered and 924,000 death cases. Furthermore, real-time reverse transcriptase-polymerase chain reaction (RT-PCR) test is believed to be highly specific. However, the test may report a false-negative rate as high as 60–70% for identifying COVID-19 which is a real clinical problem [4–6]. The physician uses an X-ray to detect COVID-19 because it presented a 90% and above accuracy, which is better than RT-PCR.

A. M. Karim
Computer Engineering Department, AYBU, Ankara, Turkey

A. Mishra (✉)
Molde University College-Specialized University in Logistics, Molde, Norway

Software Engineering Department, Atilim University, Ankara, Turkey
e-mail: alok.mishra@himolde.no

L. Garg et al. (eds.), *Healthcare Informatics for Fighting COVID-19 and Future Epidemics*, EAI/Springer Innovations in Communication and Computing,
https://doi.org/10.1007/978-3-030-72752-9_1

Besides, X-ray is easy to use than RT-PCR. But the rapid increase of COVID-19 disease between persons around the world leads to delay in diagnosis. Due to manually analysing the X-ray images and lower number of doctors compared with potential cases and tests, the physician's diagnosis becomes insufficient. In recent years, deep learning has been used in many fields such as computer security, computer vision and medical image classification [7–10].

Dealing with COVID-19, several robust academic research studies are presented depending on deep learning techniques to automatically recognise the disease by examining CT and X-ray images. Nowadays, approaches based on deep learning have been applied in chest X-ray analysis in a short time. It was preferred over chest CT scanning because of its low ionising emissions and transportability.

Wang et al. [11] present a convolutional neural network (CNN) to recognise COVID-19 diseases from analysing chest X-rays. The network was trained on 13,975 chest X-ray sample images. The method presented 98.9% recognition accuracy. In another study, authors presented a deep neural network-based technique nCOVnet, an alternative to fast screening, to recognise COVID-19 by analysing the X-rays of patients [12]. Zebin et al. [13] experimented on CNN architecture with VGG-16, ResNet50 and EfficientNetB0 pre-trained on ImageNet dataset to recognise COVID-19 by examining chest X-ray images. These three backbones achieved accuracies of 90%, 94.3% and 96.8%, respectively [13]. In another study based on machine learning methods, new Fractional Multichannel Exponent Moments (FrMEMs) applied a feature extractor. The process is parallelised with a multicore computational framework. Manta Ray Foraging Optimization algorithm which is dependent on differential evolution is applied to optimise the feature selection process. The presented method is evaluated by two COVID-19 X-ray datasets and realised accuracy rates of 96.09% and 98.09% for the first and second datasets, respectively [14]. Based on the ResNet-101 CNN structure, a CNN model is pre-trained to detect objects from a million images and then is trained to recognise anomaly in chest X-ray tests. The technique's performances in terms of AUC, sensitivity, specificity and accuracy are 0.82, 77.3%, 71.8% and 71.9%, respectively [15].

On the other hand, after analysing the previous studies, we can present the following contributions in our study:

- Developed novel method combining conic functions classifier based on local binary patterns and factor analysis.
- The proposed method results are evaluated using a confusion matrix to visualise the obtained results.
- The proposed method presented remarkable results as compared with the previous studies.

1.2 Proposed Framework

This section proposes a novel framework based on LBP, factor analysis and conic functions classifier. The X-ray images are prepared and become an input to the LBP, which extracted features, and the extracted features are wired to the factor analysis as a single-dimensional vector. The role of factor analysis is to select important features from the input vector to reduce the vector's size, which means reducing the execution time and removing redundancy features. Then, the factor analysis output is wired to the conic functions classifier, which classifies the labels' extracted features. The details of the framework sections are presented below.

1.2.1 Local Binary Patterns (LBP)

LBP is a texture feature extraction method presented by Kaplan et al. [16]. LBP has low complexity greyscale invariance and light insensitivity. It can extract the texture features of input images and merge all their features. The LBP protocol is straightforward. The algorithm takes the centre value of the image as a threshold, the pixel values that are greater than the centre pixel value are assigned as 1, and the other pixels that are smaller than the value of the centre pixel are assigned as 0. The algorithm of the LBP is represented mathematically in Eqs. (1.1) and (1.2):

$$\mathrm{LBP}_{P,R}(x, y) = \sum_{n=0}^{P-1} \left(2^n s\left(i_n - i_{x,y}\right)\right) \tag{1.1}$$

$$S(x) \begin{cases} 1, x \geq 0 \\ 0, x < 0 \end{cases} \tag{1.2}$$

Then, the texture feature of the LBP is indicated by $\mathrm{LBP}_{P,R}(x, y)$ with the centre pixel (x, y), neighbour pixel Pi_n and radius R indicating the grey value of (nth) neighbour pixel and the centre pixel grey value indicated by $i_{x,y}$.

The extracted features of the $\mathrm{LBP}_{P,R}(x, y)$ are listed as a matrix of arrays and then wired to the factor analysis for selecting sensitive features and reducing the size of the features [17–19].

1.2.2 Factor Analysis (FA)

FA is a statistical technique applied to define the erraticism between indicated variables in less unnoticed variables named as factors. The indicated variables are modelled as linear mixtures of the factors plus the error. The FA is applied to decrease the size of the features. FA predicates the amount of erraticism in the feature due to common factors. Now, let there be a set of obvious random variables represented by *N*, and the variables are represented as $x_1, x_2 \ldots x_N$ with means μ_1, μ_2, μ_N.

Assume for some unidentified coefficients λ_{ij} and *m* unnoticed random variables F_j, where $i \in 1, \ldots, N$ and $j \in 1, \ldots, m$, where $m < N$ we have

$$x_i = \lambda_{i1}F_1 +, \ldots, +\lambda_{im}F_m + \mu_i + z_i \quad (1.3)$$

where z_i is individualistically dispersed error terms with zero mean and finite modification dissimilar for every noticeable variable. The earlier expression can also be written in matrix form:

$$x = \wedge F + \mu + z \quad (1.4)$$

where vector *x* represented the observed variables; μ represented the continuous vector of means; $\wedge$ is constant which is indicated by matrix *N*-by-*m* of factor loadings; *F* is a self-governing matrix, consistent common factors; and *z* is a vector of independently spread error terms. *x* represents the new features that are selected by FA function. Then, the selected features are wired to the classifier as a one-dimensional vector. This part aims to reduce the input features' size to reduce the computational time and decrease the execution time for the classifier [20, 21].

1.2.3 Conic Functions Classifier

In [22] Gasimov and Ozturk presented conic functions as a classifier to separate two groups of features. A conic function $g : R^n \to R$, as a mathematical model, is presented in Eq. (1.5):

$$g_{(w,\xi,\gamma)}(x) = (w, (x - c)) + \xi \parallel x - c\|_p - \gamma \quad (1.5)$$

In Eq. (1.5), $x, w, c \in R^n$ and $p, \xi, \gamma \in R$, where *x* is the features that wired from the factor analysis (data point). Aim is represented by *w*, vertex point represented by *c* and the bias represented by γ. The detail of the conic functions classifier is shown in [23]. The flowchart of the presented approach is shown in Fig. 1.1.

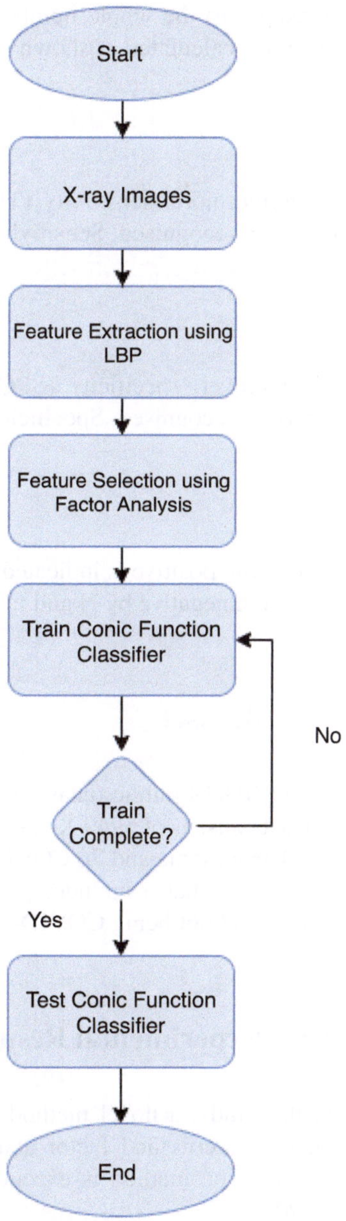

Fig. 1.1 Flowchart of the conic functions-based LBP and FA

1.3 Evaluation Parameters

In this study, several evaluation parameters are calculated to evaluate the presented method. One of the commonly used parameters in machine learning and data mining is accuracy, which represented the ratio of the correctly classified (TP + TN)

paradigm to the whole number of paradigms (TP + TN + FP + FN). Accuracy (ACC) is calculated as shown in Eq. (1.6):

$$\mathrm{ACC} = \frac{(\mathrm{TP} + \mathrm{TN})}{(\mathrm{P} + \mathrm{N})} \tag{1.6}$$

Furthermore, sensitivity (TPR) calculates the percentage of positives that are correctly recognised. Sensitivity is calculated as shown in Eq. (1.7):

$$\mathrm{TPR} = \frac{\mathrm{TP}}{(\mathrm{TP} + \mathrm{FN})} \tag{1.7}$$

Moreover, specificity (SPC) calculates the percentage of negatives that are correctly recognised. Specificity is calculated as shown in Eq. (1.8):

$$\mathrm{SPC} = \frac{\mathrm{TN}}{(\mathrm{FP} + \mathrm{TN})} \tag{1.8}$$

where true positive is indicated by TP, true negative by TN, condition positive by P, condition negative by N and false-positive rate by FPR.

1.4 Dataset

A COVID-19 public dataset [24] is applied to test the presented framework. This dataset consists of 5949 X-ray images for 2839 patient cases involving 1583 normal, 4290 pneumonia and 76 COVID-19 infection cases. The main serious matter in this database is that it includes pneumonia that is the infection produced by bacterial effects and not being COVID-19.

1.5 Experimental Results

In this study, a novel method combines conic functions classifier based on local binary patterns and factor analysis for COVID-19 detection by analysing X-ray images. The method is executed using MATLAB 2020 in a machine with 8 GB RAM.

The dataset is divided automatically in our framework in the first stage as follows: 70% for train and 30% for test sets. There are two critical issues in the dataset; the first issue is that the dataset consists of different sizes of images. This problem is normal and is common in all X-ray images, and the framework is designed to avoid this problem where each input image is 397 × 446 × 3. This step aims to fix the size of all inputs because the machine learning techniques cannot analyse the different sizes of input images. The second issue which is the unbalanced datasets is also a big challenge that reduces each model's performance, but our model is not affected with this problem.

In the second stage, the RGB images are converted to greyscale images. This conversion aims to reduce the computation time's size, and the LBP deals only with greyscale images. This means dividing each image size to three, which leads to the reduction of the computation time by 1/3, which becomes 397 × 446. Figure 1.2 shows the input X-ray to our proposed method.

In the third stage, the LBP is applied to encode local texture information in which the two-dimensional images are converted to one-dimensional array with a small size of elements. Only 59 features are extracted from the input image.

Table 1.1 presents the evaluation parameters ACC, TPR and SPC of the developed framework which is a competitive COVID-19 infection recognition method. It is shown that the presented conic functions classifier-based LBP and FA model is the competitive method as it has better and reliable true positive and true negative values as compared with several methods. Furthermore, the presented method has lower false-negative and false-positive values. Consequently, the presented method can powerfully recognise COVID-19 cases.

The proposed method is also compared with several studies presented in the previous studies and is shown in Table 1.2.

Fig. 1.2 X-ray image

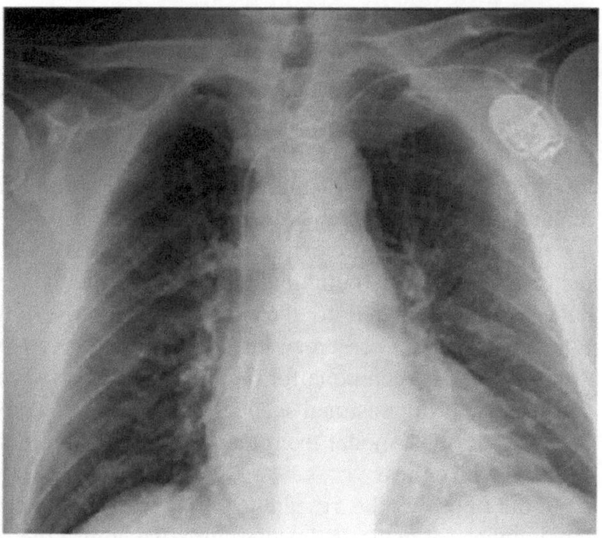

Table 1.1 Confusion matrix of the proposed method

Class	*n* (truth)	*n* (classified)	Accuracy (%)	Precision	Recall	F1 score
Pneumonia	999	1000	99.54	1.0	1.0	1.0
Normal	500	500	99.61	0.99	0.99	0.99
COVID-19	27	26	99.8	0.96	0.93	0.94

Table 1.2 Comparison of the proposed method against popular methods in the literature

Ref	Method	Acc (%)
[25]	Tailored CNN	92.3
[26]	DenseNet	88.90
[27]	Capsule networks	95.7
[28]	ResNet50	96.2
[29]	DarkNet-19-based CNN	87.02
[30]	Transfer learning with Xception Net	96.6
[31]	Customised CNN architecture	96.67
Our method	LBP + FA + conic functions classifier	99.59

By analysing Table 1.2, the results show that the proposed method presented better results than other state-of-the-art studies. The presented method applied classical techniques such as LBP and FA, presenting remarkable results with low datasets. On the other hand, deep learning techniques require a large number of data to achieve better results, and they are very expensive to train due to their complex data models.

1.6 Conclusions

In this paper, a new COVID-19 detection framework is developed using a conic functions classifier based on local binary patterns and factor analysis. The main problem with machine learning techniques is dealing with high-dimensional features with a low number of instances. This leads to overfitting in the model or low rate in the testing of the model. We are aiming to use feature extraction and feature selection techniques to avoid overfitting. This study's critical contribution is combining the feature extraction technique LBP with feature selection technique factor analysis. This combination leads to effective extracted features from input data which are wired to the classifier. Moreover, we conclude that the conic functions classifier presented fast and accurate results with fewer training datasets. Thus, this lowly technique for dividing the given two finite point disjoint groups A and B in the n-dimensional space is proposed. The combination of these techniques produces a robust model that presented remarkable outcomes compared with other well-known studies.

In the future works, researchers may apply the presented methods in fields with low numbers of datasets. Furthermore, we advise the researchers to combine conic functions classifier with deep learning techniques such as CNN, deep sparse auto-encoder, LSTM and RNN.

References

1. E.A. Severo, J.C.F. De Guimarães, M.L. Dellarmelin, Impact of the COVID-19 pandemic on environmental awareness, sustainable consumption and social responsibility: Evidence from generations in Brazil and Portugal. J. Clean. Prod. **286**, 124947 (2020). https://doi.org/10.1016/j.jclepro.2020.124947. ISSN 0959-6526
2. W. Heo, A. Rabbani, J.E. Grable, An evaluation of the effect of the COVID-19 pandemic on the risk tolerance of financial decision makers. Financ. Res. Lett. **2020**, 101842 (2020). https://doi.org/10.1016/j.frl.2020.101842. ISSN 1544-6123
3. F. Altuntas, M.S. Gok, The effect of COVID-19 pandemic on domestic tourism: A DEMATEL method analysis on quarantine decisions. Int. J. Hosp. Manage. **92**, 102719 (2022). https://doi.org/10.1016/j.ijhm.2020.102719. ISSN 0278-4319
4. General Office of National Health Committee, Of a Program for the Diagnosis and Treatment Notice on the Issuance of Novel Coronavirus (2019-nCoV) Infected Pneumonia (trial sixth edition) (2020-02-18). http://www.nhc.gov.cn/yzygj/s7653p/202002/8334a8326dd94d329df351d7da8aefc2.shtml?from=timeline. Accessed 24 Feb 2020
5. M. Chung, A. Bernheim, X. Mei, et al., CT imaging features of 2019 novel coronavirus (2019-nCoV). Radiology (2020). https://doi.org/10.1148/radiol.2020200230
6. P. Huang, T. Liu, L. Huang, et al., Use of chest CT in combination with negative RT-PCR assay for the 2019 novel coronavirus but high clinical suspicion. Radiology (2020). https://doi.org/10.1148/radiol.2020200330
7. P. Puri, N. Comfere, L.A. Drage, H. Shamim, S.A. Bezalel, M.R. Pittelkow, M.D.P. Davis, M. Wang, A.R. Mangold, M.M. Tollefson, J.S. Lehman, A. Meves, J.A. Yiannias, C.C. Otley, R.E. Carter, O. Sokumbi, M.R. Hall, A.G. Bridges, D.H. Murphree, Deep learning for dermatologists: Part II. Current applications. J. Am. Acad. Dermatol. (2020). https://doi.org/10.1016/j.jaad.2020.05.053. ISSN 0190-9622
8. Y. Tian, F. Saiji, A descriptive framework for the field of deep learning applications in medical images. Knowl. Based Syst. **210**, 106445 (2020). https://doi.org/10.1016/j.knosys.2020.106445. ISSN 0950-7051
9. C. Stefano, S. Shanmukh, C. Federico, Applications of deep learning in dentistry. Oral Surg. Oral Med. Oral Pathol. Oral Radiol. (2020). https://doi.org/10.1016/j.oooo.2020.11.003. ISSN 2212-4403
10. Z. Tong, J. Gao, D. Yuan, Advances of deep learning applications in ground-penetrating radar: A survey. Construct. Build. Mater. **258**, 120371 (2020). https://doi.org/10.1016/j.conbuildmat.2020.120371. ISSN 0950-0618
11. R. Lu, X. Zhao, J. Li, P. Niu, B. Yang, H. Wu, et al., Genomic characterisation and epidemiology of 2019 novel coronavirus: Implications for virus origins and receptor binding. Lancet **395**(10224), 565–574 (2020)
12. H. Panwar, P.K. Gupta, M.K. Siddiqui, R. Morales-Menendez, V. Singh, Application of deep learning for fast detection of COVID-19 in X-rays using nCOVnet. Chaos Solitons Fractals **138**, 109944 (2020). https://doi.org/10.1016/j.chaos.2020.109944
13. T. Zebin, S. Rezvy, COVID-19 detection and disease progression visualization: Deep learning on chest X-rays for classification and coarse localization. Appl. Intell. (2020). https://doi.org/10.1007/s10489-020-01867-1
14. M.A. Elaziz, K.M. Hosny, A. Salah, M.M. Darwish, S. Lu, et al., New machine learning method for image-based diagnosis of COVID-19. PLoS One **15**(6), e0235187 (2020). https://doi.org/10.1371/journal.pone.0235187
15. M.Z.C. Azemin, R. Hassan, M.I.M. Tamrin, M.A.M. Ali, COVID-19 deep learning prediction model using publicly available radiologist-adjudicated chest X-ray images as training data: Preliminary findings. Int. J. Biomed. Imag. **2020**, 8828855 (2020). https://doi.org/10.1155/2020/8828855
16. K. Kaplan, Y. Kaya, M. Kuncan, H.M. Ertunç, Brain tumor classification using modified local binary patterns (LBP) feature extraction methods. Med. Hypotheses **139**, 109696 (2020). https://doi.org/10.1016/j.mehy.2020.109696. ISSN 0306-9877

17. K. Kaplan, Y. Kaya, M. Kuncan, M.R. Minaz, H.M. Ertunç, An improved feature extraction method using texture analysis with LBP for bearing fault diagnosis. Appl. Soft Comput. **87**, 106019 (2020). https://doi.org/10.1016/j.asoc.2019.106019. ISSN 1568-4946
18. J. Tang, Q. Su, B. Su, S. Fong, W. Cao, X. Gong, Parallel ensemble learning of convolutional neural networks and local binary patterns for face recognition. Comput. Methods Progr. Biomed. **197**, 105622 (2020). https://doi.org/10.1016/j.cmpb.2020.105622. ISSN 0169-2607
19. A. Güner, Ö.F. Alçin, A. Şengür, Automatic digital modulation classification using extreme learning machine with local binary pattern histogram features. Measurement **145**, 214–225 (2019). https://doi.org/10.1016/j.measurement.2019.05.061. ISSN 0263-2241
20. D. Salas-Gonzalez, J. Górriz, J. Ramírez, I. Illán, M. López, F. Segovia, et al., Feature selection using factor analysis for Alzheimer's diagnosis using F18-FDG PET images. Med. Phys. **37**(11), 6084–6095 (2010). https://doi.org/10.1118/1.3488894
21. M. Usman, S. Ahmed, J. Ferzund, A. Mehmood, A. Rehman, Using PCA and factor analysis for dimensionality reduction of bio-informatics data. Int. J. Adv. Comput. Sci. Appl. **8**(5) (2017). https://doi.org/10.14569/ijacsa.2017.080551
22. R.N. Gasimov, G. Ozturk, Separation via polyhedral conic functions. Optim. Methods Softw. **21**(4), 527–540 (2006)
23. E. Çimen, A random subspace based conic functions ensemble classifier. Turk. J. Electr. Eng. Comput. Sci. **28**(4), 2165–2182 (2020). https://doi.org/10.3906/elk-1911-89
24. J.P. Cohen, P. Morrison, L. Dao, COVID-19 image data collection. arXiv.2020, https://github.com/ieee8023/covid-chestxray-dataset
25. L. Wang, A. Wong, COVID-Net: A tailored deep convolutional neural network design for detection of COVID-19 cases from chest radiography images. ArXiv 2200309871 (2020)
26. X. Li, D. Zhu, COVID-Xpert: An AI powered population screening of COVID-19 cases using chest radiography images. ArXiv:200403042 1–6 (2020)
27. P. Afshar, S. Heidarian, F. Naderkhani, A. Oikonomou, K.N. Plataniotis, A. Mohammadi et al., -Caps: A capsule network-based framework for identification of Covid-19 cases from X-ray images. ArXiv Prepr ArXiv200402696 1–4 (2020)
28. M. Farooq, A. Hafeez, "COVID-ResNet: A Deep Learning Framework for Screening of COVID19 from Radiographs", ArXiv:2003.14395, 2020
29. T. Ozturk, M. Talo, E.A. Yildirim, U.B. Baloglu, O. Yildirim, U. Rajendra Acharya, Automated detection of COVID-19 cases using deep neural networks with X-ray images. Comput. Biol. Med. **121**, 103792 (2020)
30. A.I. Khan, J.L. Shah, M.M. Bhat, Coronet: A deep neural network for detection and diagnosis of COVID-19 from chest x-ray images. Comput. Methods Prog. Biomed. **196**, 105581 (2020)
31. L. Wang, A. Wong, COVID-Net: A tailored deep convolutional neural network design for detection of COVID-19 cases from chest radiography images. arXiv preprint arXiv:2003.09871 (2020)

Chapter 2
A Real-Time Review of Social Health Protection and Health Informatics Support for COVID-19 Outbreak

Chokri Arfa, Ilker Dastan, Kamel Barkaoui, and Borgi Taoufik

2.1 Introduction

As of June 12, 2020, a total of 195 countries have planned or introduced social protection measures in response to coronavirus (COVID-19). Social assistance transfers are the most widely used class of interventions of the social protection response. A total of 621 measures were recorded, accounting for 60% of the response. Significant action in social protection and labor market-related measures and cash transfer programs are intervened to support the social assistance [1]. As a globally and unprecedented crisis with devastating effects, COVID-19 has required urgent and rapid actions.

Developing countries are facing shocks on the economy through a decrease in growth, loss of jobs, and household income as well as on the health system. More financial resources are needed for health and for enhancing the Social Health Protection (SHP). In these countries, the economic crisis is affecting vulnerable groups in terms of living and access to healthcare services. COVID-19 preparedness

C. Arfa (✉)
The National Institute of Labour and Social Studies, University of Carthage, Ariana, Tunisia

I. Dastan
The World Health Organization, Regional Office for Eastern Mediterranean, Cairo, Egypt
e-mail: dastani@who.int

K. Barkaoui
Conservatoire National des Arts et Metiers, Computer Science Department, Lab. Cedric, Paris, France
e-mail: barkaoui@cnam.fr

B. Taoufik
Computer Center of the Ministry of Health, Tunis, Tunisia
e-mail: taoufik.borgi@rns.tn

L. Garg et al. (eds.), *Healthcare Informatics for Fighting COVID-19 and Future Epidemics*, EAI/Springer Innovations in Communication and Computing,
https://doi.org/10.1007/978-3-030-72752-9_2

and response should prioritize health and increase fiscal space for health to mobilize additional resources and to guarantee the SHP through both schemes of social health coverage and medical assistance. The management of health requires to move toward more flexibility and better coordination between stakeholders to ensure continuity of care and timely act for the increased demand [2, 3]. New methods and technics of service delivery and SHP are required to maintain essential health packages for infected and non-infected patients as well as needy population during the pandemic. It is crucial that poor and vulnerable people or people with disability or chronic conditions can access to healthcare services during the pandemic for both emergency and primary healthcare. They should protect them from the burden of health financing, mainly due to the lack of suitable health coverage or assistance.

SHP is in general designed for the health system to ensure funding and to protect the users socially and financially. SHP should manage schemes in a single pool with a defined benefits package and strategic purchasing of healthcare services to ensure protecting the whole population from the burden of health financing and thus improving access, health status, and well-being [4, 5]. Obviously, a robust health delivery system within the framework of a well-functioning regulatory authority is the backbone for SHP. The invaluable presence of consistent and trustworthy information systems for generating data and evidence that can be achieved only through the optimal utilization of support's informatics is mandatory for effective SHP. One of the ways of ensuring medical follow-up, monitoring use of resources, reduction of wastage, and duplication of tests is to use interoperable electronic or digital systems for health and social information exchange [6].

In this chapter, we present the valuable findings and a conception of informatics tools for data generation, exchange, and support for SHP. With regard to SHP, the book talks of improving availability of medical and social data in generic, dynamic, flexible, highly interactive, and respond to user's changes of health information. It means how to improve the management of diseases in digital information systems and improve access to quality healthcare services. The chapter incorporates the issues of SHP in the time of COVID-19 crisis.

2.2 A Review of COVID-19 Outbreak and Its Economic and Social Effects

As of July 2020, the pandemic has worldwide more than 13 million confirmed cases and 596.37 deaths [7]. Its effects are unprecedented economic crisis and recession. In fact, travel restrictions, self-isolation, and social distancing measures have negative effects on all sectors, and they have negatively impacted all sectors and have caused losses of jobs and revenues [8]. Health inequities are increased likely from the negative economic effects of the pandemic and its responses such as lockdown and confinement restrictions. However, these measures can have a profound negative impact on individuals and societies and disproportionately affect disadvantaged groups, people in precarious situations, migrants, and refugees. Vulnerable households are more likely to be affected [8]. The pandemic reveals extreme inequalities and the huge gap such as between the wealthy and the rest of society and for those living in crowded conditions. Then, the poorest people will face terrible economic difficulties [9].

2.2.1 The Economic Impacts

In the developing countries, the economic effects of the pandemic will be substantial. It is predicted that GDP real growth will be reduced by average more than 3% in 2020. Growth rates of these countries are expected to be less than observed over the global financial crisis 2008–2009 [10] and the oil price decrease in 2015 [11]. In EMR, the World Bank estimates that the growth downgrade will be 3.7 %, reflecting the double shocks of COVID-19 costs and sharp decrease of oil prices [4, 12]. GDP is predicted to contract in the Middle East and Central Asia by approximately 3%, in countries like Lebanon and Sudan, by 2% and 7%, respectively, [13, 14]. The economic downturn would likely be felt more strongly in developing countries due to the lack of social security, the high degree of informality, and the limited ability of governments to aid vulnerable groups during the crisis [10]. The COVID-19 has caused a decline in oil prices from January to mid-March 2020. In the EMR, the estimated loss was about $11 billion [15, 16]. The countries exporting oil will suffer from the decreases in both global demand and prices. The UNESCWA estimates, at the current oil prices, that the EMR region will lose daily 550 USD million, while oil importers' gains are minor compared with the losses in exports [17]. The countries that import oil in the region will have further problems due to a decrease in remittances and investment and capital flows. As a result, the pandemic has severely impacted all economic sectors and leads to a prolonged and deep recession and sharp economic volatility [18].

Failure to contain the epidemic will further disrupt the economy and disproportionately affect the poorer sections of society [19]. EMR is also characterized by an exceptional level of migration, displacement, and mobility and is home to the world's largest population of refugees and internally displaced persons. A worst-case healthcare system is in Libya, Syria, and Yemen, due to wars and conflicts, and consequently, the exposure to the pandemic is much greater. Health systems in the region suffer from deficiencies that may subsequently undermine their response to the COVID-19 outbreak, including low production capacity (shortage in intensive care units and beds, ventilators, medical staff) and low public spending, which could complicate all COVID-19 responses.

As a result of the closure of firms, suspend and suppression of salaries and total lockdowns for at least 2 months, unemployment rates, which have historically affected the young population and women in the region, are likely to go up. In 2019, the unemployment rate for youth was 26.9% vs. 9.8% total unemployment. The unemployment rate for men was 7.7%, while it was 18.1% for female employees [20]. ILO predictions show that the pandemic will destroy approximately 10.3% of working hours in the region during the second and third quarters of the year 2020, and this is equal to 6 million full-time workers. Consequently, the decline of revenue and the loss of jobs will increase vulnerability and poverty.[1] It is predicted that the informal sector makes up for 68.6% of the Arab region's total employment, and this figure is 58.1% in Northern Africa. Due to the containment and lockdown measures, access to markets especially for farmers in agriculture has been limited, which decreased the demand for certain areas such as tourism and domestic work.[2] Furthermore, since these segments are usually not covered in social insurance schemes, social protection coverage is generally low.

The vulnerable groups include in general low-skilled and income persons, those working on the informal sector, migrants, refugees, and those working on the informal economy. For instance, migrants and refuges experience the economic and psychosocial impacts of COVID-19, and therefore, they have a higher risk of losing their jobs and being pushed to financial health hardship, during and after this pandemic.

2.2.2 *The Social Impacts: Vulnerability, Poverty, and Inequality*

The pandemic has disrupted the economy and disproportionately affected the poorer sections of society [5, 19]. With the loss of jobs and income, poverty is predicted to go up by 8.3 million more people in the MENA and Arab States region,[3]of which half are children.[4]Additional 1.9 million people are at risk of becoming undernourished.[5]UNU-WIDER researchers predict that there might be a 10% decrease in per capita income, which is likely to increase existing poverty monitored in the MENA and Arab States area since 2013, reaching as high as 8.9%

[1]Refers to the ILO's definition of Arab States. The ILO has identified a number of key economic sectors that will be particularly hit by the crisis and hence experience high levels of unemployment. Those sectors include accommodation and food services, manufacturing, real estate and business activities, and wholesale and retail trade. ILO Monitor: COVID-19 and the world of work. Third edition (ILO, 2020).

[2]See also Impact of public health measures on informal workers livelihoods and health (WIEGO, 2020).

[3]Mitigating the impact of COVID-19: Poverty and food insecurity in the Arab region (ESCWA, 2020).

[4]Between a rock and a hard place, COVID-19 doubles the burden for millions of children in the Middle East and North Africa Region (UNICEF, 2020).

[5]Idem.

and 24.1% for the US$1.9/day and US$3.2/day poverty lines, respectively, meaning levels as high as in 1990.[6]

The cited effects of the COVID-19 generated the increase of social inequalities which already observed and measured even before the crisis at the developing countries.[7]About 55 million people require humanitarian aid in the MENA/Arab States region, and 26 million of these people are uprooted from their homelands (refugees and displaced persons[8]) because of wars and armed conflicts in Arab countries (Syria, Palestine, Yemen, Sudan, Iraq, and Libya (see footnote 4)). This region has an exceptional level of migration, displacement, and mobility with the high proportion of refugees and displaced persons in the world. A worst-case health system is in Libya, Syria, and Yemen, due to wars and conflicts, and consequently, the exposure to the pandemic is much greater. Health systems in the region suffer from deficiencies that may subsequently undermine their response to the COVID-19 outbreak, including low capacity (shortage in intensive care units and beds, ventilators, medical staff) and low public spending, which could complicate all COVID-19 responses. In addition, persons with disability, chronic diseases and elderly could be considered as vulnerable groups. They are in general weakly protected by the social programs that are exacerbated in the time of COVID-19, due to exclusion from work[9] and in the disruption of social protection and needy health scheme.

2.3 A Review of Health Systems and Social Health Protection: Challenges and Potential Needs

2.3.1 Health Systems

In developing countries, health systems are poorly governed and underfunded, and these compound the other issues listed in the six WHO building blocks [21, 22]. In line with these building blocks, poor governance is highlighted by the inability to sufficiently respond to the population needs, and the resulting concerns about equity, efficiency, and quality [23]. Rabbani and Hashmani [24] show that healthcare service's delivery fails to provide the essential package. Public health facilities are insufficiently equipped with curative-oriented care, to deal with the massive influx of infected patients.

[6]https://www.wider.unu.edu/sites/default/files/Publications/Working-paper/PDF/wp2020-43.pdf.

[7]https://wir2018.wid.world/part-2.html.

[8]Mitigating the impact of COVID-19: Poverty and food insecurity in the Arab region (ESCWA, 2020).

[9]Disability Inclusive Social Protection Response to COVID-19 crisis (UNPRPD, ILO, UNICEF, International Disability Alliance, Embracing Diversity, 2020).

Health financing is insufficient and fragmented in terms of collection of revenue and in risk pooling. The purchasing is not sufficiently strategic which exhibits the use of set incentives for service providers to maximize efficiency and quality of health. The fragmentation is high since a greater share of health expenditure (on average, more than 50% [25]) is derived directly from out of pocket. Thus, a significant proportion of the population experiences difficulties accessing healthcare services and financial protection against health risks [26]. There are wide variations between countries in the quality of health information system. All of them lack a comprehensive and developed and well-functioning system that can provide in a timely and reliable manner health information. There is a crucial demand of regular information on socioeconomic, demographic, epidemiological, health services utilization... for the decision-making.

Health system fails to deliver responsive services and continuous treatment [27] due to lack of efficient use of resources and lack of data and visibility of users and their requirements and needs. Users of public health facilities usually experience long wait times, lack of staff, privacy, and confidentiality, and existing informal payments [28, 29]. The public sector is underfunded, understaffed, and ill-equipped. There is a shortage of primary care physicians and specialists, combined with, presumably, an uneven distribution between urban and rural areas. The medical density is estimated under the global average with four health personnel per 1000 people [26–28].

2.3.2 Social Health Protection

SHP means that public authorities should guarantee that all persons can satiate their health needs and adequately access to healthcare services in the country, without any limiting factor such as the ability to pay. Inadequate SHP system with lack of social assistance to mitigate the effects of economic recession and unemployment will push further households to poverty.

Countries are already battling with low levels of health spending and health financial protection and are ill-prepared for the high treatment costs of NCDs. Moreover, there are wide variations in current levels of total current health expenses (CHEs) as a percentage of GDP), ranging from 3 to 12%. In this middle-class or lower middle-class region, the largest share of current health expenditure is private, and mostly out of pocket (OOP), household spending. It is well established that public health spending is the road to Universal Health Coverage (UHC) [30], yet countries in the region remain reliant on OOP as the primary financing source [31]. A considerable body of literature highlights that a high level of OOP expenditures can have severe negative impacts on health financial protection for households.

Social protection systems are mostly based on Social Insurance Schemes (SISs) and Social Assistance (SA). Employees of old age of public and formal private sectors are covered by social insurance schemes. SA is especially cash transfers, food vouchers, and access to basic health services, which have become more common recently [32]. They are of great importance in COVID-19 pandemic since they can be used to (1) eliminate financial obstacles, (2) insure that infected persons will not loss income, (3) support workers in informal sectors to afford needs and ensure food security, and (4) enhance solidarity and social cohesion and prevent social tensions. The COVID-19 pandemic has induced human threats as the virus is rapidly spread and affecting the lives of billions. Effective responses require in practice a timely action based on an evidence-based and well-communicated approach and a partnership spirit and social solidarity.

2.3.3 Preparedness and Responses

The developing countries are currently facing uncertainty about the progress of the COVID-19, a situation that requires clear preparedness and response. These countries have adopted budgetary measures based mainly on domestic funding, but donor funding would still play a significant role. The situation is even bleaker in low-income countries such as in Afghanistan, with its dubious health system preparedness capacity. COVID-19 also affects the refugees, migrants, and internally displaced populations and has severe implications for fragile and conflict-torn states.

A priority will be to expand the scope and capacity of the health system and mobilize additional resources. It require solid and strong informatics supports to generate timely and useful information in order to ensure effective responses [31, 32]. The COVID-19 outbreak imposes measures to strengthen health financing and remove financial barriers. A foremost concern is to review the managerial process of the pandemic through a coherent and efficient information system and to ensure the health protection of vulnerable groups. These groups are facing a causal nexus of deficient preventative care, high risk of health, and impaired welfare due to the high OOPs. Consequently, they are exposed to catastrophic health payments and impoverishment [33].

2.4 Informatics Supports for the COVID-16 Responses: Knowledge Sharing and Information Exchanges

Developing countries should rely on digitization to shape and support their social and health financing strategy which should include needy groups and thus none left behind. Digitization is based on a wide range of technologies from simple applications on mobile such as tablets or smartphones to Big Data that brings data from different sources and different formats. The Big Data provides a set of tools to address the triple problems, called the 3V rule [34]. It contains a large size of structured or unstructured data from different sources with a level of achieved velocity, namely the frequency of creation, of collection, and of data sharing.

However, Big Data development depends on evolution of storage technologies in correlation with the deployment of cloud computing characterized by a large calculation and storage capacity thus allowing parallel processing as well as the development of unstructured databases with regard to the Hadoop, MongoDB, Cassandra, or Redis database management systems. As a constantly progressing environment, Big Data is always seeking to optimize the performance of tools, and new solutions are frequently derived for several complex issues.

The use of Big Data to fight against the spread of the coronavirus has made possible to cross-reference data issued from several sources such as the computerized medical record, the telephone operators for the geolocation of people, facial recognition, and the processing of video surveillance images by artificial intelligence. Public authorities can easy localize in real time infected people, track their displacements and notify other persons that may have encountered them. Public authorities can also use this data to follow-up and provide psychological assistance and financially protect vulnerable groups in seeking healthcare services.

Here is a need to identify the needy population, including those affected by the pandemic. Social programs, including health assistance, are already available in many developing countries. However, they are considered working with deficient information systems and ineffective mechanisms of identifying and targeting vulnerable groups. Developing countries still rely national surveys to generate information about needy population. These surveys are very expensive, not yearly implemented and not suitable to generate data of needy population in due time.

The use of Big Data technologies to routinely and timely collect demographic, socioeconomic, and health data of the population and vulnerable groups allows to overcome may difficulties. It could be achieved through a desegregation of solid indicators that describe well the households. Practically, crossing data from different sources such as civil status, social security, fiscality, land conservation, transport, employment, banks, company of the electricity, and gas supplier and through open data of various institutions will be available a rich dataset of households. Then, it will be possible to calculate a weighted score of household's standards of living. A specific score threshold will allow to easily and timely identify needy groups that are eligible for financial aid and for free access to healthcare services.

Various data issued from different sources should be linked. This process can be using the interoperability platform that makes feasible exchanging and recovering of data through international standards and norms and in data formats and communication protocols. The implementation of interoperability platform constitutes an important lever for socioeconomic development as it will be possible to permanently identify, monitor, evaluate, and generate information of the needy groups in time and after the COVID-19.

Interoperability is crucial for making communication between various and heterogeneous IT systems (Fig. 2.1). It will help to ensure the secure data exchange through various information systems of public and private institutions and to generate a reliable and complete database of needy groups. In this respect, interoperability can be fixed through a web service platform, which in turn, facilitate communication of applications in different programming languages and allow data sharing without

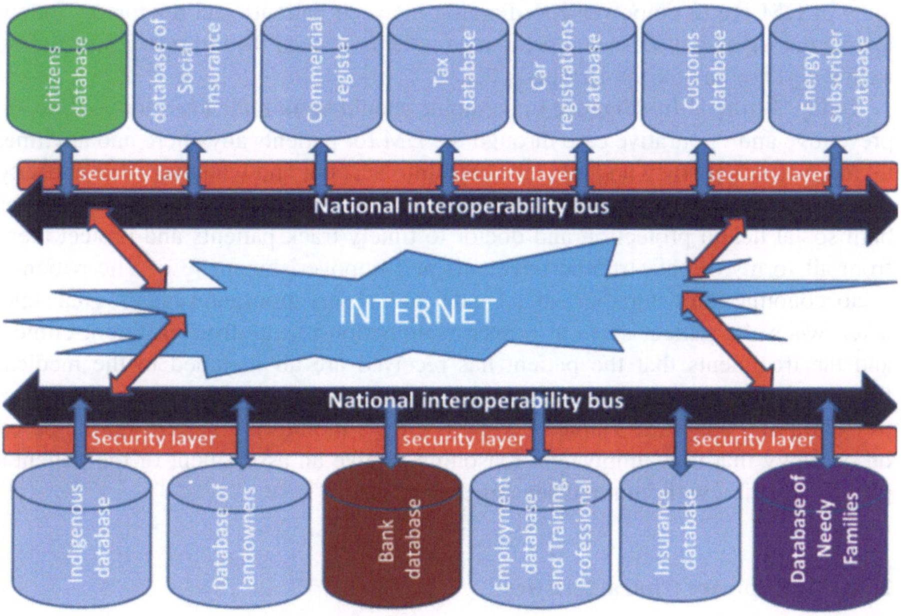

Fig. 2.1 General architecture of data exchange interoperability

mollifying the different information systems. The advantages of a web service are (1) easy access via the internet network, (2) functionalities invoked by the client through the HTTP protocol, (3) multiplatform not depending on the technologies used for the information systems, and (4) easy data sharing by multiple clients. The use of a web service by a client triggers an action with a server. Indeed, the client can request from the server who reply with response in the known format beforehand. Thus, interoperability based on web services is a promising technique allowing to overcome obstacles of heterogeneous and communication of information systems with low costs.

2.4.1 Hapicare: A Healthcare Monitor System with Self-adaptive Coaching and Probabilistic Reasoning

During COVID-19 (coronavirus) outbreak, patients who have chronic diseases [35, 36] are confined in their houses and can seek for home care if inpatient care is not required. In low- and middle-income settings, COVID-19 has hit countries with both health and economic and unprecedented fallout of financing health and the weak health information system. In such countries, there are many attempts to create "disease management (DM)." DM is a system of coordinated healthcare interventions and communications for patient with chronic conditions. The main aims of DM are to empower coordination between patients and doctors to follow up and manage the disease and prevent complications and then improve life quality, saving costs of healthcare services.

Today, Artificial Intelligence in medicine should sustain the need for continuous preventive and/or curative care through the DM for patients anywhere and anytime, taking patient's privacy and ethical norms into account and whatever their capacity to pay or their socioeconomic situation. A smart monitoring system is needed for both social health protection and doctor to timely track patients and protect them from all forms of catastrophic payments and impoverishment [37]. The patient's socioeconomic characteristics, social and health observations, and events, vital signs taken when the patient stays at home, examination results from different clinics, and the treatments that the patient has received are all included in the medical file, the common model of monitoring. For this goal to be achieved, we propose to exploit and adapt the Hapicare system [38], a monitoring system that is based on ontology that uses ambivalent reasoning to give an assessment of the patient's present situation with minimal sensing actions.

2.4.1.1 Hapicare Characteristics

- Within an ontology, there is a probabilistic reasoning system that interacts with Bayesian belief network with non-monotonic production rules.
- Actions based on Bayesian network are selected to cut down the sensing actions in order to evaluate the patient's situation.

An IoT monitoring system converts the sensor's data into ontological facts and the other way around, converting ontological facts to actions that are either reactive or sensing.

2.4.1.2 Design and Architecture of Hapicare System

The monitoring system relies on working memory of expert knowledge, on monitoring principles, and on Bayesian deduction process of information patient. First, the system receives the information from the patients, gathered from the daily life and the self-evaluation. Suitable reactions are suggested by the system. Figure 2.2 displays the suggested system that is boxed with double line, and it interacts with the real world through Cloud. Data conversion, ontology, a perception layer, Bayesian belief network, and rule engine are included.

Perception layer is the first level, and here, sensors, self-evaluations, and examinations gather all the information. All this data is sent and kept in a Cloud. Ontology is the following layer, and it standardizes the data representation for reusability and homogeneity. The system is operating on ontology. Consequently,

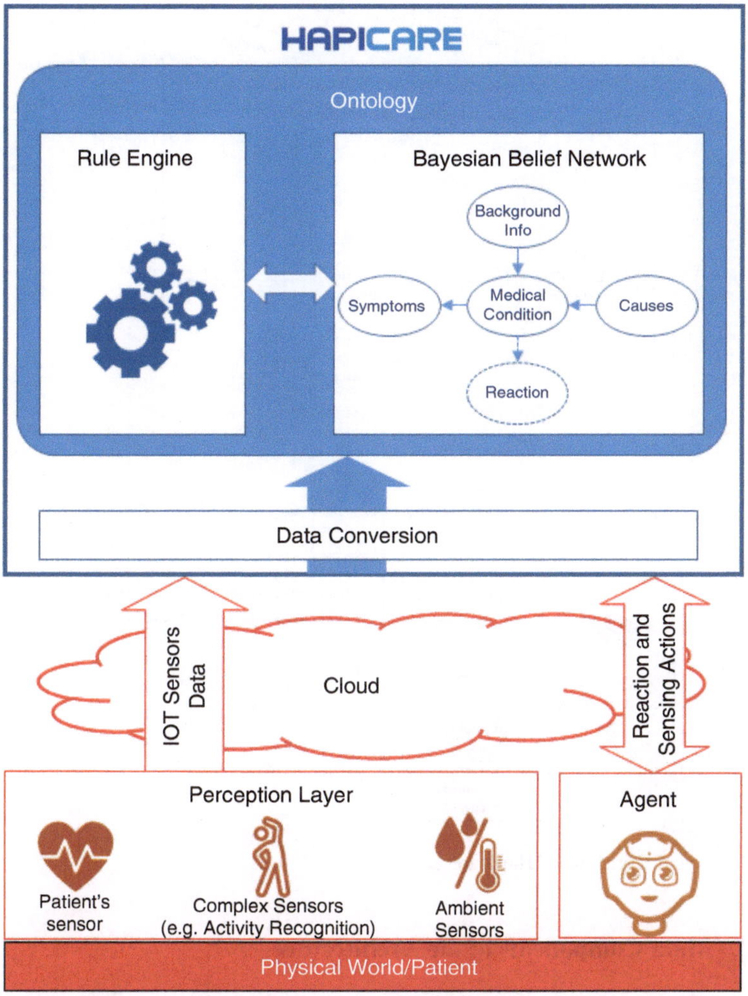

Fig. 2.2 Overview of the Maidis Hapicare platform architecture

a "data conversion" level is needed to represent the information on the ontology. The next level is Bayesian belief network and its rationales over the contextual information on probabilistic reasoning. It gives suitable responses. Rule engine is the next component, which is responsible for managing the probabilistic reasoning and gives context-based data. The final part is agent, and it provides the interaction with the patients. It asks the patient to take sensing actions, gives advice, notes his/her symptoms, and listens to his/her answers.

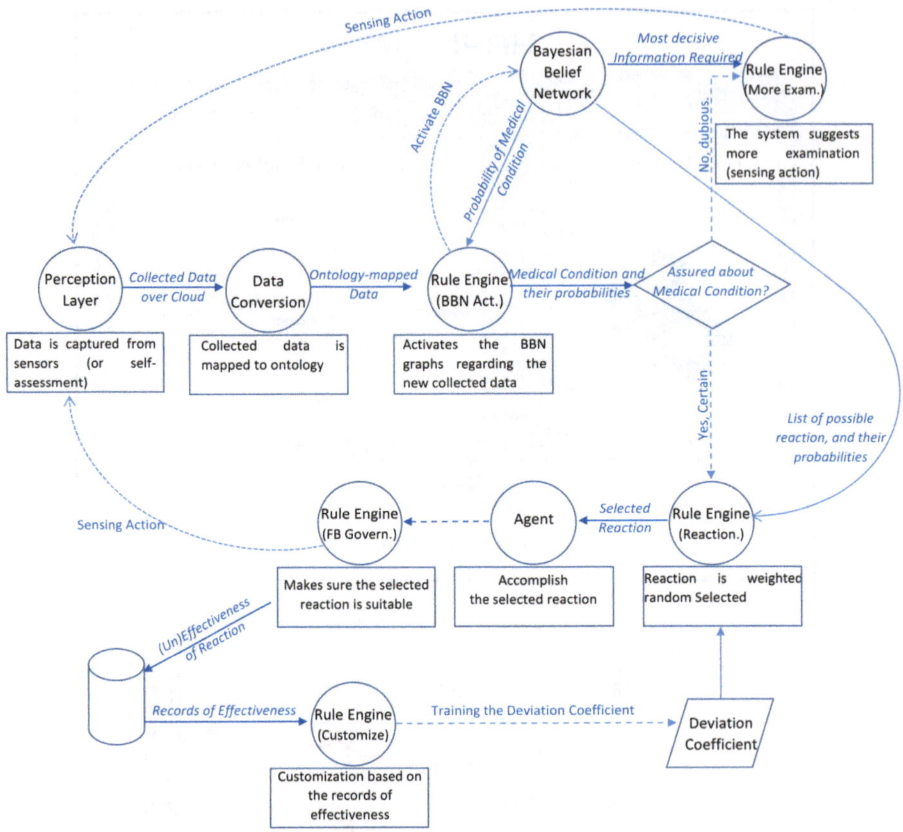

Fig. 2.3 Typical workflow of Hapicare

2.4.1.3 Main Components of the Architecture

The main components of the architecture are

Ontology

Formal specification of a shared conceptualization is called ontology [39], and therefore it facilitates formal representation of information and their relevance [40]. Ontology is used in all the levels or layers of Hapicare, meaning that the information should be demonstrated with the use of an ontology. This part is shown as the full box incorporating the core of the system in Fig. 2.3. The two classifications of information for modeling are (1) socioeconomic and medical data and (2) sensor data. The first one has patients' health history that shows medical conditions, prescriptions, and all the other relevant medical information.

Bayesian Belief Network (BBN)

Medical information is saved as BBN. Each diagram contains five groups of nodes:

- Socioeconomic and Medical Condition: the objective of the Bayesian probabilistic estimation is the node.
- Reasons: the occurrences that influence the likelihood of a medical condition are the nodes of this group
- High Risks: Patient's medical history that influences the likelihood of a medical condition is the nodes.
- Symptoms: the nodes of this group are the events that are observed.

The BBN is produced based on medical experts and general statistics. The BBN calculates the possibilities of an illness depending on reasons or observations. Equations (2.1) and (2.2) present these two, respectively, [41]. In the previous one, ni are derived from groups High Risks and Causes. In the equations, *mc*, *n*, *v*, and *b* represent medical condition, nodes of graph, the values of nodes, and observation.

$$P(mc = X) = \sum (P(mc = X|n_{1..n} = v_{1..n}) \prod_{i=1}^{n} P(n_i = v_i)) \tag{2.1}$$

$$P(mc = X|N = b) = \frac{P(N = b|mc = X).P(mc = X)}{P(N = b)} \tag{2.2}$$

Workflow

These components work together, and as soon as the new information is perceived by the perception layer, the workflow begins. A usual work and information flow in the system are shown in Fig. 2.2. The components are shown with their names in circles and a box of their description below. Solid and dashed arrows show the transmission of data and work between components.

In the last few years, the significance of healthcare has attracted a lot of attention. When the preferences of patients and the time and the cost of hospitalization are taken into account, a smart monitoring system is needed to track their homestays with no interference. With this aim, we propose Hapicare, an IoT sensor-based system to gather detailed data about the patients. It also has reasoning to evaluate the context and make decisions with background data and the information it has gathered. Moreover, in addition to reasoning to reinforce uncertainty in the information, it is reconfigured to probabilistic reasoning.

2.4.2 *HapiChain: A Blockchain-based Framework for Patient-Centric Telemedicine*

Health systems have economic and financial challenges that are aggravated during the COVID-19 crisis. Telemedicine, which uses intelligent systems with reduced cost for comprehensive healthcare, is highly advised; however, there are some reliability and security concerns about data and process. We propose HapiChain, a blockchain-based framework for patient-centric telemedicine [42]. HapiChain uses blockchain technology to make security, scalability, and reliability of social health protection and medical workflows better. HapiChain is not only patient-centered but also will help the managers of health system to gather enough data for improving the delivery of healthcare services. The present blockchain-based approaches in healthcare can be categorized into two main classes: Secure Storage and Secure Workflow.

Medical files are stored electronically. Then, Secure Storage approach is reassuring and beneficial for the medical systems. However, unlike Secure Workflow approaches, they do not use some features of blockchain technology such as accountability and adaptability of medical workflows. Secure Workflow methods emphasize protecting telemedicine services as a whole.

In HapiChain, there are two embedded telemedicine services: telemonitoring and teleconsultation. For telemonitoring, Hapicare works as healthcare monitoring system with self-adaptive coaching using probabilistic reasoning. It is completed after consultation that uses blockchain technology. Data of the multiple agents (such as doctors, patients, laboratory's technicians...) are are shared via internet network. The security and reliability of teleconsultation are given a great importance. Also, there are three main layers in the HapiChain framework: interface layer, DApp layer, and blockchain layer. For the first level, Hapicare is used to communicate with the users such as patients and doctors. The second one is the DApp procedure layer (smart contracts and distributed storage), required for security and scalability of HapiChain. The third layer is implemented exploiting the InterPlanetary File System (IPFS). Ethereum blockchain is utilized as a platform of DApps in the blockchain layer.

2.4.2.1 Blockchain Technology

Blockchain technology is from Decentralized Ledger Technology (DLT) [43]. DLT is a unity of reproduced, common, and synchronous data, and this data can be shared without going through a central administration or a data storage center. Blockchain has a connected list of blocks. Every one of these blocks contains a copy of data when they are exchanged through a peer-to-peer network. Hash values and digital signatures are used to chain these blocks to the previous ones, and a previous block cannot be modified without changing all the blocks in the chain structure [44].

Bitcoin uses blockchain technology, and it was this peer-to-peer anonymous cash system that brought blockchain in the limelight [45].

After blockchain technology was famous, various fields started using it. Structured scripting for application development is then needed. As a result, and related to the next phase of blockchain technology, there have been some changes like including smart contracts and scripts that are carried out after specific transactions have happened. So as to implement extra transactions as soon as transaction has occurred, such as imposing transaction of tax-paying on the transaction of a buy, smart contracts can be used.

Buterin [46] is an open-source blockchain-based platform featuring smart contacts. It exploits an updated model of the blockchain, consisting of a state machine during a transaction. Next state depends on the data in the previous state and the current transaction. As illustration in a cash system, the states are balance data of different entities, and they are updated by a transaction "transfer amount X from sender A to receiver B;" such that, in the next state, the balance of entity A is reduced by X, while the balance of entity B has been increased by the same amount. In Ethereum, in order to create smart contracts, there is a language called Solidity. Solidity code method can be traced through transactions. Storing too much data may not be effective despite the fact that there are not any restrictions for storage [46]. To overcome such restrictions, InterPlanetary File System (IPFS) [47] is commonly used. Extensive contents of data can be reached easily through IPFS, which is a shared file platform. Since each information has an address of its own and shared through peer-to-peer network, it can be retrieved directly.

2.4.2.2 Teleconsultation

In teleconsultation, there are two agents: a doctor and a patient, and they share sources such as prescription and consultation reports. On the other hand, in HapiChain service, Hapicare is also included as the third party with its sensor data, context-based information, and diagnosis reports.

In the teleconsultation workflow,

- Firstly, the patient requests an appointment that has been suggested by Hapicare. To do it, the patient goes through the available slots created by physicians. The workflow happens during the teleconsultation session and starts when the appointment starts. Figure 2.1 illustrates the simple version of the workflow. As soon as the patient joins the doctor's virtual room, the consultation starts. At this time, doctor is selected by the patient and then the video consultation starts. Doctors can also call in a patient a couple of times with possible viewing of some primary information on the waiting room. During this consultation, the patient's EHRs along with Hapicare sensor data, context-based data, and reports can be accessed. Thus, the patient can share his/her concerns, and the doctor can ask questions for diagnosis or even ask for additional investigations

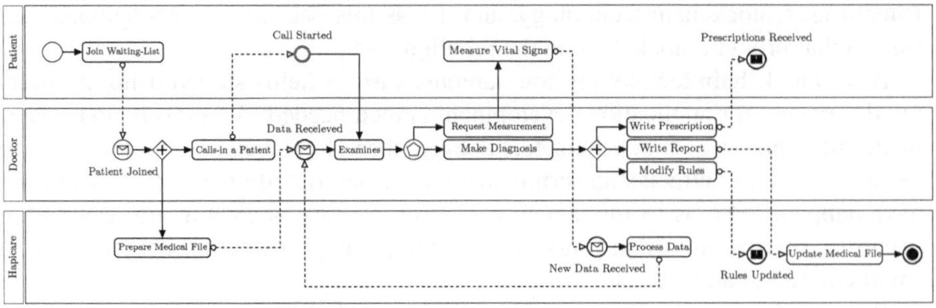

Fig. 2.4 The simplified process model of a teleconsultation session

for better diagnosis and decision. Live investigation using IoT sensors can be transferred to the doctor via Hapicare. At the end, invoice and prescription will be delivered to the patient. Prescriptions are not just medication. They could include additional investigations such as laboratory examination or directing the patient to a specialist. Moreover, Hapicare rules can be updated depending on new observations.

The teleconsultation workflow is not the same for all cases. As the system is evolving, prescriptions can be sent directly to the pharmacies instead of the patients. Moreover, knowing that each case is different, other processes might be joined to the teleconsultation, like the appeal for other advices or diagnosis or the security of data, which is a big challenge. In face-to-face consultation, medical files are often stored digitally. Blockchain technology is thus used to ensure safety of data manipulation and interception that are generated through the teleconsultation. All these inputs are considered during designing dynamicity of the workflow (Fig. 2.4).

Regarding modularity and security, the HapiChain, a blockchain-based framework for patient-centric telemedicine, is used. An outline of its structure is shown in Fig. 2.2. We have chosen blockchain since it gives simplicity and flexibility in developing Distributed Applications (DApps) [46]. It is implemented in the platform layer to enhance smart contracts and distributed storage. Smart contracts are the basics of HapiChain as they have solidity codes to access to the storage and to ensure the workflow process. HapiChain contains two roles: (1) users such as physicians, patients, and Hapicare system and (2) administrators to configure HapiChain. The smart contracts of HapiChain are listed in the following classes:

- **Source of Authentication**: HapiChain is designed using an interface layer in order to avoid unauthorized requests and thus to allow only predefined sources of requests. In the Ethereum platform, there is no limitation of execution by default. Unauthorized sources of requests should be explicitly programed. The HapiChain administrator will have overseen authorized requests. HapiChain declines all requests unless specified by Hapicare.

- **Request Integrity**: HapiChain should include a process to verify that the received request is an authentic request from the authorized source. In other words, it needs to know that requests have not tampered such as physician and patient are well identified in the request. A digital signature is used to validate integrity. In Hapicare, the request parameters are hashed before transmission. Then, in HapiChain, the hash value is again computed and compared to the one received. In tampering cases, the hash values will not match and HapiChain will drop the request.
- **User Authentication**: Ensuring the identity of the user is vital prior to access control. The Hapicare user is identified and the identification is validated in the set of smart contracts. Hapicare does the authentication through physician login. In HapiChain, before processing the physician requests, he/she will need to be identified and registered in the list of authorized physicians. The HapiChain administrator can update, check, and/or delegate the list to the Hapicare administrator.
- **Access Control**: The medical files provide the most important information to the health system. A set of Solidity codes secures the confidentiality and integrity of these files. Access control is customized for each patient. The access control codes are categorized under two sub-headings:
  - **Read Medical File**: During telemonitoring, a medical file for diagnosis is constantly used by Hapicare, but it is not necessary to reach all the medical files. During the teleconsultation, the physician should also reach the medical files.
  - **Modify Medical File**: The medical file shall be modified if needed, by his/her physician for an allowed time.

HapiChain has a dynamic access control, ensured through the read and modify medical files. A mapped access control is defined for all the process and prior to any requests: from the identification number to the list of allowed requests.

In practice, the request contains the patient's identification number, the medical file (monitoring or consultation), request type (read or modify), and access period. For the telemonitoring, the Hapicare system can access only to monitor medical files of all patients for an infinite time, and his/her administrator can define the access controls. Since the medical files can get bigger, it is nearly impossible to keep them in the blockchain. Therefore, IPFS is used to store data for better scalability [48] and anonymized and encrypted before storage for data confidentiality and privacy. Moreover, when the smart contracts verify that the "modify" request is permitted, the new data in a storage node will be saved by IPFS, and the address is saved for future accesses. If Hapicare has not specifically chosen the type of new data for monitoring, the type will be consultation. In retrieval cases, the items are loaded from the stored addresses. The Hapicare system acts as an interface for communication with physicians and patients. This layer communicates with smart contracts through the Application Programming Interfaces (APIs) (Fig. 2.5).

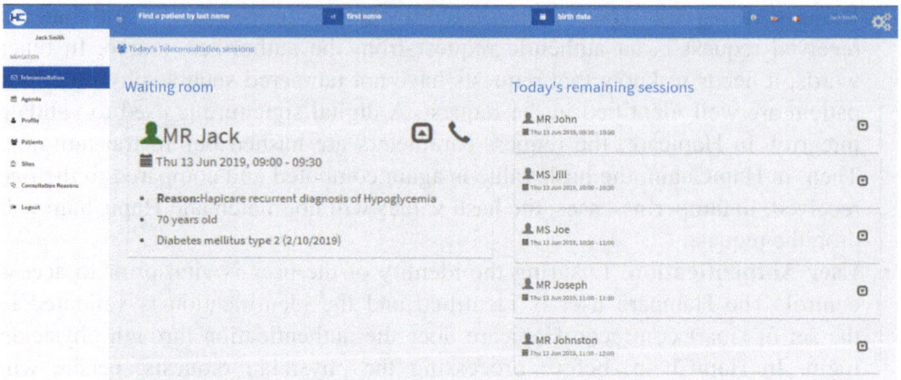

Fig. 2.5 A view of virtual waiting room

2.5 Conclusion

Informatics support is a set of mechanisms with electronic health records and information systems, which facilitate referrals of patients with severe signs and symptoms of coronavirus and those with needs of social protection. In the time of the COVID-19 crisis, countries are facing increase in vulnerability due to lost of jobs and incomes. Consequently, households are experiencing catastrophic health expenditure and impoverishment. Social protection is a major factor of coordinated policy response while resolving crisis, which also enables patients to reach health services as well as supporting job and income security for the ones who are most affected. The crisis has emphasized the significance of ensuring suitable information and informatics tools to support the universal health coverage.

This chapter presents the main informatics supports to improve the social health protection policies to the COVID-19 outbreak and provides tools to ensure enough and coherent evidences. We covered the management of the socioeconomic and health characteristics of patients, their living location using Hapicare, and its role as a blockchain-based framework for telemedicine which is patient-centric. Together, these informatics supports help in providing characteristics and feedback from patients and doctors, which are very useful information for the social health protection.

References

1. U. Gentilini et al., Social protection and jobs responses to COVID-19 (2020)
2. World Health Organization, Coronavirus disease COVID19, situation report, 182 (2020)
3. G. Gabutti et al., Coronavirus: update related to the current outbreak of COVID-19 (2020), pp. 1–13

4. R. Arezki et al., How transparency can help the Middle East and North Africa. The World Bank (2020)
5. R. Baldwin, B.W.d. Mauro, *Economics in the Time of COVID-19* (CEPR Press, London, 2020)
6. S.N. Sarbadhikari, Public Health Informatics and Universal Health Care, The role of public health informatics in providing universal health care (UHC). Int. J. Med. Sci. Public Health **2**(2), 162–164 (2013)
7. M. Nicola et al., The socio-economic implications of the coronavirus pandemic (COVID-19): a review. Int. J. Surg. **78**, 185 (2020)
8. M. Makoni, Keeping COVID-19 at bay in Africa. Lancet Respir. Med. **8**(6), 553–554 (2020)
9. V. Covello, R. Hyer, *COVID-19: Simple Answers to Top Questions, Risk Communication Guide*. Association of State and Territorial Health Officials, Virginia (2020)
10. W.J. McKibbin, R. Fernando, The global macroeconomic impacts of COVID-19: seven scenarios (2020)
11. International Moneatory Fund, Middle East and Central Asia: Confronting the COVID-19 Pandemic in the Middle East and Central Asia (2020)
12. R. Arezki et al., Middle East and North Africa Economic Update, April 2020: How Transparency Can Help the Middle East and North Africa. The World Bank (2020)
13. L.N.-N.I.J.E.O. Farhan, COVID-19 (2020), p. 1
14. I.M. Fund, World Economic Outlook: The Great Lockdown W.E.O. Reports, Editor (2020)
15. M. Karamouzian, N. Madani, COVID-19 response in the Middle East and north Africa: challenges and paths forward. Lancet Glob. Health **8**(7), e886–e887 (2020)
16. ESCWA, COVID-19 Economic Cost to the Arab Region, U. Nations, Editor. (2020)
17. ESCWA, COVID-19 Economic Cost to the Arab Region (2020)
18. J. Furman, Protecting people now, helping the economy rebound later, in *Mitigating the COVID Economic Crisis: Act Fast and Do Whatever It Takes*, ed. by R. Baldwin, B. Weder di Mauro. Center for Economic Policy and Research (CEPR Press, Washington, DC, 2020), p. 191
19. R. Baldwin, B.W. di Mauro, *Economics in the Time of COVID-19*. 1 CEPR Press, 2020. VoxEU.org
20. International Labor Organization, Regional Economic Outlook: Middle East and Central Asia. Washington, DC (2020)
21. World Health Organization, *Monitoring the Building Blocks of Health Systems: A Handbook of Indicators and Their Measurement Strategies* (World Health Organization, Geneva, 2010)
22. WHO, *Monitoring the Building Blocks of Health Systems: A Handbook of Indicators and Their Measurement Strategies* (WHO, Geneva, 2010)
23. K. Mate et al., Review of Health Systems of the Middle East and North Africa Region. Int. Enc. Public Health **2017**, 347 (2017)
24. F. Rabbani et al., Hospital management training for the Eastern Mediterranean Region: time for a change? J Health Organ. Manag. **29**, 965–972 (2015)
25. E.Z. Asbu et al., Health status and health systems financing in the MENA region: roadmap to universal health coverage. Glob. Health Res. Policy **2**(1), 25 (2017)
26. A.S. Yazbeck, T.S. Rabie, A. Pande, Health sector reform in the Middle East and North Africa: prospects and experiences. Health Syst. Reform. **3**(1), 1–6 (2017)
27. D. Cotlear et al., Going universal: how 24 developing countries are implementing universal health coverage from the bottom up. The World Bank (2015)
28. S. Jabbour et al., *Public Health in the Arab World* (Cambridge University Press, Cambridge, 2012)
29. World Bank, *Fairness and Accountability: Engaging in Health Systems in the Middle East and North Africa* (World Bank, Washington, DC, 2013)
30. V.Y. Fan, W.D. Savedoff, The health financing transition: a conceptual framework and empirical evidence. Soc. Sci. Med. **105**, 112–121 (2014)
31. H. Elgazzar et al., Who pays? Out-of-pocket health spending and equity implications in the Middle East and North Africa (2010)
32. A.C. Machado et al., Overview of non-contributory social protection programmes in the Middle East and North Africa (MENA) region through a child and equity lens. Research Report (2018)

33. World Health Organization, Strengthening health financing systems in the Eastern Mediterranean Region towards universal health coverage: health financing atlas (2019)
34. N. Elgendy, A. Elragal. Big data analytics: a literature review paper, in *Industrial Conference on Data Mining* (Springer, Cham, 2014)
35. World Health Organization, Global report on diabetes (2016)
36. C.E. Zelaya et al., QuickStats: age-adjusted percentage of adults aged$\geq$ 18 years who were never in pain, in pain some days, or in pain most days or every day in the past 6 months, by employment status-national health interview survey, United States, 2016 (vol. 66, pg 796, 2016). Morb. Mortal Wkly. Rep. **66**(44): 1238–1238 (2017)
37. Worl Health Organization, Tracking universal health coverage: first global monitoring report (World Health Organization, Geneva, 2015)
38. H. Kordestani et al., Hapicare: healthcare monitoring system with self-adaptive coaching using probabilistic reasoning, in *2019 IEEE/ACS 16th International Conference on Computer Systems and Applications (AICCSA)* (IEEE, Piscataway, 2019)
39. W.N. Borst, Construction of engineering ontologies for knowledge sharing and reuse (1999)
40. N.D. Rodríguez et al., A fuzzy ontology for semantic modelling and recognition of human behaviour. Knowl. Based Syst. **66**, 46–60 (2014)
41. J. Rohmer, Uncertainties in conditional probability tables of discrete Bayesian Belief Networks: a comprehensive review. Eng. Appl. Artif. Intell. **88**, 103384 (2020)
42. H. Kordestani, K. Barkaoui, W. Zahran, HapiChain: a blockchain-based framework for patient-centric telemedicine, in *IEEE International Conference on Serious Games and Applications for Health (SeGAH)* (IEEE, Piscataway, 2020)
43. H. Natarajan, S. Krause, H. Gradstein, Distributed ledger technology and blockchain. World Bank (2017)
44. M. Nofer et al., Blockchain. Bus. Inf. Syst. Eng. **59**(3), 183–187 (2017)
45. S. Nakamoto, A. Bitcoin, A peer-to-peer electronic cash system (2008)
46. V. Buterin, A next-generation smart contract and decentralized application platform. White Paper **3**(37) (2014)
47. J. Benet, IPFS-content addressed, versioned, P2P file system (DRAFT 3) (2014)
48. Q. Xia et al., MeDShare: trust-less medical data sharing among cloud service providers via blockchain. IEEE Access **5**, 14757–14767 (2017)

Chapter 3
Active Learning-Based Estimation of COVID-19 Pandemic: A Synergetic Case Study in Selective Regions Population

Arijit Chakraborty, Sajal Mitra, Dipankar Das, Debnath Battacharyya, Debashis De, Sankar Prasad Mondal, and Anindya J. Pal

3.1 Introduction

The COVID-19 pandemic induced by the 2019-novel coronavirus (2019-nCoV) causes common health-related disorders ranging from flu to acute respiratory syndromes [1–3]. The 2019-nCoV microorganism is inducted in the CoV family without any previous trace until the recent times. The variants of CoV such as Middle East respiratory syndrome coronavirus (MERS-CoV) and severe acute respiratory syndrome coronavirus (SARS-CoV) cause infectious outbreaks in Saudi Arabia and China, respectively, in the recent past [4]. The SARS-CoV-2, also known as 2019-nCoV, is a novel virus, and several patients with symptoms of viral pneumonia identified epidemiologically are linked with the Wuhan city of China

A. Chakraborty (✉) · D. Das
Bachelor of Computer Application Department, The Heritage Academy, Kolkata, India

S. Mitra
Department of Computer Science and Engineering, Heritage Institute of Technology, Kolkata, India

D. Battacharyya
Department of Computer Science and Engineering, K L Deemed to be University, KLEF, Guntur, India

D. De
Department of Computer Science and Engineering, Maulana Abul Kalam Azad University of Technology, Kolkata, India

S. P. Mondal
Department of Applied Science, Maulana Abul Kalam Azad University of Technology, Kolkata, India

A. J. Pal
University of Burdwan, Burdwan, India

L. Garg et al. (eds.), *Healthcare Informatics for Fighting COVID-19 and Future Epidemics*, EAI/Springer Innovations in Communication and Computing,
https://doi.org/10.1007/978-3-030-72752-9_3

in December 2019 [5]. Since then, the COVID-19 adversely affected every aspect of the human civilization. This outbreak circulated mostly through facial and oral tracts [6]. A confirmed case of COVID-19 positive can infect a minimum of three other persons, and its symptoms can be seen within a fortnight. In this context, the categories of the 2019-nCoV outbreak in a society are as follows:

1. **Stage 1**, also known as *imported transmission*: In this stage, individuals who have been tested positive for COVID-19 with a travel history in COVID-19-infected foreign countries imported it back to their host country. It incorporates all the nations except the epicenter (China) which started reporting cases of COVID-19.
2. **Stage 2** referred to as *local transmission*: In this stage, the infection is transmitted from one person with a travel history in the epidemic country to another person in the non-epidemic country. The trajectory of the virus spread extended from the source individual to all other infected individuals.
3. **Stage 3** or *community transmission*: This is an alarming stage because the transmission spreads into a community and the chain of transmission of the virus becomes hard to trace, i.e., the virus keeps circulating within a society.
4. **Stage 4** or *pandemic*: This is a fatal stage of the outbreak, where the outbreak becomes epidemic with a prolonged resurfacing in a country.

Presently, most of the countries of the world couldn't escape this global outbreak and positioned at either of these COVID-19 stages. Therefore, necessary preventive measures must be exercised to break this outbreak chain, which warrants a regular supply of the COVID-19 preventive logistics in severely affected countries. Till now, there is no known cure for this pandemic except prevention. Therefore, it is imperative to design a robust model to estimate the spread of the contagious 2019-nCoV to help the administration develop a unified framework to fight the COVID-19 epidemic.

In this context, authors of [7] introduced an optimization model, namely, FPASSA-ANFIS, to project the COVID-19 spread in China. Al-qaness et al. [7] used the WHO dataset consisting of COVID-19 positives in China between 21 January 2020 and 18 February 2020. They estimate the outbreak pattern of 10 days up the line using their model, which is an improvisation of the adaptive neuro-fuzzy inference system (ANFIS) utilizing the flower pollination algorithm (FPA) and the salp swarm algorithm (SSA). They optimized the performance of ANFIS by fine-tuning the parameters of ANFIS using FPASSA. The performance of the FPASSA-ANFIS model is compared to eight different models in terms of coefficient of determination (R^2), RMSE, mean absolute percentage error (MAPE), root mean squared relative error (RMSRE), mean absolute error (MAE), and computing time. FPASSA model outperformed other existing models with $R^2 = 0.9645$, RMSE = 5779, MAPE = 4.79, RMSRE = 0.07, MAE = 4271, and computing time = 23.30. Additionally, Al-qaness et al. [7] tested their proposed model with the US and China's weekly influenza datasets and achieved encouraging results.

In their paper, authors of [8] employed a time-series model to generate a daily estimation of the COVID-19 outbreak. The authors considered the dataset of the

WHO, National Health Commission of China, and Johns Hopkins University. Elmousalami and Hassanien [8] used time-series models, namely, moving average (MA), weighted moving average (WMA), and single exponential smoothing (SES) to measure the performance of forecasting in terms of RMSE, mean squared error (MSE), MAPE, and mean absolute deviation (MAD). They observed that the SES model outperforms other time-series forecasting methods. Consequently, Elmousalami and Hassanien [8] concluded that the SES model is the best-fit candidate for the day-level forecasting of confirmed, recovered, and death cases induced by COVID-19. Following which, Elmousalami and Hassanien [8] considered the SES model for trend analysis with a confidence interval of 95% and forecasted up to more than 200,000 confirmed cases, 140,000 recovered cases with a ratio of 95.6%, and 7000 death cases with a 3.5% ratio globally by 9 April 2020. Their model also revealed with a 95% confidence interval a double-fold rise in the no. of confirmed cases by April 2020 in Egypt. This forecasting model also recommended that the no. of COVID-19-affected cases rises exponentially, i.e., at more than 25% per day worldwide, in countries that do not obey social distancing and lockdowns as precautionary measures against this outbreak. In another work, the authors of [9] used time-series models to forecast the infection outbreak of hepatitis A virus in Turkey. They employed ARIMA, multilayer perceptron (MLP), and time delay neural networks (TDNN) to train the models using a dataset of 13 years and concluded that the MLP method outperformed other models in forecasting hepatitis A outbreak. Zhao et al. [10] estimated the MERS and SARS outbreak using the serial interval (SI) method. Additionally, the authors also estimated the outbreak of 2019-nCoV in China based on the value of the basic reproduction number denoted by R_0 in a range [2.24, 3.58] at a 95% confidence level. Table 3.1 outlines the use of goodness-of-fit statistics in estimating pandemic outbreaks.

Currently, countries such as China and Italy are well-positioned in an alarming pandemic (Stage 4). Therefore, it becomes necessary to determine the adversity of this pandemic in these countries, including India, by 13 April 2020 to decide the outbreak pattern in India. In this context, we considered the WHO [11] dataset of COVID-19 from 21 January to 23 March 2020. However, no single estimation method based on a small dataset can be reasonably concluded as the best-fit candidate because of the inherent imprecision and noise associated with a small dataset. Thus, we employed a plethora of estimation methods to obtain a decisive outcome. This publication elucidates the use of the goodness-of-fit statistics, curve-fitting method, and support vector machine-based regression (SVR) in estimating the adversity of this contagious outbreak in India by 13 April 2020.

3.1.1 Motivation of the Work

The COVID-19 epidemic caused by the 2019-nCoV is fundamentally a single-strand RNA microorganism. This microbe is noble in nature and not known to us until the recent times, and the progress of this global pandemic supplements unfolding

Table 3.1 Goodness-of-fit statistics in a pandemic [7–10]

Authors	Forecasting method		Forecasting disease	Performance of best-fit candidate based on					
	Statistical	Time series	COVID-19	R^2	R_0	RMSE	MAPE	MAD	Computing time
Al-qaness et al. [7]	✓	✓	✓	✓		✓	✓	✓	✓
Elmousalami et al. [8]	✓		✓			✓	✓	✓	
Ture [9]		✓				✓			
Zhao et al. [10]		✓	✓		✓				
Our method	✓	✓	✓	✓		✓			

new traits of the 2019-nCoV. The incubation period is the time duration between exposure to this fatal virus and visible symptoms incurred by individuals. The average incubation period of COVID-19 ranges between 5 and 14 days. During this pre-symptomatic period, the infected individuals are potentially contagious in spreading this fatal microbe, and a multifold increase in COVID-19-infected specimens mainly circulated through the facial and oral pathways [6]. However, a significant no. of COVID-19 patients with moderate symptoms have not presented to the clinics, thereby limiting us with only a handful of information about the catastrophe. The stated scenario motivated us to present this publication as follows:

- To inform policymaking officials and health experts about the COVID-19 pandemic situation in densely populated countries like China and India and Italy (the worst-affected country) by 13 April 2020 to take innovative and effective countermeasures to restrict the outbreak of this unpropitious epidemic. The reason for choosing the estimation by 13 April 2020 is because most of these nations are under strict social restrictions as a preventive measure till 14 April 2020.
- Estimating the fatality of the COVID-19 outbreak in China and Italy apart from India can help decision-makers to quantify the supply of preventive logistics to counter COVID-19 in China, Italy, and India.

3.1.2 Novelties of the Work

The availability of a small COVID-19 pandemic dataset makes it astonishingly challenging for us to decide on the appropriate estimation model to predict the fatality of 2019-nCoV in China, Italy, and India. This small-scale data imprecision and uncertainty restricted us to choose any specific estimator in portraying the COVID-19 situation in these countries by 13 April 2020. Moreover, an inherent challenge in using small-scale data is that it often overfits the training samples, thereby offering biased outcomes. In contrast, using a plethora of estimation techniques helps in convincingly determining the best-fit estimation candidate. Consequently, we included some widely accepted curve-fitting methods such as linear, cubic, and quadratic curves to determine the best-fit curve in terms of goodness-of-fit statistics and the SVR-based estimation method to depict the pandemic scenario in China, Italy, and India.

3.1.3 Schematic Diagram of the Proposed Work

In Fig. 3.1, the schematic diagram of the proposed work for determining the candidate model of the COVID-19 is shown.

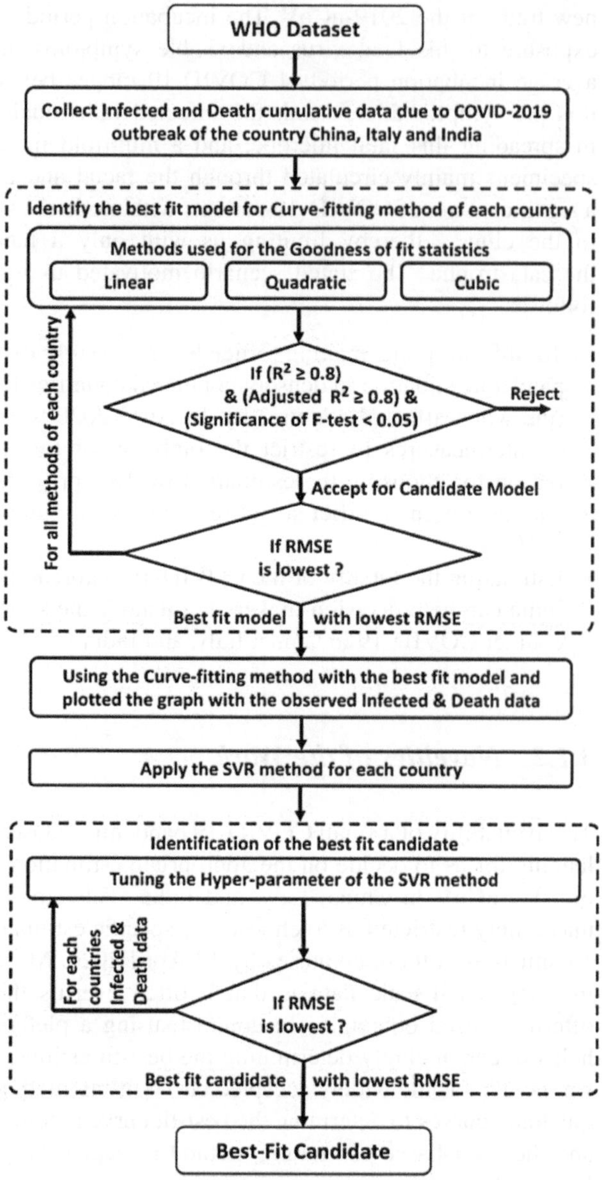

Fig. 3.1 Determination of the best-fit estimation model

3.2 Preliminary Statistical Concept

3.2.1 *The Goodness-of-Fit Statistics*

The coefficient of correlation (R^2) is a measure of association between two and more variables in an interval of [0, 1]. However, R^2 is scale intuitive, and R^2 value increases proportionally with model enhancement wherein $R^2 = 1$ indicates a perfect fit. The adjusted R^2 statistic uses the R^2 statistic and adjusts it for the no. of independent variables considered in an estimation model. Like R^2, an adjusted R^2 value close to 1 confers a more considerate fit [12–14]. F-test is used to assess the statistical significance of the model. F-test's significantly less than the significance level denoted by α indicates a better fit of the model than the intercept-based model [15]. The closeness between the observed and predicted values, i.e., the model's quality, can be measured from the RMSE value wherein a low value of RMSE implies a better fit [14].

3.2.2 *Curve Fitting*

The use of a curve-fitting technique is a widely accepted estimation approach where a curve that fits most of the samples is employed for out-sample predictions. In this context, Kafazi et al. [16] used the curve-fitting technique for energy forecasting, whereas Donmez et al. [17] used a similar approach to forecast the electricity demand. In another work, Srikanth et al. [18] compared the performance of polynomial curve-fitting, ARIMA, and ANFIS methods and concluded that the polynomial curve outperformed the other two methods. Jalil et al. [19] employed the polynomial and Gaussian fits to develop a forecast model of solar radiation. Descriptions of the curves employed for the COVID-19 estimation are given in Eqs. (3.1)–(3.3).

1. **Linear equation-based model**

$$Y = a_0 + a_1 \times t \tag{3.1}$$

2. **Quadratic polynomial-based model**

$$Y = a_0 + a_1 \times t + a_2 \times t^2 \tag{3.2}$$

3. **Cubic polynomial-based model**

$$Y = a_0 + a_1 \times t + a_2 \times t^2 + a_3 \times t^3 \tag{3.3}$$

In Eqs. (3.1)–(3.3), Y denotes time-series values; t denotes time; and a_0, a_1, a_2, and a_3 denote regression coefficients.

The goodness-of-fit statistics used in this publication are as follows:

1. R^2.
2. Adjusted R^2.
3. Significance of F-test.
4. RMSE of held-out training data (10%).

3.2.3 Support Vector Regression

Support vector machine (SVM) extended as a regression approach resulted in SVR [20]. The SVR method is fundamentally similar to SVM in constructing a hyperplane with the maximal margin. However, in SVR, an additional small threshold is introduced, which approximates the SVM method's outcome.

For a given set $S = \{(x_i, y_i) \mid \forall\, i \in [1, N]\}$, where S is the training space such that $S \subseteq T$, where $T = R^d$, the SVR method with a small ζ bound aims to find a function $f(x)$ with a maximum permissible error of ζ, i.e., the upper bound on deviations from the actual targets y_i must be ζ. The rudimentary form of the function $f(x)$ is described in Eq. (3.4).

$$y = f(x) = W^T \times X + b \tag{3.4}$$

In Eq. (3.4), W is the weight vector and b is the bias factor.

The principal goal of the SVR method is to realize the degree of flatness, i.e., the actual y_i should not deflect more than ζ, and this can be safeguarded by including the concept of convex optimization proposed by Vapnik [21] with the objective function described in Eq. (3.5).

$$\text{minimize } \frac{1}{2}\|W\|^2$$

$$\text{subject to} \begin{cases} y - W^T X - b \leq \zeta \\ y - W^T X + b \leq \zeta \end{cases} \tag{3.5}$$

In real life, to accommodate the errors, the concept of slack variables denoted by ε_1 and ε_2 is introduced, and accordingly Eq. (3.5) is adjusted to Eq. (3.6).

$$\text{minimize } \frac{1}{2}W^2 + C \times \sum_{i=1}^{N} \varepsilon_{1i} + \varepsilon_{2i} \tag{3.6}$$

$$\text{subject to} \begin{cases} y - W^T X - b \leq \zeta + \varepsilon_1 \\ y - W^T X + b \leq \zeta + \varepsilon_2 \\ \varepsilon_1, \varepsilon_2 \geq 0 \end{cases}$$

In Eq. (3.6), C is a positive constant, which is an acceptable tolerance measure beyond the deviation ζ.

In the SVR method, the choice of kernel function is critical, and we considered the normalized polykernel. For a polynomial of degree γ, the polykernel and normalized polykernel are described in Eqs. (3.7) and (3.8).

$$K_\gamma \left(\overrightarrow{y_1}, \overrightarrow{y_2}\right) = \left(\overrightarrow{y_1}^T, \overrightarrow{y_2} + 1\right)^\gamma \tag{3.7}$$

$$K_{\text{Norm}\gamma} \left(\overrightarrow{y_1}, \overrightarrow{y_2}\right) = \frac{K_\gamma \left(\overrightarrow{y_1}, \overrightarrow{y_2}\right)}{\sqrt{\left(\overrightarrow{y_1} \cdot \overrightarrow{y_1}\right)} \sqrt{\left(\overrightarrow{y_2} \cdot \overrightarrow{y_2}\right)}} \tag{3.8}$$

In Eqs. (3.7) and (3.8), $\overrightarrow{y_1}$ and $\overrightarrow{y_2}$ are input vectors.

3.3 Methodology for Solving the Proposed Problem

3.3.1 Fitting the Problem with the Said Proposed Methods

The reason for performing principal analysis of the COVID-19 adversities in China, Italy, and India with curve-fitting techniques and the SVR method is because the collection of data usually is measured at an equal interval of time in the time-series forecasting approach. The characteristics of time series are as follows:

- Trends.
- Incorporating fluctuations including seasonal and cyclical.
- Accommodation of irregular components in the dataset.

The trend analysis of the time-series data helps us to understand the general average tendency of the data, whereas the regression analysis is employed to identify the best-fit line or curve that describes the data most. Therefore, to predict future values, extrapolation of the best-fit line or curve is widely recognized as one of the most straightforward approaches. The advantage of employing the SVR method is that its computation complexity does not depend on the input space dimension. Also, the SVR has superior generalization ability with high prediction efficiency.

3.3.2 A Pseudo Code for Candidate Model (CM) Selection

Input Conventional curve-fitting models, i.e. Linear, Cubic, and Quadratic
Machine Learning (ML) based estimation: SVR
Candidate Model (CM) Set: θ = {Linear, Cubic, Quadratic, SVR}

Output Winner: θi with min. Ri, where Ri is the RMSE of ith member of θ

```
For each candidate θi∈ θ, ∀I∈[1,3]                              //Candidate models
  If R² ≥ 0.8 AND Adjusted R² ≥ 0.8 AND F-test <0.05 then // 95% Confidence
       Store Ri in R
  End if
End for
Set min← 0
For each Ri ∈ R                                                 // ith RMSE value
  If min < Ri
       Store Ri in min
  End if
End for
Set min_SVR←min. RMSE of SVR                                    // θ4: SVR
If min_SVR > min then
       Store min_SVR in min
End if
```

3.4 Discussion of the Problem with Numerical Data

3.4.1 Dataset Used for the Problem

WHO renders the global report of the 2019-nCoV outbreak archived from 21 January 2020 [11]. This paper's empirical outcomes are based on this publicly available daily situation report of the 2019-nCoV consisting of the information about the no. of people affected and who died globally due to the 2019-nCoV epidemic. Consequently, we build our datasets by considering the data of China, Italy, and India from 21 January 2020 to 23 March 2020, i.e., a total of 63 days.

We adopted the R package version 201-12-12r77564 [22–24] and WEKA 3.8.1 [25] package in our experiment for obtaining the best-fit model to forecast the COVID-19 outbreak in China, Italy, and India. The R package is used to implement the curve-fitting methods, whereas the WEKA package is employed to implement the SVR method and fine-tune the polykernel parameter.

3.4.2 Numerical Results

We considered the WHO dataset consisting of 63 pieces of information about the no. of COVID-19 infections and deaths in China, Italy, and India as in-sample specimens to determine these countries' candidate curves. The statistical measures R^2, adjusted R^2, and RMSE remain the determinants to identify the candidate models for each of these countries. Consequently, R^2, adjusted R^2, and RMSE that are achieved for these three countries are listed in Table 3.2. The blue highlighted cells in Table 3.2 indicate the lowest RMSE corresponding to the R^2 and adjusted R^2 of a particular country.

Remark 3.1 It is evident from the goodness-of-fit statistics listed in Table 3.2 that China has the lowest RMSE value of 1613.54 for the quadratic model, and Italy and India have the lowest RMSE values of 7136.51 and 91.27, respectively, for the cubic model. Thus, the quadratic model becomes the best fit for China, whereas the cubic model is the best fit for Italy and India.

The candidate curves for cumulative infected data of the COVID-19 outbreak in China, Italy, and India are as follows:

1. **Country: China**
   - Candidate models: linear, quadratic, and cubic
   - Model selected: **quadratic**
2. **Country: Italy**
   - Candidate models: quadratic and cubic
   - Model selected: **cubic**
3. **Country: India**
   - Candidate models: quadratic and cubic
   - Model selected: **cubic**

Table 3.2 Goodness-of-fit statistics of cumulative infected data

	China			Italy			India		
	Linear	Quadratic	Cubic	Linear	Quadratic	Cubic	Linear	Quadratic	Cubic
R^2	0.86583	0.955119	0.973203	0.545506	0.887133	0.986957	0.551366	0.890936	0.985995
Adj. R^2	0.86339	0.953457	0.971686	0.535626	0.882117	0.986067	0.541821	0.886194	0.985062
F test	354.9274	574.5927	641.6084	55.21144	176.8498	1109.773	57.76243	187.8849	1056.067
Sig. of F test	1.18E-25	4.03E-37	1.28E-41	2.07E-09	4.82E-22	1.85E-41	1.01E-09	7.36E-23	1.06E-41
RMSE	27372.37	1613.54	21555.54	32811.98	18986.44	7136.51	195.83	137.32	91.27

In Table 3.3, the mathematical model of the best in-sample curve fits achieved by us for these three countries is listed.

Remark 3.2 It is apparent from Table 3.3 that even though cubic curve becomes the best fit for both Italy and India, the coefficient of the highest polynomial term is 1.56 for Italy and 0.01 for Italy and India, respectively, which indicates a higher chance that Italy witnesses a rise in COVID-19 adversities steeper than India.

Accordingly, using best curves as listed in Table 3.3, the in-sample observed values of the cumulative COVID-19 infections in China, Italy, and India are shown in Figs. 3.2, 3.3, and 3.4.

Remark 3.3 From Fig. 3.2, it is evident that the quadratic estimate of the no. of cumulative infection in China by 23 March is close to 80,000, and Fig. 3.3 reveals that the cubic estimate of the no. of cumulative infection in Italy by this date is 60,000, whereas Fig. 3.4 shows that for India, the cubic estimate of the no. of cumulative COVID-19-infected people is approximately 220.

Table 3.3 Best-fit model of cumulative infected data in China, Italy, and India

Country	Model	Description
China	Quadratic	$y = -21{,}016.34 + 4001.90 \times t - 38.23 \times t^2$
Italy	Cubic	$y = -4109.10 + 1271.51 \times t - 85.46 \times t^2 + 1.56 \times t^3$
India	Cubic	$y = -27.42 + 8.53 \times t - 0.53 \times t^2 + 0.01 \times t^3$

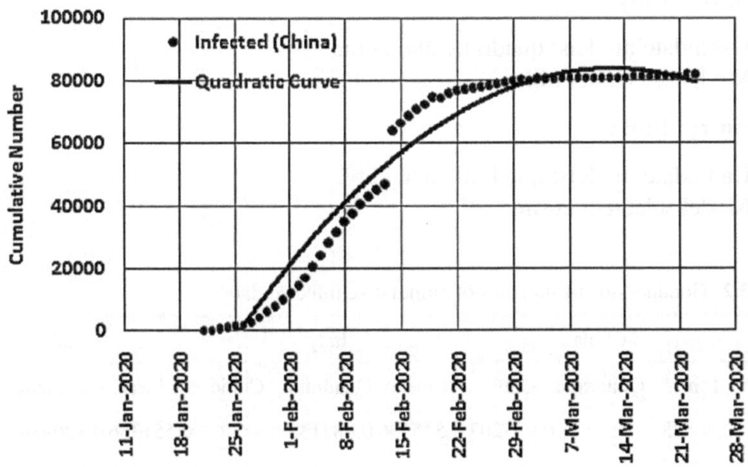

Fig. 3.2 Quadratic curve of cumulative infected data of China

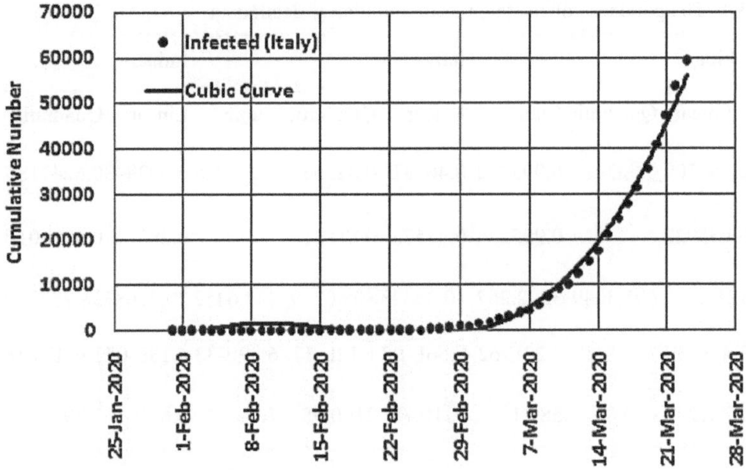

Fig. 3.3 Cubic curve of cumulative infected data of Italy

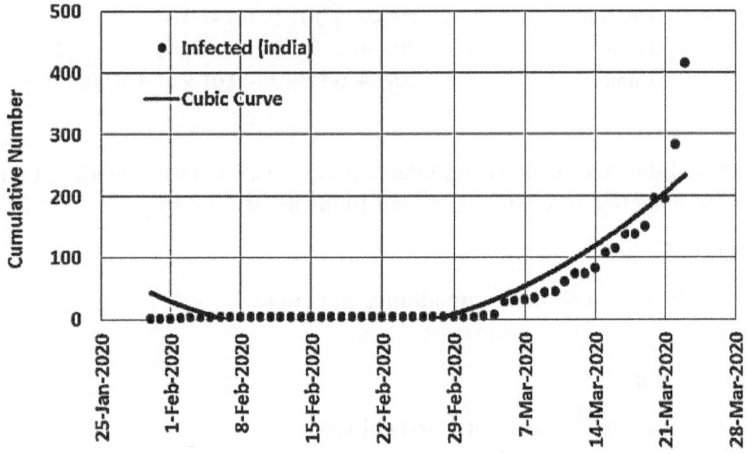

Fig. 3.4 Cubic curve of cumulative infected data of India

Table 3.4 shows the goodness-of-fit statistics in terms of R^2, adjusted R^2, and RMSE of the estimates achieved using the in-sample cumulative death data of China, Italy, and India listed.

Remark 3.4 In Table 3.4, the blue highlighted cells indicate the lowest RMSE against the maximal R^2 and adjusted R^2 for each of these countries. Consequently, the quadratic curve with $R^2 = 0.96$ and RMSE $= 480.3$ is the best fit for China, whereas cubic curve with $R^2 = 0.97$ and RMSE $= 1099.12$ and $R^2 = 0.84$ and RMSE $= 1.02$ become the best fit for COVID-19-induced human casualties in Italy and India, respectively.

Table 3.4 The goodness-of-fit statistics of cumulative death data

	China			Italy			India		
	Linear	Quadratic	Cubic	Linear	Quadratic	Cubic	Linear	Quadratic	Cubic
R^2	0.956709	**0.962412**	0.995482	0.46731	0.823558	**0.967999**	0.302948	0.624718	**0.839478**
Adj. R^2	0.955922	**0.961019**	0.995226	0.45573	0.815717	**0.965817**	0.288117	0.608401	**0.828776**
F test	1215.48	691.3049	3892.257	40.35423	105.0209	443.6452	20.42683	38.28722	78.44503
Sig. of F test	3.47E-39	3.36E-39	4.23E-62	8.56E-08	1.12E-17	6.89E-33	4.18E-05	1.62E-10	6.67E-18
RMSE	759.12	**480.3**	589.17	3210.78	2160.95	**1099.12**	3.6	2.39	**1.02**

Table 3.5 Best-fit model of cumulative deaths in China, Italy, and India

Country	Model	Description
China	Quadratic	$y = -696.84 + 107.19 \times t - 0.64 \times t^2$
Italy	Cubic	$y = -508.10 + 150.95 \times t - 9.61 \times t^2 + 0.16 \times t^3$
India	Cubic	$y = -0.65 + 0.19 \times t - 0.01 \times t^2 + 0.0002 \times t^3$

Based on Table 3.4, the best candidate curves for cumulative death toll due to the COVID-19 pandemic in China, Italy, and India are as follows:

1. **Country: China**
   - Candidate models: linear, quadratic, and cubic
   - The model selected: **quadratic**
2. **Country: Italy**
   - Candidate models: quadratic and cubic
   - The model selected: **cubic**
3. **Country: India**
   - Candidate models: cubic
   - The model selected: **cubic**

Consequently, Table 3.5 lists the best curve fits for no. of deaths in China, Italy, and India.

Remark 3.5 Similar to model descriptions in Table 3.3, the cubic curves as listed in Table 3.5 for Italy and India reveal that the coefficient of the highest polynomial term is 0.16 for Italy and 0.0002 for India, respectively, which indicates that the death toll induced by COVID-19 is lesser than the infected persons in Italy because 0.16 is much lesser than 1.56, i.e., the coefficient of the highest polynomial term

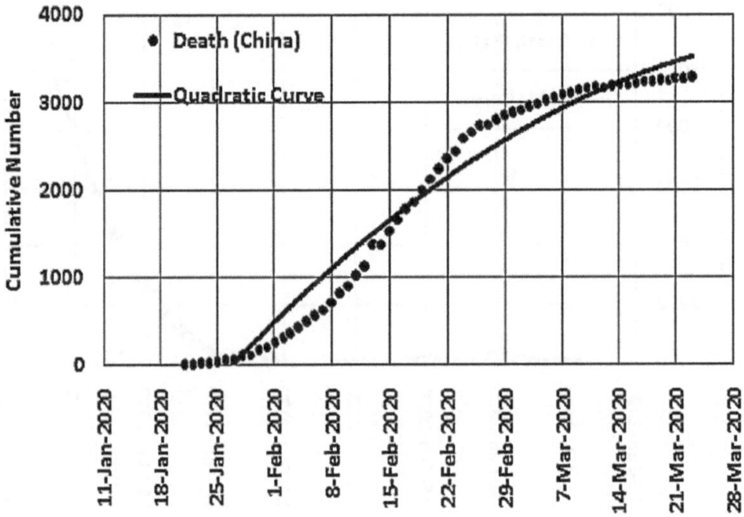

Fig. 3.5 Quadratic curve of cumulative death data of China

in infected curve. However, in case of India, the death toll is much lesser than the infectants because the coefficient of t^3 for India is 0.0002, a negligibly small value.

Therefore, the best curves listed in Table 3.5 estimate the in-sample observed values of the cumulative COVID-19 deaths in China, Italy, and India as shown in Figs. 3.5, 3.6, and 3.7.

Remark 3.6 From Fig. 3.5, it is apparent that the quadratic estimate of the no. of cumulative deaths in China by 23 March is close to 3500, whereas Fig. 3.6 shows that cubic estimates of the no. of cumulative deaths in Italy by this date are close to 5500, and lastly, Fig. 3.7 reveals that for India, the cubic death estimate is close to 6.

3.4.2.1 SVR Estimates

Notwithstanding the results achieved by curve-fitting-based estimates, we also employed the SVR method because of its ability to fit small-sized data. However, the choice of kernel function is critical in the SVR method's performance, yet choosing a perfect context-specific kernel is a fascinating investigation in SVR-based applications, and it resembles to be selected discretionary, so far [26]. In this context, we chose SVR-polykernel, described in Eqs. (3.7) and (3.8), and the meta-description of the SVR method employed in this publication is as follows:

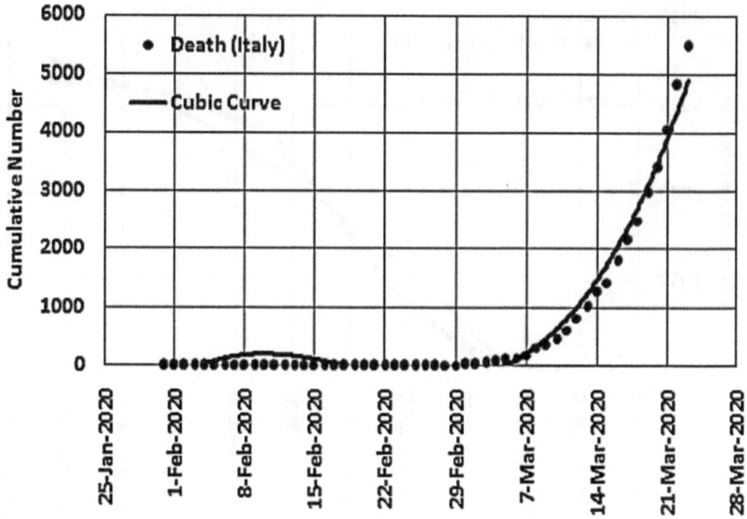

Fig. 3.6 Cubic curve of cumulative death data of Italy

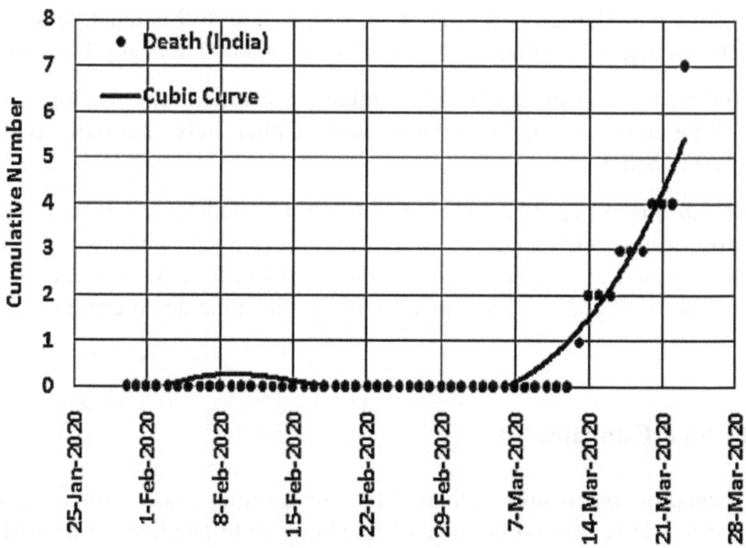

Fig. 3.7 Cubic curve of cumulative death data of India

Method	Support vector regression
Kernel	Polynomial kernel
Batch size	100
Complexity	1.0
Filter	Normalized training data
Training data normalized	SVR-sequential minimal optimization algorithm (SMO) adaption of the stopping criterion [27]
Hyper-parameter	Exponent value

3.4.2.2 Parameter Tuning

The hyper-parameter tuning of the SVR method is essential as the default parametric values do not always yield the best estimation performance. We obtained the RMSE of the estimation for both the no. of infections and the no. of deaths using WHO-based in-samples for SVR-polykernel. The SVR model trained on 90% of the in-samples for estimating 10% of the held-outs is as follows:

Country	Total observations (in days)	Training set (in days)	Held-out training set (10%) (in days)
China	63	57	6
Italy	53	48	5
India	54	49	5

After that, we fine-tuned the SVR method's exponent parameter by plotting the exponent parameter against RMSE for each of these countries, listed in Tables 3.6 and 3.7.

In Table 3.6, the lowest RMSE and its corresponding exponent for each of these countries are marked bold.

The country-wise fine-tuned exponents of the SVR method for the no. of infections are as follows:

1. **Country: China**
   - Tuned exponent value, 0.57; lowest RMSE, 19.50
2. **Country: Italy**
   - Tuned exponent value, 1.06; lowest RMSE, 373.76
3. **Country: India**
   - Tuned exponent value, 0.56; lowest RMSE, 2.77

Table 3.6 Hyper-parameter tuning table of cumulative infected data of China, Italy, and India

China		Italy		India	
Exponent	RMSE	Exponent	RMSE	Exponent	RMSE
0.50	773.6011	1.02	4459.398	0.50	37.8248
0.51	698.7735	1.03	4090.386	0.51	31.8646
0.52	662.2886	1.04	3207.172	0.52	25.1343
0.53	487.3975	1.05	1366.772	0.53	19.1418
0.54	592.4651	**1.06**	**373.7574**	0.54	11.3192
0.55	406.7633	1.07	650.6875	0.55	6.9786
0.56	67.1413	1.08	749.3844	**0.56**	**2.7686**
0.57	**19.5035**	1.09	1662.993	0.57	4.5568
0.58	210.9696	1.10	2427.523	0.58	9.8725
0.59	199.8567	1.11	2918.487	0.59	14.3362

Table 3.7 Hyper-parameter tuning table of cumulative death data of China, Italy, and India

China		Italy		India	
Exponent	RMSE	Exponent	RMSE	Exponent	RMSE
0.33	14.1041	0.95	4942.67	**0.50**	**1.327**
0.34	15.5837	0.96	3151.201	0.51	1.4179
0.35	8.2859	0.97	1776.605	0.52	1.4425
0.36	16.6798	0.98	963.034	0.53	1.5278
0.37	**0.8026**	0.99	241.6418	0.54	1.6127
0.38	2.3594	**1.00**	**23.9207**	0.55	1.6507
0.39	3.4758	1.01	334.2492	0.56	1.7042
0.40	8.8868	1.02	764.1755	0.57	1.7764
0.41	18.7469	1.03	974.0423	0.58	1.8667
0.42	39.8646	1.04	1259.953	0.59	1.9543

In Figs. 3.8, 3.9, and 3.10, the hyper-parameter tuning of SVR model for cumulative infected data is presented.

Table 3.7 lists parameter tuning of exponent in the SVR method for the cumulative death tolls in China, Italy, and India. The bold marked cells in Table 3.7 indicate the lowest RMSE and its corresponding exponent of SVR for each country.

A country-wise fine-tuned exponents of the SVR method for the no. of deaths are as follows:

1. **Country: China**
   - Tuned exponent value, 0.37; lowest RMSE, 0.80
2. **Country: Italy**
   - Tuned exponent value, 1.00; lowest RMSE, 23.92
3. **Country: India**
   - Tuned exponent value, 0.50; lowest RMSE, 1.33

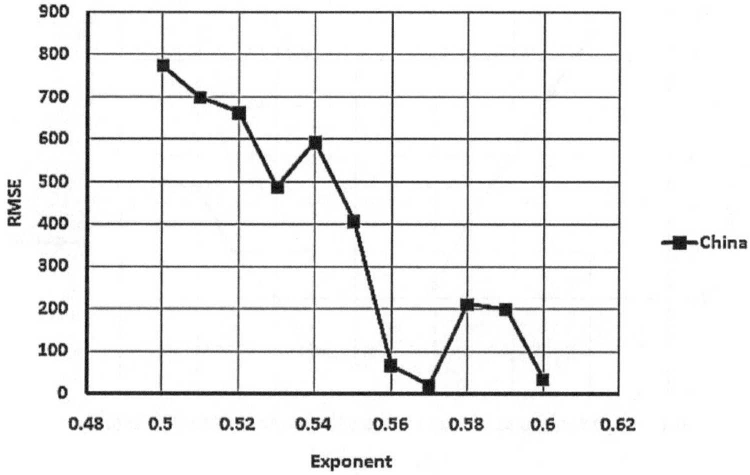

Fig. 3.8 Hyper-parameter tuning of SVR model of cumulative infected data of China

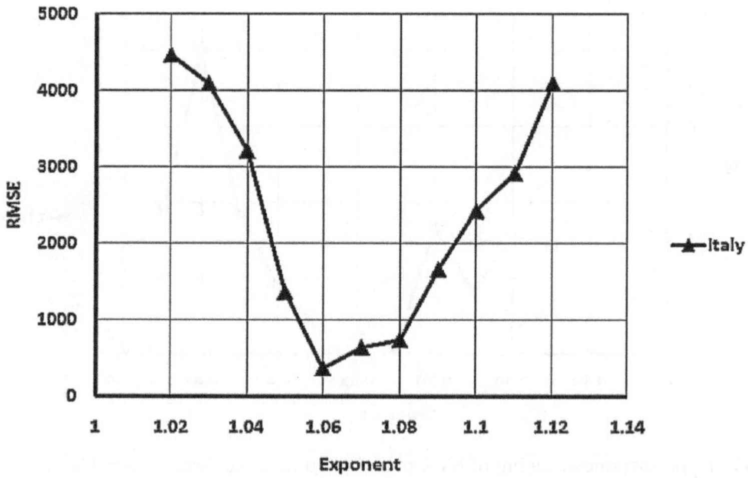

Fig. 3.9 Hyper-parameter tuning of SVR model of cumulative infected data of Italy

In Figs. 3.11, 3.12, and 3.13, the hyper-parameter tuning of SVR model for cumulative no. of deaths in China, Italy, and India is shown.

3.4.3 Out-Sample Estimation

We performed out-sample estimates of the no. of COVID-19 infection by 13 April 2020, in China, Italy, and India. The out-sample estimates for these countries

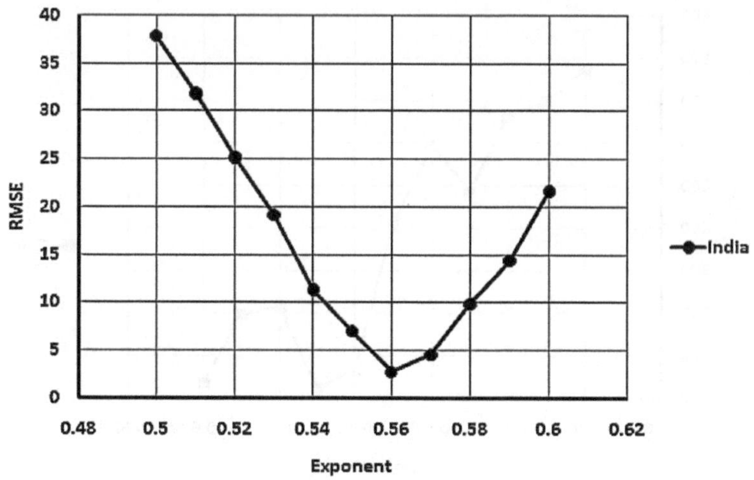

Fig. 3.10 Hyper-parameter tuning of SVR model of cumulative infected data of India

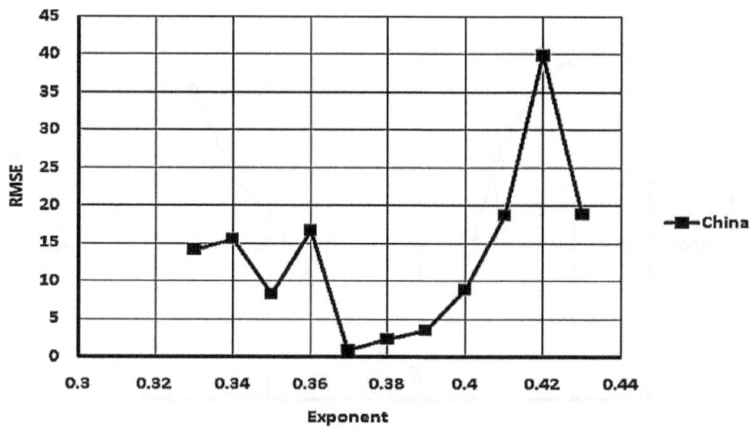

Fig. 3.11 Hyper-parameter tuning of SVR model of cumulative death data of China

are listed in Tables 3.8, 3.9, and 3.10 and shown in Figs. 3.14, 3.15, and 3.16, respectively, whereas in-sample prediction for the no. of infection up to 23 March 2020, in China, Italy, and India is shown in Figs. 3.17, 3.18, and 3.19, respectively.

Remark 3.7 In Table 3.8, it is apparent that the SVR model estimate of the no. of COVID-19 infection in China by 13 April is 89,074, whereas Table 3.9 reveals the estimated no. of cumulative infection in Italy in that period is 514,832. Finally, from Table 3.10, it appears that the predicted no. of cumulative infection in India is 19,437.

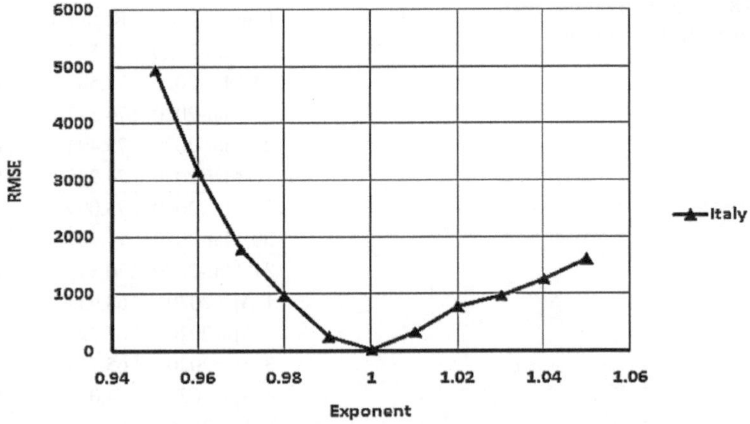

Fig. 3.12 Hyper-parameter tuning of SVR model of cumulative death data of Italy

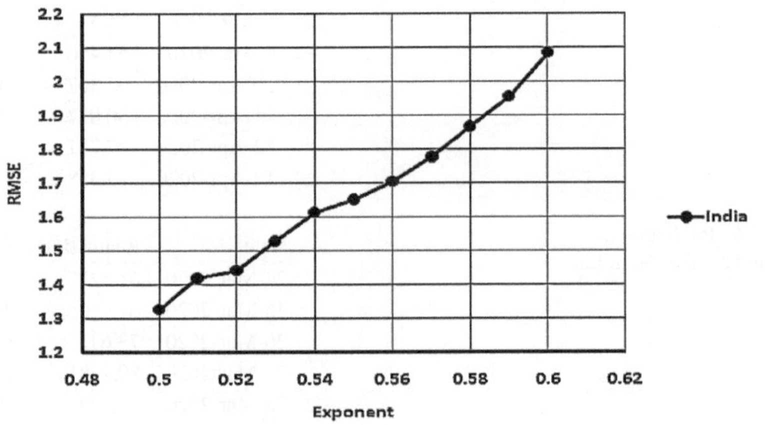

Fig. 3.13 Hyper-parameter tuning of SVR model of cumulative death data of India

Remark 3.8 Figures 3.17, 3.18, and 3.19 show the observed COVID-19 infection in China, Italy, and India, respectively, by 23 March 2020.

Remark 3.9 Figures 3.14, 3.15, and 3.16 show that the predicted no. of COVID-19 infection in China, Italy, and India by 13 April 2020 in China, Italy, and India will be 89,074, 514,832, and 19,437, respectively.

The SVR method offers out-sample estimates of death tolls up to 13 April 2020 in these countries based on in-sample death tolls up to 23 March listed in Tables 3.11, 3.12, and 3.13 and shown in Figs. 3.20, 3.21, and 3.22, respectively. The SVR-based

Table 3.8 Prediction of cumulative infection in China

Date	Regression	SVR
24-Mar-2020	78,513	81,718
25-Mar-2020	77,583	81,883
26-Mar-2020	76,577	82,083
27-Mar-2020	75,494	82,313
28-Mar-2020	74,335	82,570
29-Mar-2020	73,099	82,851
30-Mar-2020	71,787	83,167
31-Mar-2020	70,398	83,536
1-Apr-2020	68,933	83,934
2-Apr-2020	67,392	84,334
3-Apr-2020	65,774	84,732
4-Apr-2020	64,079	85,123
5-Apr-2020	62,308	85,510
6-Apr-2020	60,461	85,896
7-Apr-2020	58,537	86,280
8-Apr-2020	56,537	86,666
9-Apr-2020	54,460	87,063
10-Apr-2020	52,307	87,486
11-Apr-2020	50,077	87,956
12-Apr-2020	47,771	88,485
13-Apr-2020	45,388	89,074

Table 3.9 Prediction of cumulative infection in Italy

Date	Regression	SVR
24-Mar-2020	61,523	66,493
25-Mar-2020	67,410	74,323
26-Mar-2020	73,642	82,878
27-Mar-2020	80,228	92,365
28-Mar-2020	87,179	102,812
29-Mar-2020	94,502	114,118
30-Mar-2020	102,208	126,392
31-Mar-2020	110,305	139,665
1-Apr-2020	118,804	154,193
2-Apr-2020	127,714	170,260
3-Apr-2020	137,043	188,048
4-Apr-2020	146,802	207,480
5-Apr-2020	157,000	228,908
6-Apr-2020	167,645	252,526
7-Apr-2020	178,749	278,628
8-Apr-2020	190,319	307,609
9-Apr-2020	202,365	339,941
10-Apr-2020	214,898	376,148
11-Apr-2020	227,925	416,864
12-Apr-2020	241,456	462,798
13-Apr-2020	255,502	514,832

Table 3.10 Prediction of cumulative infection in India

Date	Regression	SVR
24-Mar-2020	327	589
25-Mar-2020	359	848
26-Mar-2020	394	1252
27-Mar-2020	430	1798
28-Mar-2020	468	2481
29-Mar-2020	509	3348
30-Mar-2020	551	4356
31-Mar-2020	596	5466
1-Apr-2020	643	6657
2-Apr-2020	692	7908
3-Apr-2020	744	9175
4-Apr-2020	798	10,437
5-Apr-2020	855	11,677
6-Apr-2020	914	12,875
7-Apr-2020	976	14,016
8-Apr-2020	1040	15,094
9-Apr-2020	1107	16,103
10-Apr-2020	1177	17,041
11-Apr-2020	1250	17,908
12-Apr-2020	1325	18,706
13-Apr-2020	1403	19,437

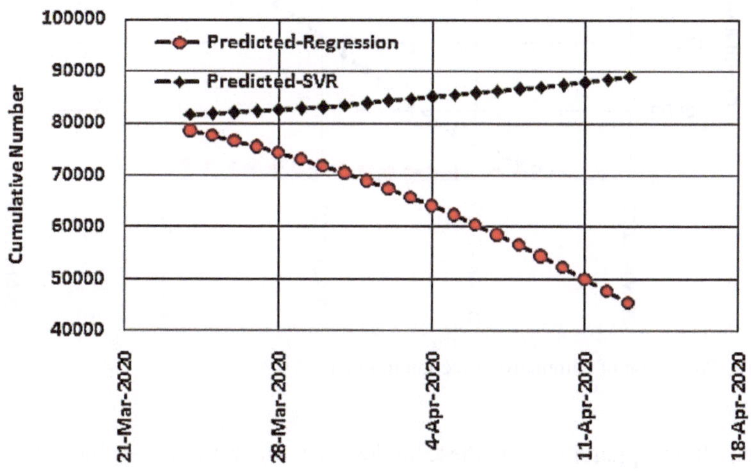

Fig. 3.14 Prediction of cumulative infection in China

in-sample death tolls in China, Italy, and India are shown in Figs. 3.23, 3.24, and 3.25, respectively.

Remark 3.10 In Tables 3.11, 3.12, and 3.13, the predicted death obtained from the regression and the SVR model of the country, China, Italy, and India, respectively,

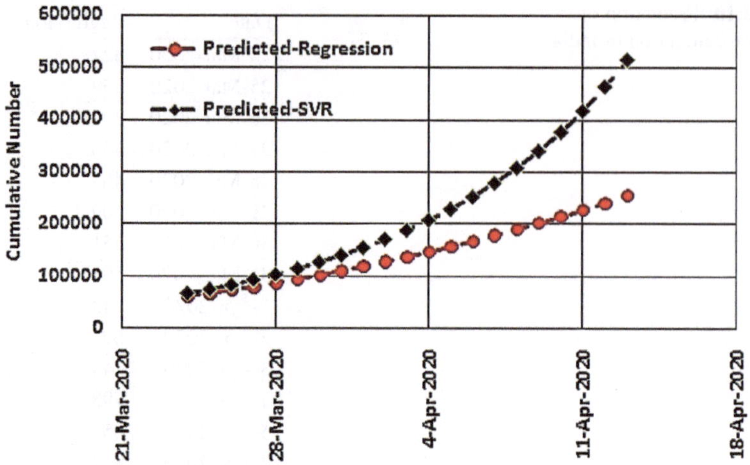

Fig. 3.15 Prediction of cumulative infection in Italy

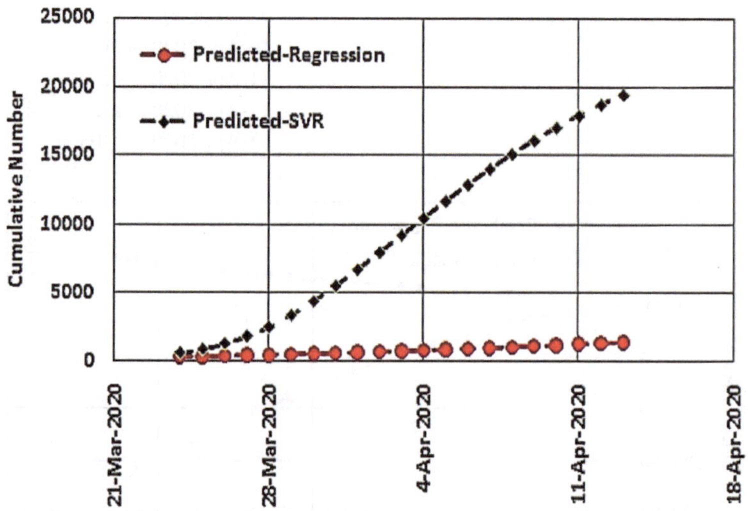

Fig. 3.16 Prediction of cumulative infection in India

is listed. It is apparent from these tables that the estimates achieved using the SVR method are close to real-time no. of deaths, particularly in China and India, and outperformed the conventional regression estimates. In contrast, the regression estimates performed better in approximating the no. of death tolls in Italy till 13 April 2020.

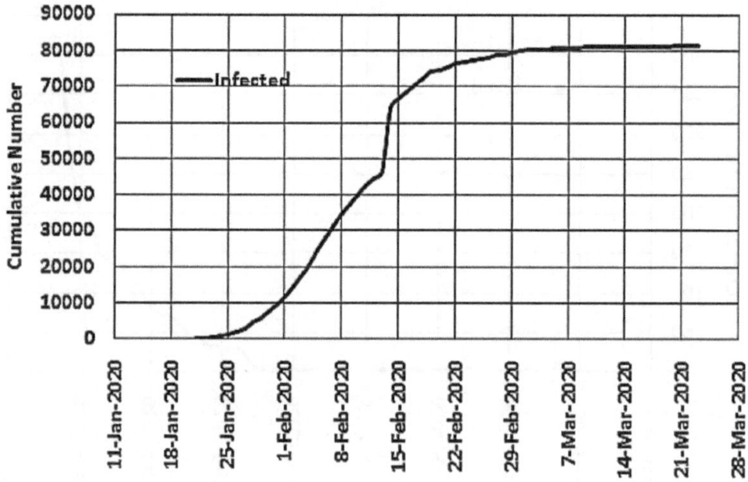

Fig. 3.17 Cumulative infection in China

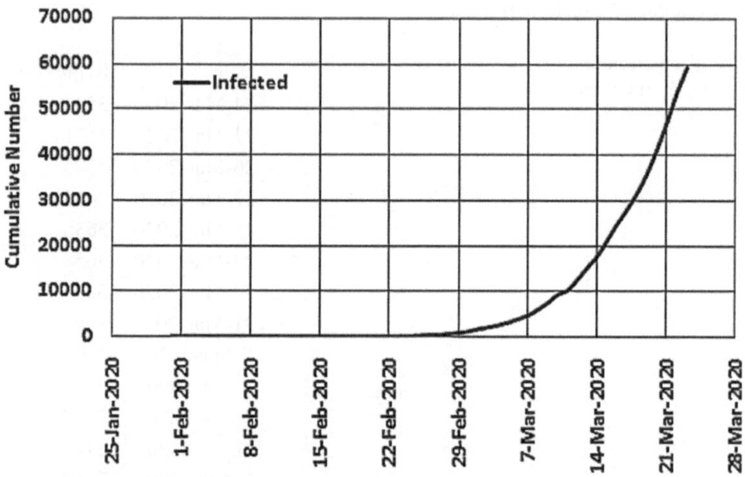

Fig. 3.18 Cumulative infection in Italy

3.5 Time Complexity Analysis

We considered linear, quadratic, and cubic curve-fitting techniques and the SVR method in estimating the catastrophe. The asymptotic analysis is critical in estimating the performance of algorithms independent of machine-specific constants. Therefore, complexity analysis of curve-fitting and SVR methods is crucial for perceiving the upper bound of theoretical time taken by these methods in offering the estimates of the COVID-19 outbreak in China, Italy, and India.

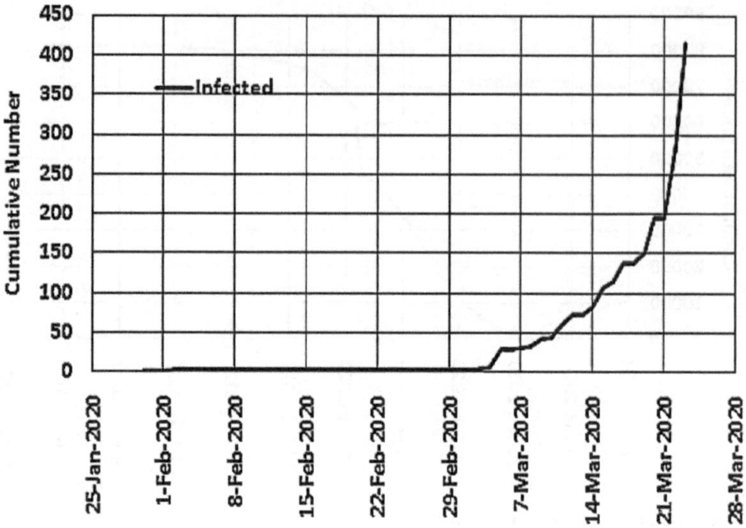

Fig. 3.19 Cumulative infection in India

Table 3.11 Prediction of cumulative death in China

Date	Regression	SVR
24-Mar-2020	3547	3287
25-Mar-2020	3571	3293
26-Mar-2020	3595	3301
27-Mar-2020	3617	3307
28-Mar-2020	3638	3314
29-Mar-2020	3658	3320
30-Mar-2020	3676	3324
31-Mar-2020	3693	3329
1-Apr-2020	3709	3335
2-Apr-2020	3724	3339
3-Apr-2020	3737	3344
4-Apr-2020	3749	3349
5-Apr-2020	3760	3355
6-Apr-2020	3769	3360
7-Apr-2020	3777	3366
8-Apr-2020	3784	3372
9-Apr-2020	3790	3378
10-Apr-2020	3794	3383
11-Apr-2020	3797	3389
12-Apr-2020	3799	3394
13-Apr-2020	3799	3400

Table 3.12 Prediction of cumulative death in Italy

Date	Regression	SVR
24-Mar-2020	5433	6249
25-Mar-2020	5998	7142
26-Mar-2020	6597	8058
27-Mar-2020	7232	9148
28-Mar-2020	7904	10,258
29-Mar-2020	8614	11,416
30-Mar-2020	9363	12,788
31-Mar-2020	10,151	14,215
1-Apr-2020	10,981	15,735
2-Apr-2020	11,852	17,388
3-Apr-2020	12,766	19,066
4-Apr-2020	13,723	20,937
5-Apr-2020	14,725	22,976
6-Apr-2020	15,773	25,095
7-Apr-2020	16,868	27,427
8-Apr-2020	18,011	29,939
9-Apr-2020	19,202	32,656
10-Apr-2020	20,442	35,697
11-Apr-2020	21,734	38,987
12-Apr-2020	23,077	42,624
13-Apr-2020	24,472	46,757

Table 3.13 Prediction of cumulative death in India

Date	Regression	SVR
24-Mar-2020	6	10
25-Mar-2020	7	16
26-Mar-2020	7	24
27-Mar-2020	8	34
28-Mar-2020	9	46
29-Mar-2020	10	59
30-Mar-2020	11	73
31-Mar-2020	11	88
1-Apr-2020	12	104
2-Apr-2020	13	119
3-Apr-2020	14	133
4-Apr-2020	16	147
5-Apr-2020	17	159
6-Apr-2020	18	170
7-Apr-2020	19	180
8-Apr-2020	20	189
9-Apr-2020	22	197
10-Apr-2020	23	204
11-Apr-2020	25	210
12-Apr-2020	26	215
13-Apr-2020	28	220

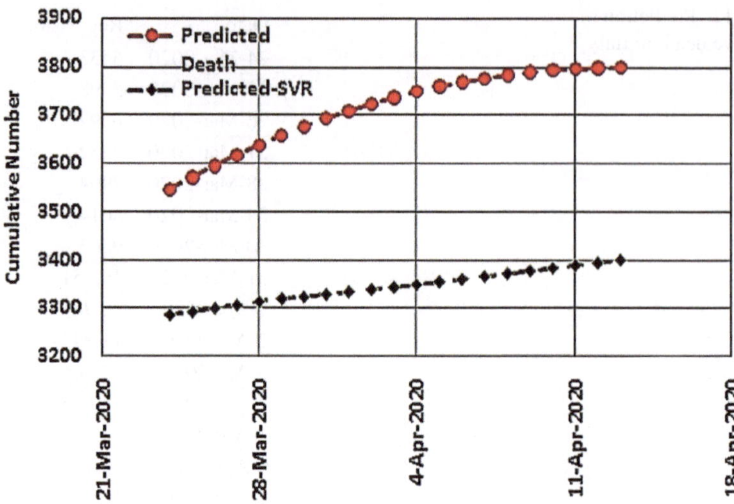

Fig. 3.20 Estimation of cumulative death in China

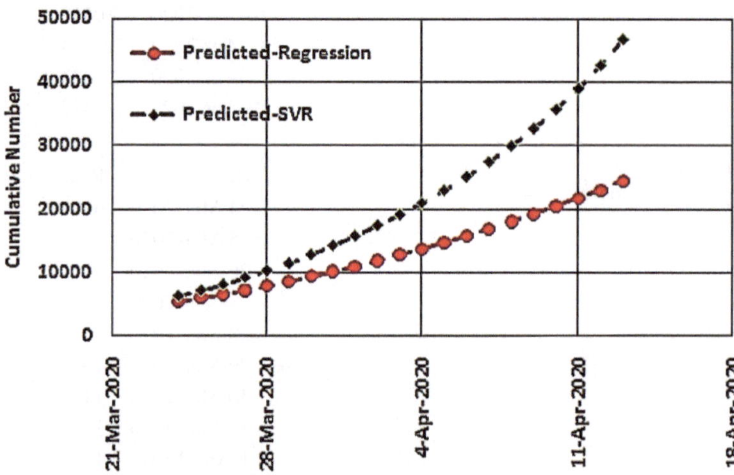

Fig. 3.21 Estimation of cumulative death in Italy

3.5.1 Time Complexity of the Curve-Fitting Models

The linear model is guided by Eq. (3.1), and the worst-case time complexity becomes $O(a_0 + a_1 \times t) \approx O(t)$. Similarly, the quadratic model is guided by Eq. (3.2), and the time complexity is $O(a_0 + a_1 \times t + a_2 \times t^2) \approx O(t^2)$, and lastly, the cubic model is guided by Eq. (3.3) and has a time complexity of $O(a_0 + a_1 \times t + a_2 \times t^2 + a_3 \times t^3) \approx O(t^3)$. Although $O(t) \ll O(t^2) \ll O(t^3)$,

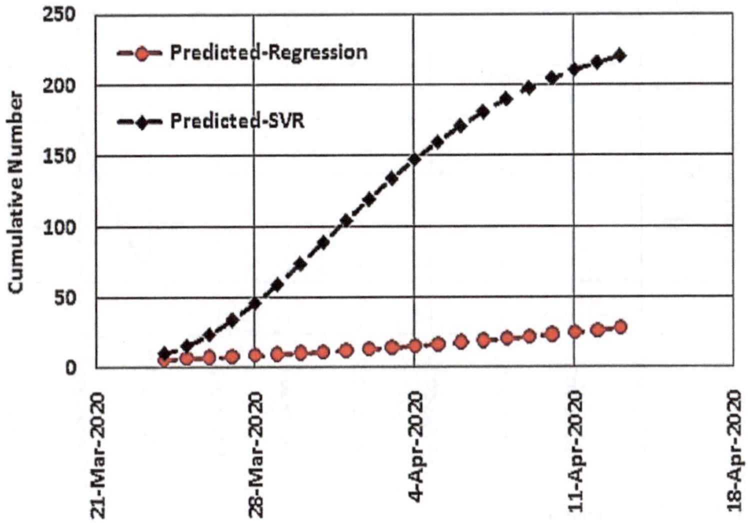

Fig. 3.22 Estimation of cumulative death in India

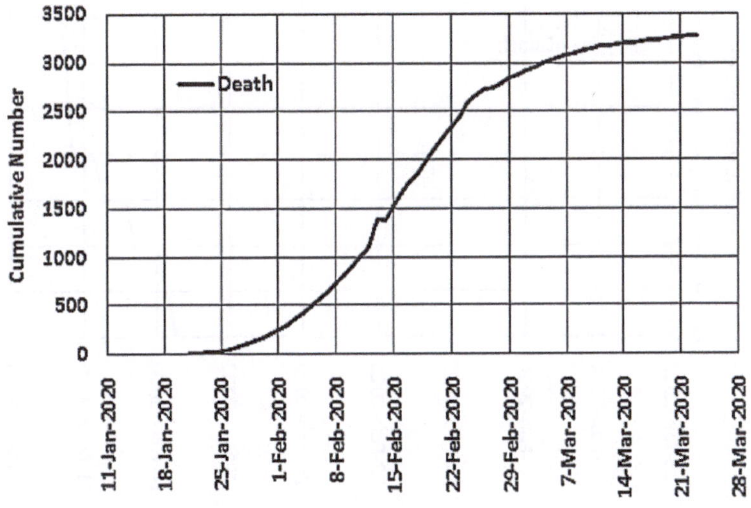

Fig. 3.23 Cumulative death in China

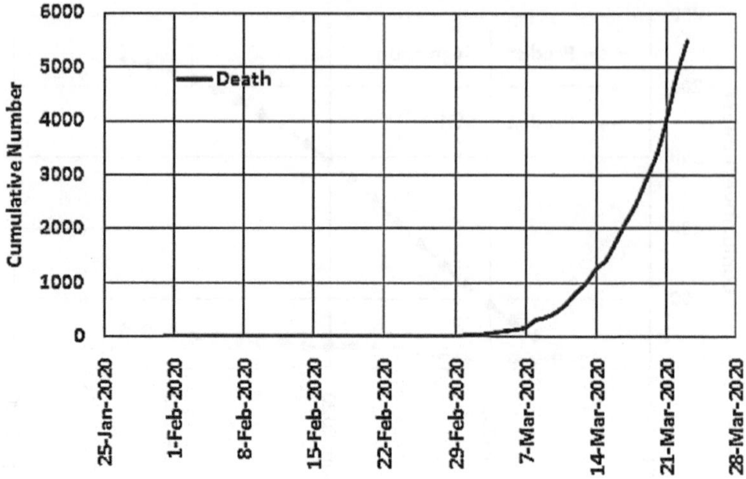

Fig. 3.24 Cumulative death in Italy

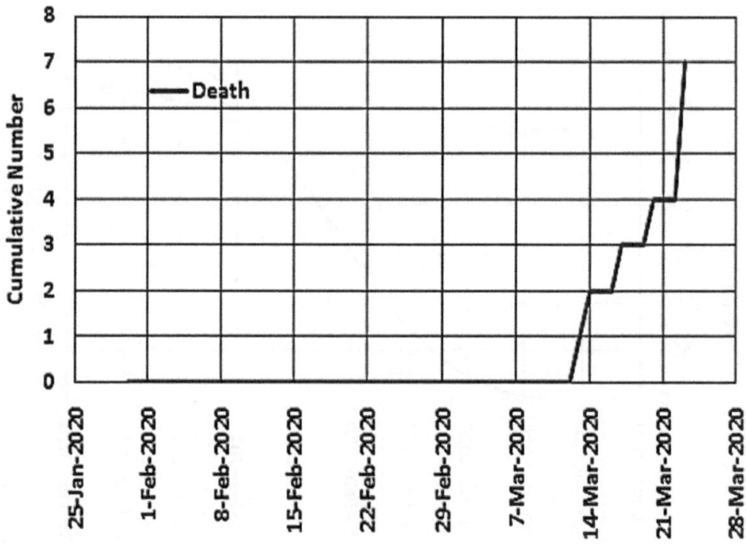

Fig. 3.25 Cumulative death in India

the linear model is observed to be inadequate in our work and doesn't match the exponential rise of the COVID-19-affected people in these three countries.

3.5.2 Time Complexity of the SVR Method

An upper bound on the time complexity of the SVR method is guided by $O(n^2 \times f + n^3)$, for training the model using large no. of samples, whereas for prediction, the time complexity becomes $O(n^{'} \times f)$, where n is the no. of training samples, f is the no. of features, and $n^{'}$ is the no. of support vectors. Since this publication considered a small dataset rendered by WHO and two features, namely, no. of affected people and no. of people who died, the upper bounds on the time complexities of training and prediction are modified as $O(n^2 \times f + n^3) \approx O(n^2 \times 2 + n^3) \approx O(n^3)$ and $O(n^{'} \times f) \approx O(n^{'})$.

3.5.3 Time Complexity of Selecting the Best-Fit Candidate

The algorithm to select the best-fit candidate is primarily limited to the problem of finding the candidate with the lowest RMSE out of the four estimation methods considered in this paper. For m, no. of methods where $m = 4$, the upper bound on the time complexity of choosing the one with the lowest RMSE is reduced to $O(m - 1)$.

In our work, the SVR outperformed the curve-fitting methods in terms of lowest RMSE. Consequently, the upper bound on the total time complexity of selecting the best-fit candidate and predicting the adversity caused by this outbreak becomes $O(m - 1) + O(n^3) + O(n^{'}) \approx O(n^3) + O(n^{'})$.

3.6 Recommendation for Controlling the Spread of COVID-19 Outbreak Based on the Proposed Study

The outcomes obtained by the SVR method to depict the COVID-19 scenario in China, Italy, and India is satisfactory; however, the role of trend analysis using curve-fitting methods cannot be ignored to estimate the pattern of a pandemic outbreak. In this context, Yang et al. [28] proposed the use of time-series forecasting methods such as the early aberration reporting system (EARS), the cumulative SUM (CUSUM), ARIMA, and the Holt-Winters algorithm, for quick detection of infectious outbreaks in Korea. In another work, authors of [29] employed a statistical model, namely, the susceptible-infectious-recovered-dead (SIRD) model, to estimate the COVID-19 outbreak in the Hubei region of China. The SIRD model outperformed the linear regression method in terms of the estimated average

Table 3.14 Disease outbreak estimation methods [28–30]

Authors	Forecasting method		Forecasting disease	
	Statistical	Time series	Pandemic	COVID-19
Yang et al. [28]	✓	✓	✓	
Anastassopoulou et al. [29]	✓		✓	✓
Kuniya [30]	✓		✓	✓
Our work	✓	✓	✓	✓

Table 3.15 Comparative result between SVR and Worldometers estimates

Country	Infected (SVR)	Real-time infected (up to 12 April 2020)	Deaths (SVR)	Real-time deaths (up to 12 April 2020)
China	89,000	82,160	3400	3341
Italy	514,832	159,516	46,757	20,465
India	19,437	10,453	220	358

value of the basic reproduction number (R_0) of 2019-nCoV. Additionally, the SIRD model suggested a slowdown of the outbreak at the end of February 2020 in the Hubei province. In a similar work, Kuniya [30] proposed a statistical model, namely, the susceptible-exposed-infectious-recovered (SEIR), to predict the pandemic peak of COVID-19 in Japan. The SEIR model used a least squares-based method with Poisson noise and estimated the adversity of the pandemic in terms of R_0. Their model predicted that Japan reaches the epidemic peak by the mid of summer 2020. An outline of pandemic estimation methods adopted by Yang et al., Anastassopoulou et al. and Kuniya [28–30] is listed in Table 3.14.

This publication employed curve-fitting and SVR methods to estimate the pandemic status in three countries, namely, China, Italy, and India. Accordingly, we observed that the SVR method offers better estimates than linear regression and outperformed the time-series forecasting methods in terms of RMSE, R^2, and adjusted R^2 in China and India. A summary of comparisons between the SVR-based estimates and real-time Worldometers statistics [31] is listed in Table 3.15.

Remark 3.11 In Table 3.15, it is apparent that China will witness 89,000 and 3400 COVID-19 infections and deaths, respectively, by 13 April 2020, against a very close match of 82,160 and 3341 infections and deaths, respectively, by 12 April 2020 as rendered by [31]. As for Italy, the SVR method recommends that there will be 514,832 and 46,757 COVID-19 infections and deaths, respectively, by 13 April 2020 against 159,516 and 20,465 infections and deaths, respectively, by 12 April 2020 given by [31]. Lastly, for India, the SVR method estimated a 19,437 infections and 220 deaths by 13 April against real-time 10,453 and 358 infections and deaths, respectively, by April 12.

The estimation result achieved for Italy indicates that the SVR-based in-sample estimation yielded higher RMSE than China and India and becomes unfit for Italy, whereas the regression-based estimates confer 255,502 COVID-19 infections and

24,472 deaths by 13 April 2020 against real-time statistics of 159,516 infections and 20,465 deaths in Italy by 12 April 2020. Consequently, based on these outcomes, we recommend the use of the following:

- SVR method fits close to the COVID-19 outbreak patterns for highly populous countries such as China and India.
- For a relatively less dense country such as Italy, the use of traditional time-series forecasting methods can be a reasonable choice where the SVR method becomes incompetent.

3.7 Conclusion and Future Scope

The unfortunate outbreak of the COVID-19 epidemic unfavorably struck the liveliness of the human race. This unprecedented situation warrants effective countermeasures to stop the expansion of this deadly outbreak. The virus is novel without any trace before, which makes it incredibly challenging for us to estimate its adversity. Apart from it, a relatively small dataset is publicly available to discover a robust estimation model to measure the misfortune which resulted from the COVID-19, where the use of any single estimation method is unconvincing because a small-scale data consisting only of 63 in-samples often leads to imprecise and overfit estimates. Consequently, this publication annotated the use of the SVR method and trend analysis techniques such as curve fitting to determine the best-fit estimation candidate in terms of RMSE to represent the trouble to be induced by this global outbreak in China, Italy, and India in a specified period. Based on our observations, the quadratic polynomial becomes the best fit to predict the cumulative no. of deaths and infections in China, whereas cubic polynomial is the best-fit candidate to estimate the adversities in Italy and India, respectively. The quadratic curve fit for China supports the fact that it witnessed a fall in the no. of cases, whereas the recent spikes induced by the COVID-19 justify cubic fit in the no. of affected and death in Italy and India.

Nonetheless, these curve-fitting methods are wearisome and labor-intensive. As such, we employed the SVR method because of its input space-independent nature in the estimation of COVID-19 misfortunes. However, the SVR method's performance depends on the choice of kernel function and parameter tuning, wherein we fine-tuned the exponent of the SVR-polykernel to achieve optimal estimates in terms of minimum RMSE based on R^2 and adj. R^2 between the no. of affected and dead specimens. Based on the outcomes, we conclude that the SVR method outperformed the curve-fitting methods in terms of RMSE of out-of-sample estimates in China and India. However, the practical outcome of this pandemic is time-variant and depends on other yet socioeconomic determinants. Therefore, we used a plethora of estimation models utilizing a small dataset to achieve close estimates to help authorities in formulating counter-strategies to combat COVID-19.

References

1. V.D. Menachery, B.L. Yount Jr., K. Debbink, S. Agnihothram, L.E. Gralinski, J.A. Plante, R.L. Graham, T. Scobey, X.Y. Ge, E.F. Donaldson, S.H. Randell, A. Lanzavecchia, W.A. Marasco, Z.L. Shi, R.S. Baric, A SARS-like cluster of circulating bat coronaviruses shows the potential for human emergence. Nat. Med. **21**(12), 1508–1513 (2015). https://doi.org/10.1038/nm.3985
2. N. Zhu, D. Zhang, W. Wang, X. Li, B. Yang, J. Song, X. Zhao, B. Huang, W. Shi, R. Lu, P. Niu, F. Zhan, X. Ma, D. Wang, W. Xu, G. Wu, G.F. Gao, W. Tan, A novel coronavirus from patients with pneumonia in China, 2019. N. Engl. J. Med. (2020). https://doi.org/10.1056/NEJMoa2001017
3. C. Huang, Y. Wang, X. Li, L. Ren, J. Zhao, Y. Hu, L. Zhang, G. Fan, J. Xu, X. Gu, Z. Cheng, T. Yu, J. Xia, Y. Wei, W. Wu, X. Xie, W. Yin, H. Li, M. Liu, Y. Xiao, H. Gao, L. Guo, J. Xie, G. Wang, R. Jiang, Z. Gao, Q. Jin, J. Wang, B. Cao, Clinical features of patients infected with 2019 novel coronavirus in Wuhan, China. Lancet **395**(10223), 497–506 (2020). https://doi.org/10.1016/S0140-6736(20)30183-5
4. A.M. Zaki, S.V. Boheemen, T.M. Bestebroer, A.D.M.E. Osterhaus, R.A.M. Fouchier, Isolation of a novel coronavirus from a man with pneumonia in Saudi Arabia. N. Engl. J. Med. **367**(19), 1814–1820 (2012). https://doi.org/10.1056/NEJMoa1211721
5. R. Lu, X. Zhao, J. Li, P. Niu, B. Yang, H. Wu, W. Wang, H. Song, B. Huang, N. Zhu, Y. Bi, X. Ma, F. Zhan, L. Wang, T. Hu, H. Zhou, Z. Hu, W. Zhou, L. Zhao, J. Chen, Y. Meng, J. Wang, Y. Lin, J. Yuan, Z. Xie, J. Ma, W.J. Liu, D. Wang, W. Xu, E.C. Holmes, G.F. Gao, G. Wu, W. Chen, W. Shi, W. Tan, Genomic characterisation and epidemiology of 2019 novel coronavirus: Implications for virus origins and receptor binding. Lancet **395**(10224), 565–574 (2020). https://doi.org/10.1016/S0140-6736(20)30251-8
6. J. Gale, *Coronavirus May Transmit Along Fecal-Oral Route*, Xinhua Reports, 3rd (2020)
7. M.A.A. Al-qaness, A.A. Ewees, H. Fan, M.A.E. Aziz, Optimization method for forecasting confirmed cases of COVID-19 in China. J. Clin. Med. **9**(3), 674 (2020). https://doi.org/10.3390/jcm9030674
8. H.H. Elmousalami, A.E. Hassanien, Day level forecasting for coronavirus disease (COVID-19) spread: Analysis, modeling and recommendations. Quant. Biol. (2020) https://arxiv.org/abs/2003.07778v1
9. M. Ture, I. Kurt, Comparison of four different time series methods to forecast hepatitis A virus infection. Expert Syst. Appl. **31**(1), 41–46 (2006). https://doi.org/10.1016/j.eswa.2005.09.002
10. S. Zhao, Q. Lin, J. Ran, S.S. Musa, G. Yang, W. Wang, Y. Lou, D. Gao, L. Yang, D. He, M.H. Wang, Preliminary estimation of the basic reproduction number of novel coronavirus (2019-nCoV) in China, from 2019 to 2020: A data-driven analysis in the early phase of the outbreak. Int. J. Infect. Dis. **92**, 214–217 (2020). https://doi.org/10.1016/j.ijid.2020.01.050
11. WHO | Novel Coronavirus – China, Situation report archived from WHO, https://www.who.int/emergencies/diseases/novel-coronavirus-2019/situation-reports. Accessed 23 Mar 2020
12. https://in.mathworks.com/help/curvefit/evaluating-goodness-of-fit.html?s_tid=gn_loc_drop
13. https://www.theanalysisfactor.com/assessing-the-fit-of-regression-models
14. https://towardsdatascience.com/wth-are-r-squared-and-adjusted-r-squared-7b816eef90d9
15. https://statisticsbyjim.com/regression/interpret-f-test-overall-significance-regression
16. E. Kafazi, R. Bannari, A. Abouabdellah, M.O. Aboutafail, J.M. Guerrero, Energy production: A comparison of forecasting methods using the polynomial curve fitting and linear regression, in *International Renewable and Sustainable Energy Conference (IRSEC)*, (IEEE Press, Tangier, 2017), pp. 1–5. https://doi.org/10.1109/IRSEC.2017.8477278
17. A.H. Donmez, Y. Karakoyun, Z. Yumurtaci, Electricity demand forecast of Turkey based on hydropower and windpower potential. Energy Sources Part B Econ. Plan. Policy **12**(1), 85–90 (2017). https://doi.org/10.1080/15567249.2015.1084401

18. P. Srikanth, D. Rao, P. Vidyullatha, Comparative analysis of ANFIS, ARIMA and polynomial curve fitting for weather forecasting. Indian J. Sci. Technol. **9**(15), 1–6 (2016). https://doi.org/10.17485/ijst/2016/v9i15/89814
19. M.A.A. Jalil, S.A.A. Karim, Z. Baharuddin, M.F. Abdullah, M. Othman, Forecasting solar radiation data using Gaussian and polynomial fitting methods, in *Sustainable Electrical Power Resources Through Energy Optimization and Future Engineering*, (Springer, Singapore, 2018), pp. 11–24. https://doi.org/10.1007/978-981-13-0435-4_2
20. M. Awad, R. Khanna, *Support Vector Regression, Efficient Learning Machines* (Apress, Berkeley, CA, 2015). https://doi.org/10.1007/978-1-4302-5990-9_4
21. V. Vapnik, A. Lerner, Pattern recognition using generalized portrait method. Autom. Remote. Control. **24**(6), 774–780 (1963)
22. R.J. Hyndman, G. Athanasopoulos, C. Bergmeir, G. Caceres, L. Chhay, M. O'Hara-Wild, F. Petropoulos, S. Razbash, E. Wang, F. Yasmeen, forecast: Forecasting functions for time series and linear models, R package version 8.4 (2018), http://pkg.robjhyndman.com/forecast
23. R.J. Hyndman, Y. Khandakar, Automatic time series forecasting: The forecast package for R. J. Stat. Softw. **26**(3), 1–22 (2008). https://doi.org/10.18637/jss.v027.i03
24. R Core Team, *R: A Language and Environment for Statistical Computing* (R Foundation for Statistical Computing, Vienna, Austria, 2019) https://www.R-project.org
25. A. Smith, C. Tony, Introducing machine learning concepts with WEKA, in *Statistical Genomics Methods in Molecular Biology*, vol. 1418, (Humana Press, New York, 2016), pp. 353–378. https://doi.org/10.1007/978-1-4939-3578-9_17
26. A. Zakrani, M. Hain, A. Idri, Improving software development effort estimation using support vector regression and feature selection. IAES Int. J. Artif. Intell. **8**(4), 399–410 (2019). https://doi.org/10.11591/ijai.v8.i4.pp399-410
27. S.K. Shevade, S.S. Keerthi, C. Bhattacharyya, K.K. Murthy, Improvements to the SMO algorithm for SVM regression. IEEE Trans. Neural Netw. **11**(5), 1188–1193 (2000). https://doi.org/10.1109/72.870050
28. E. Yang, H.W. Park, Y.H. Choi, J. Kim, L. Munkhdalai, I. Musa, K.H. Ryu, A simulation-based study on the comparison of statistical and time series forecasting methods for early detection of infectious disease outbreaks. Int. J. Environ. Res. Public Health **15**(5), 1–8 (2018). https://doi.org/10.3390/ijerph15050966
29. C. Anastassopoulou, L. Russo, A. Tsakris, C. Siettos, Data-based analysis, modelling and forecasting of the COVID-19 outbreak. PLoS One **31** (2020). https://doi.org/10.1371/journal.pone.0230405
30. T. Kuniya, Prediction of the epidemic peak of coronavirus disease in Japan. J. Clin. Med. **9**(3) (2020). https://doi.org/10.3390/jcm9030789
31. https://www.worldometers.info/coronavirus/#countries. Accessed 12 Apr 2020

Chapter 4
Management of Future Outbreak Risks (Prevention, Control and Treatment)

Abhinay Thakur and Ashish Kumar

4.1 Introduction

At the beginning of December 2019, many patients with unidentified aetiology of pneumonia were reported in Wuhan City, Hubei Province, China [1]. Genetic analysis has revealed that this pneumonia, recognized as coronavirus disease 2019 (COVID-19), was triggered by severe acute respiratory syndrome coronavirus 2 (SARS-CoV-2), formerly recognized as 2019 novel coronavirus (2019-nCoV) [2]. Considering the global threat and rapid transmission of this virus, the World Health Organization on 11 March 2020 declared COVID-19 as a public health emergency of international concern. This new and emerging virus is much more similar to SARS-CoV than MERS-CoV, as both can induce pathogenesis by the same reforms [3]. SARS-CoV's transmission to humans has been confirmed from market civets, while MERS-CoV's was from camels. Additionally, the recently identified SARS-CoV-2 also tends to be transmitted through wild animals where they were sold to people in a wet market. However, the zoonotic origins of their transmission are still not evidently proved. Like SARS-CoV and MERS-CoV, this emerging SARS-CoV-2 virus is a part of the β-CoV lineage B. Based on the available date, 2019-nCoV has 3% of pathogenicity rate, which is substantially less then SARS-CoV (10%) and MERS-CoV (40%) [4, 5]. Nevertheless, the transmissibility rate of 2019-nCoV is significantly higher, i.e. R0, 1.4–5.5, as compared to SARS-CoV having R0, 2–5, and MERS-CoV having R0, <1 [6].

On 8 December 2019, Chinese officials reported the first patient showing symptoms. On 9 January 2020, WHO verified that one of the hospitalized persons was suffering from a novel coronavirus, and the first death case was documented

A. Thakur · A. Kumar (✉)
Department of Chemistry, Faculty of Technology and Sciences, Lovely Professional University, Phagwara, Punjab, India

L. Garg et al. (eds.), *Healthcare Informatics for Fighting COVID-19 and Future Epidemics*, EAI/Springer Innovations in Communication and Computing,
https://doi.org/10.1007/978-3-030-72752-9_4

on the same day [7]. The first incident outside China was observed in Thailand on 13 January. In the following few days, many other countries have reported cases of 2019-nCoV with elevated levels of infected cases and deaths [8]. As of 23 July 2020, COVID-19 has infected 213 countries and territories globally and 2 international transports with gross confirmed cases of 15,390,221, death rates of 630,537 and recoveries of 9,367,463 worldwide. The severe problems patients face in epidemic cases need timely responses from healthcare facilities. Unluckily, several conventional solutions that initiate drug production are ineffective during outbreaks; a procedure that takes years is not sufficient to support today's dying patients and firms that are being halted [9]. Studies on conscientious uses were also performed in these cases, and approvals for clinical trials were facilitated. This same scenario was prominently observed during the Ebola epidemic in 2014–2015, where a number of candidates for clinical trials were tested. Several of the treatments failed, but in the end, a vaccine was developed that was absolutely effective against the virus [10]. It must be kept in mind that finding a cure for Ebola also took years of research, and an effectively neutralized vaccine was developed and evaluated in preclinical animal trials for years, unlike the present predicament with COVID-19.

However, there has been still a lack of awareness of what is possible in the initial stages of the COVID-19 outbreak, which can be viewed as a valuable guide for the potential management of these pandemic outbreaks [11]. In this document, we will discuss various possible treatments and preventive and control measures that could be beneficial to combat against ongoing novel malignant pathogenic infections by such class of coronaviruses and can be used to plan for future outbreaks. This report may also provide useful information for future research on the relevant topics. It may help policy decision-making on strategies to address such emergencies in public health concern at regional, national and international levels [12]. Figure 4.1 illustrates the body organs infected by SARAS-CoV-2.

4.2 COVID-19 Pathophysiology

COVID-19 is a SARS-CoV-2-induced beta-coronavirus containing single-stranded RNA sequence corresponding to *Coronavirinae* subfamily, a member of *Coronaviridae* family. In Fig. 4.2, a confined structure of severe acute respiratory syndrome coronavirus 2 (SARS-CoV-2) is being shown. SARS-CoV-2 sequence analysis revealed a schematic view of other coronaviruses. Its genome was found to be similar to the coronavirus strain that provoked SARS outbreak in 2003 [13]. SARS coronavirus (SARS-CoV) has an excellently defined formulation consisting of 14 linking sequences that interact specifically with the enzyme that transforms human angiotensin. For such amino acids, eight in SARS-CoV-2 have been retained. Like the previous SARS and MERS, existing SARS-CoV-2 causes mild respiratory infections in humans. The optimal mechanism of SARS-CoV-2 remains speculative until the laboratory trials are initiated [14]. Figure 4.3 illustrates the coronavirus genome structure and comparison with MERS-CoV genome and protein.

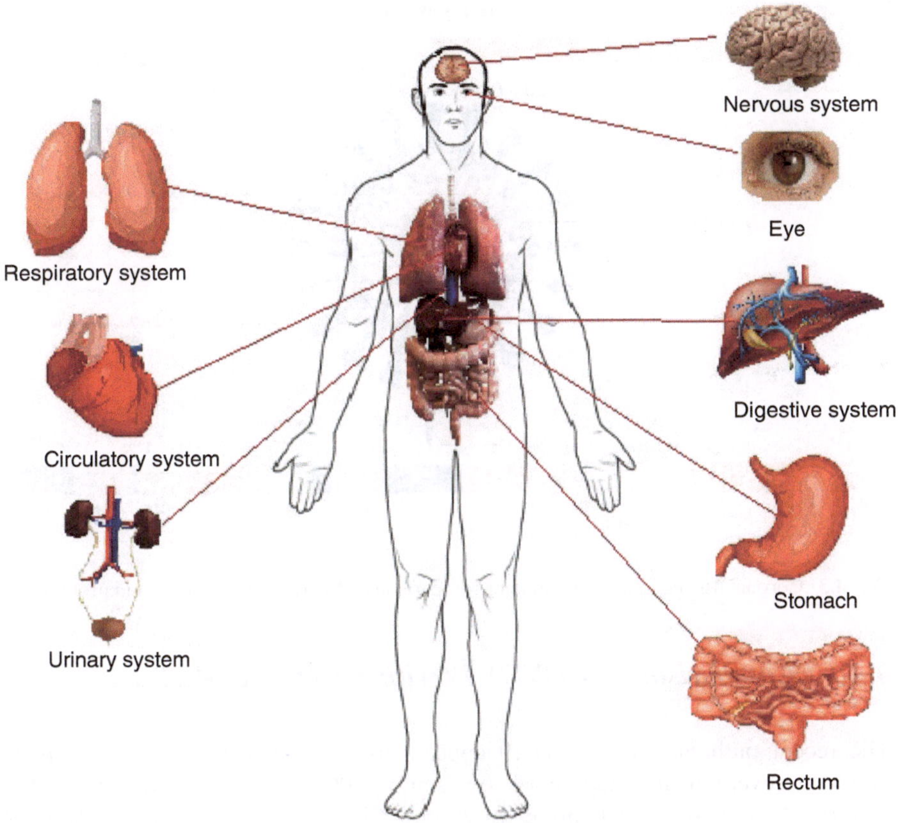

Fig. 4.1 Several organs which have been infected by COVID-19

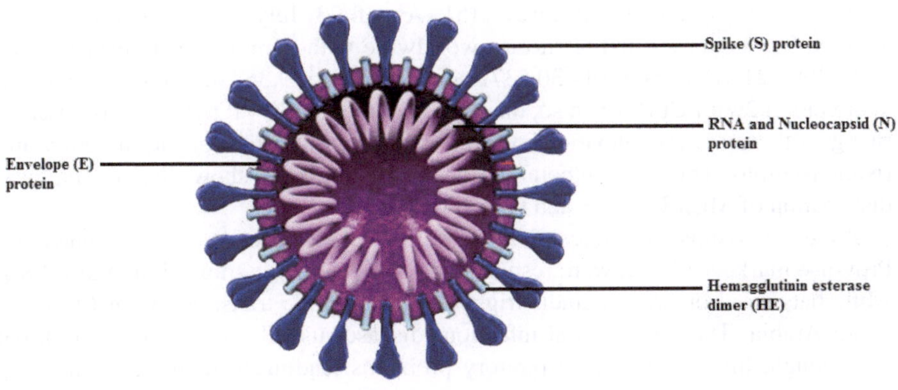

Fig. 4.2 A structure of severe acute respiratory syndrome coronavirus 2 (SARS-CoV-2)

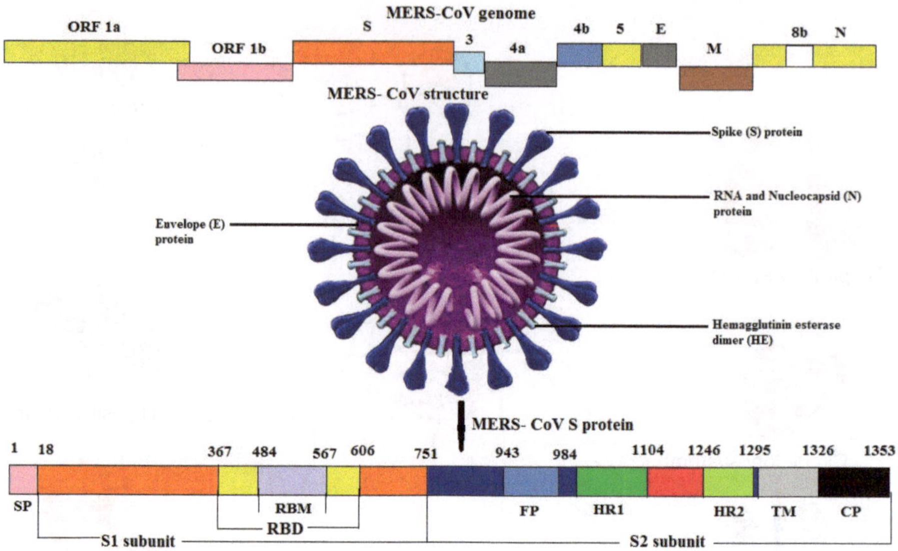

Fig. 4.3 Coronavirus genome structure and comparison of MERS-CoV genome and protein

4.2.1 Comparison of COVID-19 with SARS and MERS

The recent outbreak of COVID-19 appears to be related and distinct from the previous severe acute respiratory syndrome (2002–2003) recorded with 8096 confirmed cases and 774 fatalities in 29 countries, with an estimated 9.6% CFR. However, in the Middle East respiratory syndrome (2012–2020) merely accounted for 2519 reported case with 866 associated fatalities. Although SARS and MERS have significantly higher CFRs, COVID-19 resulted in more fatalities than the sheer number of confirmed cases [15]. As of 23 July 2020, COVID-19 has affected 213 countries and territories worldwide with cumulative confirmed cases of 15,390,221, death rates of 630,537 and recoveries of 9,367,463. It correlates into a maximum 2% of CFR. Even so, the actual number of COVID-19 cases is possibly rising as there are complexities involved in the identification of the infection and rising asymptomatic cases in communities [15]. Figure 4.4 shows the geographical distribution of MERS, SARS and COVID-19 globally.

As per transmission concern, bats by way of palm civets from Guangdong Province markets, China, were responsible for the zoonotic transmission of SARS, while bats via dromedary camels triggered the zoonotic transmission of MERS in Saudi Arabia. These three viral infectious diseases usually occur with sore throat with cough, high fever and respiratory problems leading to fatal situations [16].

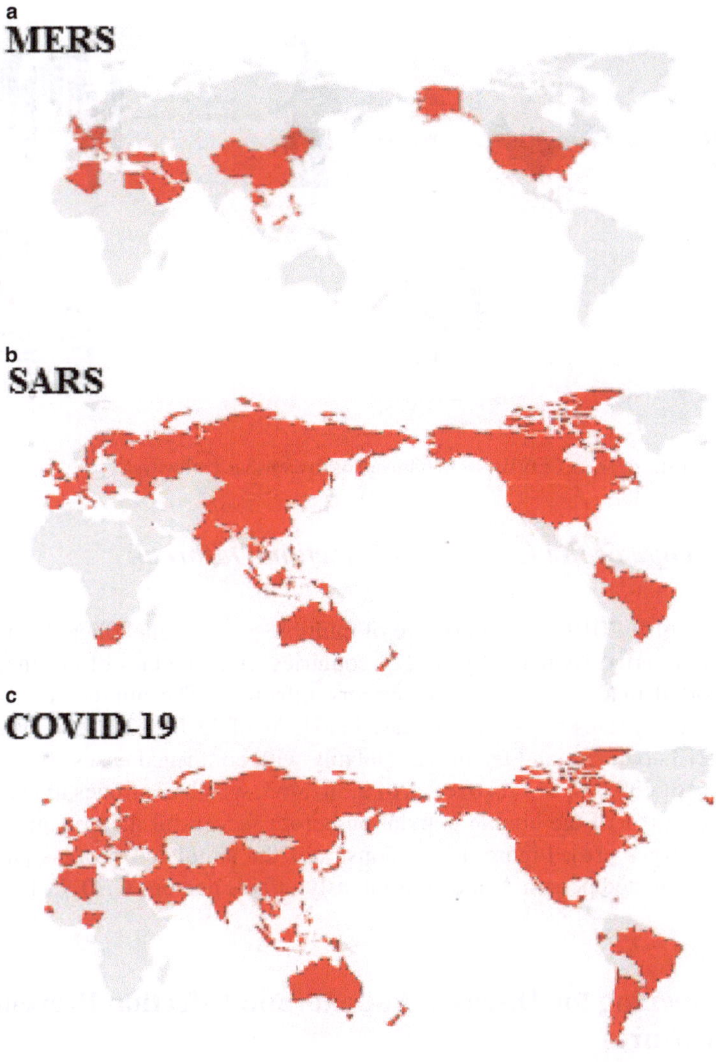

Fig. 4.4 Geographical dispersion of (**a**) MERS, (**b**) SARS and (**c**) COVID-19

Infection can be verified by examining the samples from the respiratory tract (e.g. nasal swabs), whereas symptoms, exposures and imaging of the body help in the clinical diagnosis of the patient. Supporting patient treatment is usually the normal approach, as no established effective vaccine and antiviral therapies have been reported (Fig. 4.5).

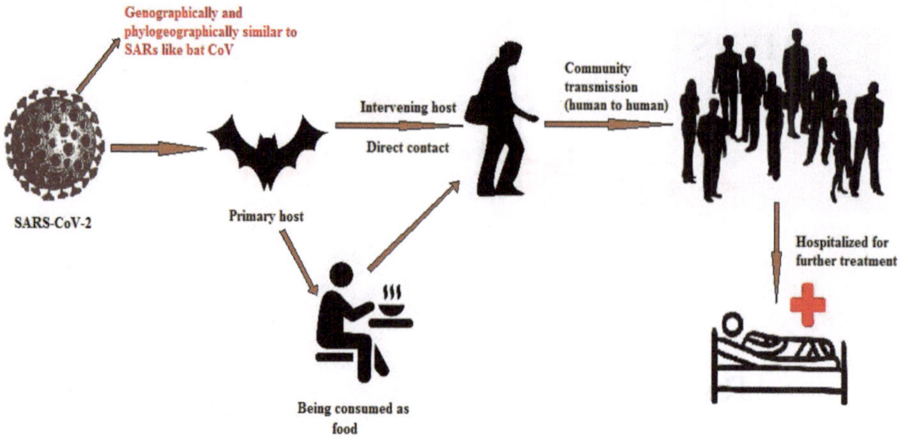

Fig. 4.5 Transmission of COVID-19 to human host by various pathways

4.2.2 Scope of the COVID-19 Infection Outbreak

Since December 2019, the occurrence of multiple cases of inexplicable pneumonia have been asserted sequentially in 213 countries. A new class of coronavirus has been reported that causes acute respiratory infection. The number of cases with higher mortality rates has so far increased [17]. As of 23 July 2020, COVID-19 has infected 213 countries and territories globally with confirmed cases of 15,390,221, death rates of 630,537 and recoveries of 9,367,463, which continues to increase and could infect 60% of the human population before successful therapy and treatment vaccine emerges [18]. Figure 4.6 demonstrates the simulated process pattern that starts with infected person A and continuously infects persons C, D, E, F and so on.

4.3 Screening for Diseased Patients and Infection Prevention Measures

4.3.1 Case Definitions

4.3.1.1 Suspected Case

An individual is a suspected case if he/she is suffering from acute respiratory disease (high fever with at least one respiratory disorder, such as asthma or dry cough); has a travel history or living in a region indicating group transmissions of COVID-19 disease, 14 days before symptoms develop; and has been in close contact with a confirmed or suspected case of COVID-19, 14 days earlier before symptom appearance, epidemiologically relating to 2019-nCoV or clustered onset infections.

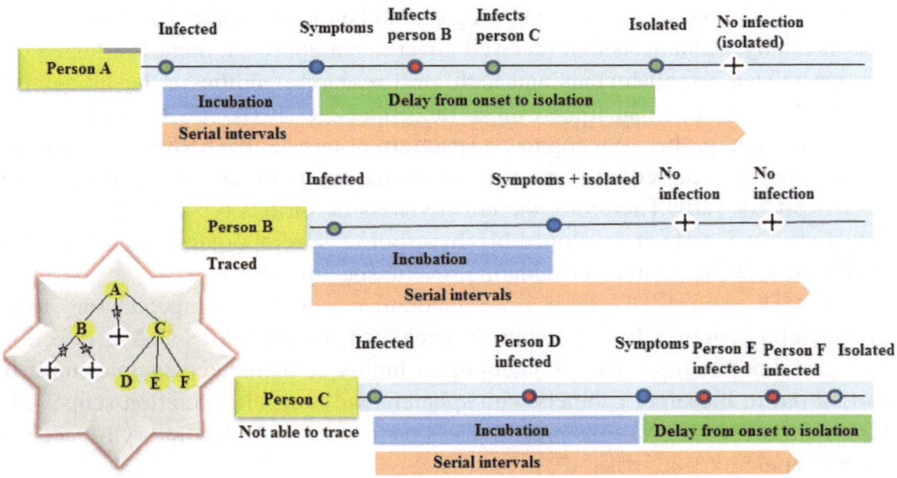

Fig. 4.6 A pattern of the simulated process that starts with an infected person A

4.3.1.2 Confirmed Case

Individuals having preceding pathogenic facts are confirmed cases: (1) positive result for SARS-CoV-2 by PCR testing for nucleic acid in respiratory or blood samples and (2) virus gene sequences showing a strong homogeneity in respiratory or blood samples to 2019-nCoV.

4.3.1.3 Close Contacts

Individuals prior to any contact before the occurrence of confirmed cases in the lack of suitable safety measures; close contact with the suspected or probable cases of COVID-19 disease; travelled to or a resident in a location where SARS-CoV-2 community transmission is currently underway [19]. Close contact with doctors and nurses and their relatives who have been treating or visiting the confirmed case or other employees within the exposed surrounding like giving direct treatment or case care.

4.4 Diagnostic Testing

SARS-CoV-2 diagnostic testing is performed mainly in specified medical laboratories. Test disruptions arise from the requirement for the administrative supervision of research at national and regional levels and the amount of time it takes to transport samples and the huge quantity of research anticipated in certain places. In the case of epidemics, more intensive monitoring should be readily available. In response to commercially viable tests that received government approval, there is a huge need for specialized establishments and high-level research facilities at health centres. Several licensed tests, such as reverse transcriptase-PCR (RT-PCR) studies, using primer sets and probes to recognize a spectrum of targets in SARS-CoV-2 genome are not widely accepted, as some may recognize other similar coronaviruses, such as SARS-CoV [20]. Therefore, the effectiveness of various types of specimens to detect viruses is not yet developed [4]. In response, several organizations including WHO and CDC recommend evaluating several specimen forms.

The CDC and WHO both issue laboratory safety recommendations when investigating samples from patients suspected of having SARS-CoV-2 infection. The guidelines suggest that the handling of highly contaminated samples must be carried out in biosafety cabinets with splatters and aerosol generation scope [21]. Figure 4.7 shows the various preparedness parameters for a laboratory to face and counter epidemic outbreaks.

4.4.1 *Aetiological Diagnosis*

Real-time reverse transcription-PCR (RT-PCR) tests in the analytical stage persist as the molecular tool of choice for aetiological treatment of SARS-CoV-2 disease though antibody-based therapies are being used as a supplementary method [22]. The WHO and US Centers for Disease Control and Prevention and several national and international scientific organizations have published relevant, comprehensive details on the production of reverse transcription-polymerase chain reaction (RT-PCR) studies that are now being adopted straightforwardly by various reference laboratories globally and undergoing specific evaluation [23].

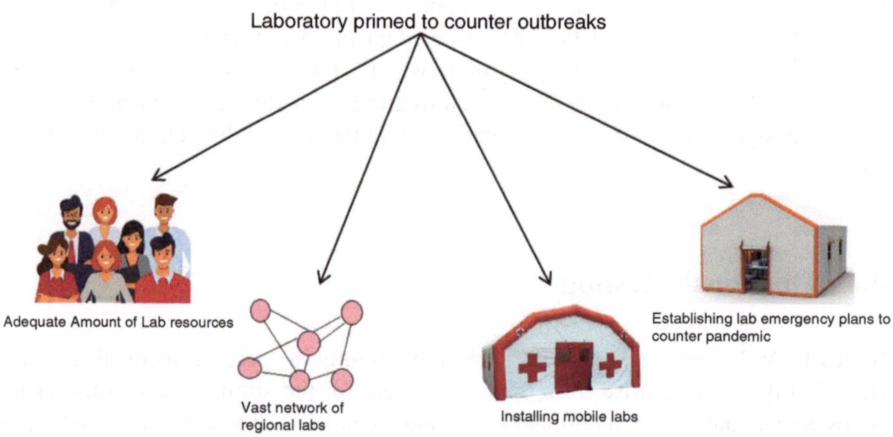

Fig. 4.7 Laboratory preparedness to face emerging outbreaks

4.4.2 Surveillance

The major objectives of COVID-19 surveillance include rapid identification, isolation, testing and management of suspected cases, recognizing and tracking contacts, directing the implementation of control measures, detecting and controlling outbreaks among vulnerable populations, assessing the effect of the pandemic on healthcare systems and community and tracking long-term epidemiological trends and innovations [24]. Comprehensive national monitoring for COVID-19 should involve, where necessary, the adaptation and strengthening of existing national systems, and the scale-up of additional monitoring capacities is required. Digital technology can be beneficial for fast monitoring, data processing and analysis. Once in operation, effective systematic monitoring should be established even in areas where there are very few cases; new cases and outbreaks of COVID-19 must be identified rapidly before the widespread transmission of disease occurs [25]. Constant COVID-19 surveillance is also crucial to understand long-term trends in the disease and the virus's evolution. Surveillance systems must be geologically detailed and cover all vulnerable individuals and communities. Surveillance should be improved for vulnerable or high-risk communities such as community-based individual surveillance, primary level surveillance and hospital-based surveillance [26].

4.4.3 Remote Patient Monitoring

Remote patient monitoring (RPM) is used to monitor and transmit vital signs from a user and provide them to clinicians with real-time insights to evaluate next actions. Wearable instruments like thermometers and pulse oximeters automatically collect data, while others (for instance, phone apps) require manual feedback [27]. The Healthcare Information and Management Systems Society noted that these digitally linked, non-invasive technologies allow clinicians to monitor heart rate, respiratory rate, temperature and other pertinent physiology for variations in disease progression and symptom progression. RPM is designed to reduce readmission rates by supporting proactive, managed care instead of responding to an avoidable issue, or waiting for months for a follow-up visit. Not only does this help patients, but it also frees busy workers to work on new cases [28]. Recently, some researches illustrated most common disorders found in COVID-19 patients, mainly lymphopenia, high levels of erythrocyte sedimentation rates (ESR) and C reactive protein (CRP) and decreased serum albumin concentration.

4.4.4 Organizational Issues

The collaborative work has been absolutely suspended or severely affected in most regions of the world. Many people are not anxious about the virus, but about their food and livelihood because they are regular wagers and survive on a regular basis. Essentials, such as food and incomes, are not accessible. However, it cannot be denied that while confronting SARS-Cov-2 outbreaks by laboratory organization with several thousand infected patients, many of those require diagnostic testing and hospitalization, the regular practice of routine and emergency testing clinical laboratories is rapidly overrun, disrupted and overloaded, so the role of medical laboratory facilities must be highly disruptive [29].

Laboratory integration, high-performance instrumentation availability and reduction in healthcare funding led to a substantial decrease in the capacity to develop evolving responses. During outbreaks such as viral infections or other biological threats, point-of-care testing (POCT) systems shall be considered to be an extremely useful resource.

4.5 Prevention

Several agencies, including the WHO and US Centers for Disease Control and Prevention (CDC), give instructions to minimize COVID-19 spread. These agencies strongly advice to restrict journey to high-risk zones, avoid direct contact with infected patients and refrain from eating meat from areas with proven COVID-19 outbreaks [30]. Precise daily handwashing is advised, and the use of face masks and PPE kits are compulsory. Bespoke Inc., a Japanese company, developed an AI-based powered chatbot (Bebot) which offers up-to-date data on outbreaks of coronavirus, preventive measures that should be taken and a symptoms checker. Below are some pre- and post-preventive measures for a person who is exposed to a suspicious environment.

4.5.1 Persons with Close Contacts and Suspicious Exposure

Individuals with close contact or suspected exposure to SARS-CoV-2 patient must follow a 14-day period of health monitoring, beginning from the last day of exposure or contact. A person monitored showing any symptoms, especially fever and respiratory problems like shortness of breath, coughing and diarrhoea, should quickly contact medical assistance. Also, contact monitoring should be conducted for the individuals who have been exposed to a suspicious environment or infected patient.

4.5.2 *Patients with Suspected SARS-CoV-2 Infection*

Individuals with a suspected infection should be isolated, monitored and treated at a hospital immediately. Doctors must make suggestions relying on patient condition. Patients with mild symptoms of infection must isolate themselves and be treated at home [31]. The body temperature of suspected infected individual staying at home should be monitored regularly by their guardians. During the home care phase, healthcare staff should conduct regular face-to-face visits (if feasible) or telephone interviews to note the patient's health progress, and, if appropriate, relevant check-up and tests should be performed.

4.5.3 *Prevention for Travellers*

International travellers must take regular precautionary measures while entering and exiting the infected regions. Also, close contact with individuals with acute respiratory infections should be prohibited, and regular cleaning of hands, particularly upon contact with sick individuals or surroundings, maintaining relevant coughing codes and avoiding direct contact with live or dead animals and bats should be observed. Passengers must also reduce unnecessary travels as much as possible [32]. If they have travelled to red areas in the last 14 days and are having fever, cough or breathing trouble, they should indeed (1) visit a doctor as soon as possible, (2) discuss all information about the latest tours and symptoms to the doctor before moving to a clinic or emergency room, (3) maintain a 2 m gap with others and (4) use a face mask to cover the mouth and nose while sneezing/coughing. Use soap and water to wash hands frequently, and, if not available, use alcohol-based hand sanitizers.

4.6 Treatment and Control

Currently, COVID-19 has no effective antiviral therapy or vaccine. Conversely, a prospective multicentre controlled clinical trial to evaluate the effectiveness and reliability of Arbidol in COVID-19 patients is currently underway [33]. First-line fever therapy requires antipyretic treatment like paracetamol and guaifenesin to cure cough. Patients with a respiratory infection, respiratory abnormality, pulmonary oedema or shocks need intensive oxygen therapy. There is still a need to follow conservative and rational antibiotic regimens. For example, the People's Republic of China's National Health Commission advises utilizing IFN-α and lopinavir. The said argument is premised on earlier investigation showing lower mortality rates for these drugs in highly infectious patients with severe acute respiratory syndrome

(SARS) [34]. Oseltamivir is another antiviral medicine widely used by healthcare professionals in China to treat patients with COVID-19 suspected infections [35].

4.6.1 Principles

Suspected and confirmed cases should be diagnosed in suitable health facilities having appropriate conditions of isolation and security. Suspected cases should be handled individually in one room; confirmed cases should be confined to the same unit; and urgent cases should be transferred to the ICU as quickly and efficiently as possible.

4.6.2 Treatment Plans

Suspected and confirmed cases must be handled with appropriate isolation and safety measures in approved hospitals. Suspected cases must be dealt with in an isolated unit, while confirmed cases must be handled in well-efficient units of the same hospital. In addition, severe patients must be admitted as early as possible into the intensive care unit. A patient must be checked for a routine check for blood level, PCT, CRP, the organs' functioning, coagulation activity, measurement of blood gas and chest imaging [36]. Safe and appropriate effective oxygen therapy should be provided, including nasal cannula, oxygen mask, high-flow nasal oxygen therapy (HFNO), non-intrusive ventilation (NIV) or intrusive mechanical ventilation. Several of the successful care approaches that the major countries have implemented are discussed below.

4.6.3 General Treatments

General treatment approaches involve complete supportive therapies maintaining an efficient level of infrastructure, ensuring consistent indoor atmosphere (water, electrolytes or another intrinsic environmental factor) and assessing vital signs (respiratory rate, heartbeat, insulin levels, pulse rate, oxygen saturation, etc.) as mentioned earlier [37–39].

4.6.4 Antiviral Therapy

The COVID-19 Treatment Advisory Committee makes guidelines based on the available evidence on the use of antiviral drugs to treat COVID-19.

4.6.4.1 Lopinavir

Lopinavir was first identified as a protease inhibitor that impedes the human immunodeficiency virus (HIV) replication and synthesis, contributing to the inclusion of non-infectious virus particles. Lopinavir was also efficiently able to bind with the SARS-CoV-2 protease endopeptidase C30 tested through molecular models. This indicates the antiviral potential of lopinavir to inhibit SARS-CoV-2 protein synthesis [40].

Moreover, various evidences reveal that when lopinavir medication is taken with other antiviral drugs, it improved the overall quality of severe SARS or MERS patients by improving ARDS [41, 42]. Even now, the NIH Panel for COVID-19 Treatment Guidelines advises against lopinavir or other HIV protease inhibitors due to their adverse pharmacodynamics and because clinical trials in COVID-19 patients did not show therapeutic significance.

4.6.4.2 Interferon-Alpha (IFN-α)

IFN-α is a subset of type I IFN family, which plays a significant role in building resistance against viral infection. IFN-α interferes directly with virus replication and stifles viral infection by encouraging innate and adaptive immunity [43]. In vitro analysis of IFN-α revealed in efficiently inhibition of SARS-CoV-2 replication. Diagnosis with and without Arbidol with IFN-α2b drastically decreased the detectable virus periods in the upper respiratory tract. It lessened the period of increased blood levels for the IL-6 and CRP inflammatory markers. In addition, a pilot drug trial showed the therapeutic utility of synthetic recombinant IFN-α for patients with SARS. Consequently, IFN-α must be listed as a therapeutic agent for COVID-19 therapy.

4.6.4.3 Ribavirin

Ribavirin, often recognized as tribavirin, is an antiviral drug for treating RSV, hepatitis C and haemorrhagic fevers [44, 45]. This is an equivalent nucleoside with significant antiviral efficacy. Ribavirin mediates the hepatitis C virus via several mechanisms including (1) innate immunity, (2) activation of inosine-5′-monophosphate dehydrogenase, (3) suppression of RNA polymerase, (4) initiation of HCV gene splicing and (5) attenuation of interferon-induced gene expression. Adding ribavirin in α-peg interferon greatly increases sustainable virologic response and reduces the risk of relapse. After the SARS incidence in Hong Kong, ribavirin has been frequently preferred to diagnose patients with or without steroids. For COVID-19 patients, ribavirin may thus be perceived as a treatment option.

4.6.4.4 Hydroxychloroquine

Hydroxychloroquine has shown to restrict in vitro replication of the SARS-CoV-2 virus. Hydroxychloroquine is also commonly used in the malaria pandemic countries to treat malaria [46]. Chloroquine and hydroxychloroquine both share identical chemical structures and associated functions. Most investigators efficiently stifle chloroquine in vitro with the CoVID-19 (SARS-CoV-2). Hydroxychloroquine is an inexpensive and effective drug that has been in use for over 70 years and is therefore effectively clinically beneficial to treat COVID-19.

4.6.4.5 Remdesivir

Remdesivir, marketed under the brand name Veklury, is a broad-spectrum antiviral drug formulated by Gilead Sciences, a biopharmaceutical firm. Remdesivir has shown to prevent replication of certain human coronaviruses associated with significant morbidity in tissue cultures, notably SARS-CoV in 2003 and MERS-CoV in the Middle East in 2012. Reportedly, the nucleoside analogue remdesivir (GS-5734) blocks SARS-CoV and MERS-CoV in vivo. A stage 1b trial of an inhaled nebulized variant was launched in late June 2020 to assess whether remdesivir could be used on an outpatient procedure and at advanced stages of the disease. Here, as a response, it poignantly blocked SARS-CoV-2 infections at minimal dose levels and showed a higher acceptability factor [47–49].

Taken in combination, these antiviral drugs are potentially viable therapeutic options for COVID-19. The following are a few things to be understood too:

1. Although there has been no placebo group in case series and case reports, one could not say whether the results are due to antiviral therapy or the essence of the recovery process or both.
2. Adverse effects such as diarrhoea, vomiting, nausea and liver damage resulting from use of these drugs should also be considered.
3. Use of more then two antiviral drugs together is not recommended, and consulting a health expert before use should be essential because not doing so can lead to unbearable side effects.
4. Yet more investigation is necessary to examine the effectiveness of existing antiviral drugs in clinical applications.

4.6.5 Cellular Therapy

4.6.5.1 Mesenchymal Stem Cells (MSCs)

MSCs can be obtained from the placenta, bone marrow and several other tissues that offer differentiation capacity and enhance active immunity and proprietary functions for recovery. MSCs, among the most commonly researched adult stem cells in regenerative medicine, provide important clinical effects for the cure of neurological, respiratory and cardiovascular problems [50]. MSCs' immune control mainly relies on immune cell activation and effector activity, suppressing lung-infiltrated cells and enhancing pulmonary oedema resolution. These cells can change the perception of innate and adaptive immune cells in specifics. They produce keratinocyte growth factor, granulocyte-macrophage colony-stimulating factor, prostaglandin E2 and IL-6 and IL-13 to promote phagocytosis and substitute alveolar macrophage that alters dendritic cell cytokine secretion and reduces the secretion of interferon-γ. All of the functions mentioned above may also be successful in COVID-19-induced ARDS [51].

4.6.5.2 Natural Killer (NK) Cells

These cells are essential for viral clearance and immunomodulation of innate immune respondents. Human NK cells lyse antibody-coated virus-infected cells through antibody-dependent cytotoxicity (ADCC) pathway. Umbilical cord blood and peripheral blood are great sources of NK cells. Because NK cells are among the key manufacturers of IFN-γ, they might be engaged in cytokine storm led by IFN, contributing to the development of inflammatory response-mediated ARDS, as well consequential COVID-19-related mortality [52, 53]. More work on the function of NK cells within COVID-19 is unquestionably necessary.

4.6.6 *Immunotherapy*

4.6.6.1 Convalescent Plasma Therapy (CPT)

Antiviral antibodies (IgA, IgG, IgM, IgD, IgE) in convalescent plasma produced by retrieved patients can efficiently cure infected patients. Viral infections like pertussis, influenza A (H5N1) and Ebola have been widely treated with CPT. Alternatively, convalescent plasma in SARS-CoV-2-infected patients can help achieve certain passive immunization [54]. The key findings based on current information are as follows: (a) CPT can decrease death rate in severely infected patients; (b) CPT can increase the neutralizing antibody titres, thereby depleting the SARS-CoV-2 RNA in patients; and (c) CPT offers a beneficial impact on clinical symptoms. Hence, to assess CPT's effectiveness in case of COVID-19 patients, well-designed multicentre clinical tests should be performed pressingly.

4.6.6.2 Monoclonal Antibodies

Neutralizing SARS-CoV-2 monoclonal antibodies has the ability for both prophylactic and therapeutic uses and could greatly help in the design and production of vaccines [55]. After discovering SARS-CoV-2 as the causal factor of COVID-19, researchers and organizations have identified monoclonal antibodies (most commonly from the B cells of patients newly recovered from SARS-CoV-2 and in some instances from patients diagnosed with the severe acute respiratory coronavirus syndrome [SARS-CoV] in 2003). The primary target of SARS-CoV-2 neutralizing monoclonal antibodies is surface spike glycoprotein, which delineates viral entries into host cells. The viral infection is induced by the interface between viral spike and angiotensin-converting enzyme 2 (ACE 2) receptor located in various cell types, thus blocking the event by neutralizing monoclonal antibodies [56, 57]. The bulk of monoclonal antibodies target the spike protein in the receptor-binding region, enabling the contact of SARS-CoV-2 on the ACE2 receptor. Moreover, based on SARS-CoV and MERS-CoV's existing awareness, possibly neutralizing antibodies may also target certain spike protein regions.

4.6.7 Traditional Chinese Medicine

Traditional Chinese medicine is derived from plant sources for the treatment of various infections. China commonly used it to cure numerous diseases for hundreds of years now. All across Western countries, Chinese medicine is progressively recognized as a type of integrative therapy. Research shows that combining Chinese medicine and Western medicine can better enhance health symptoms and well-being than just Western medicine alone [58, 59].

Baicalin is a flavone derived from *Scutellaria baicalensis*, a traditional Chinese herbal medicine. Baicalin has been shown to have antiviral efficacy by neutralization trials against ten clinically SARS-CoV-2 isolated strains. Quercetin is commonly being used as traditional Chinese Ayurvedic medicine. Lianhua Qingwen tablets or capsules were used on 284 patients with mild and moderate COVID-19 symptoms in the 23 health facilities across nine provinces. Findings demonstrate that 14-day treatment with the drug results in an increased healing rate for mild and moderate cases, helping to reduce the proportion of mild cases developing into severe cases and shorten the length of patients going from positive to negative testing. Hesperetin present in citrus fruits is stated to inhibit ACE2 and thus block severe infection of SARS-CoV-2. Quercetin has been deemed to possess antiviral impacts by inhibiting SARS-CoV-2 3CLpro and blocking SARS-CoV-2 entry into host cells. Thus, all these findings justify the vital role of Chinese medicine in COVID-19 pneumonia diagnosis and intervention.

4.6.8 Vaccines

Vaccines can be used to accelerate the development of antibodies and provide immunity against several diseases and infections when subjected to different pathogens of interest, especially in susceptible communities that are more sensitive to severe consequences, including the recent SARS-CoV-2 outbreak. The SARS-CoV was strictly controlled in 2003 and MERS-CoV was managed from inducing higher rates of mortality, the currently emerging SARS-CoV-2 is spreading aggressively with such a substantial rise in the number of cases and deaths on each passing day. There is a substantial global initiative to develop COVID-19 resistance vaccines, and as of early June 2020, at least ten vaccine agents have reached clinical trials, plus Phase II investigations. Developing vaccines includes a viral vector-based vaccine, a subunit vaccine, a virus-like particle size vaccine (VLPs), a DNA vaccine, a live attenuated vaccine (LAV) and inactivated whole-virus vaccine (IWV) [60–62].

On 23 January 2020, the Coalition for Epidemic Preparedness Innovations (CEPI) unveiled that it might financially support vaccine manufacturing projects with Inovio, University of Queensland and Moderna, an objective towards clinically testing of inventive vaccines in 16 weeks (by June 2020). Such organizations will develop the vaccines through the DNA, recombinant and mRNA vaccine frameworks. However, preliminary results of a randomized controlled, inviting-label, responsive dexamethasone clinical trials were released on 16 June 2020. Dexamethasone lessened the 28-day mortality efficiently in COVID-19 ventilated patients. Relying on these observations, the US National Institutes of Health (NIH) advised that COVID-19 patients should be given dexamethasone with artificially ventilated or necessitating supplemental oxygen supply. As it shares 79% of the genetic relationship with SARS-CoV, the protective impact of employing a reliable SARS-CoV vaccine while waiting for COVID-19 vaccine could be significant. It will involve phase-by-phase implementations of limited scale and careful supervision of vaccinations well before large-scale implementation [63, 64]. Here, Fig. 4.8 shows various factors for the treatment and management of COVID-19 outbreak.

4.7 Other Pertinent Factors in the Combat Against COVID-19 Outbreaks

Also, in identifying and containing the virus, the socio-economic effects of COVID-19 are reasonably effective for the sake of public health response to the intricacies of the outbreak [65]. WHO has declared that the international community has initiated a US$675 million preparatory and response program from February to April 2020 to mitigate the further proliferation of COVID-19. The SARS-CoV virus dragged down global production by $50 billion in 2003. The initial estimate of the world economy's cost resulting from the COVID-19 outbreak is estimated at around $360 billion [66–68].

Furthermore, information on the epidemiological characteristics, such as recognition of the animal reservoirs and the health risk of the disease, is extremely important to win the fight against such an outbreak. It is necessary to recognize the intermediate host carrying the disease for the current epidemic and prevent

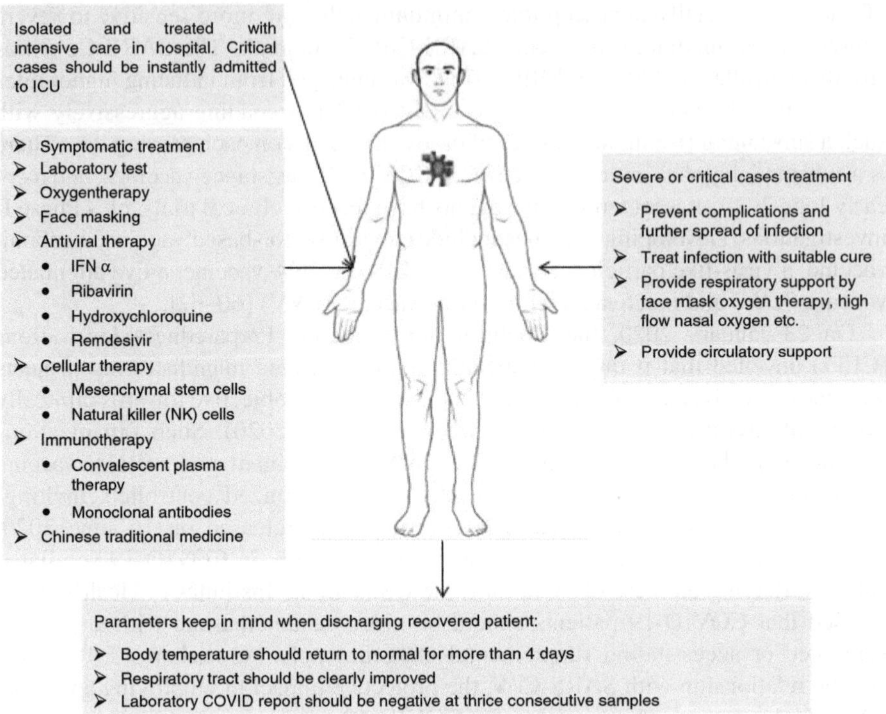

Fig. 4.8 Several factors for the treatment and management of COVID-19 outbreak

a future outbreak. The quest for a COVID-19 vaccine is equally essential, along with all the factors mentioned earlier. Although there is no recorded medication or vaccines offered for COVID-19, some therapies are known to be effective in combating COVID-19 up to some degree [69, 70].

4.8 Lessons Learned from the COVID-19 Outbreak

Comparison with the SARS outbreaks and the global response to COVID-19 has been much more consistent and reliable. However, some points need to be considered from the COVID-19 pandemic when managing potential outbreaks [71]. It is further strictly advised that the government's guidelines for a viral response should be released 1–2 weeks before the public is informed. It would help in the effective initiation of combat measures that would restrict the spread of viruses, such as monitoring suspicious cases at work and in public [72]. Furthermore, several feasible malfeasance strategies for global health should be made, people returning from high-risk regions should be adequately screened, individuals having possible health risk should be quarantined and isolated immediately, and lastly, more investment is needed to speed up the manufacturing of effective drugs and to develop appropriate interventions to control potential outbreaks of contagious diseases.

4.9 Conclusion

The current COVID-19 epidemic has indeed been declared as a global health issue. China itself demonstrated that the COVID-19 pandemic could be contained if approaches and techniques for responding to public health outbreaks are introduced early on. The count of confirmed cases has begun to thrive globally and currently measured around 15,390,221 confirmed cases, 630,537 death rates and 9,367,463 recoveries worldwide.

It is relatively straightforward that quarantine itself might not be effective in preventing COVID-19 from spreading, and one of the increasing concerns is the worldwide effect of this viral infection. To reduce the threat of infection in the community, people should be advised or recommended to wash their hands frequently, practice respiratory care (e.g. cover the face while coughing), avoid gatherings and avoid direct contact with the patient where possible. However, face masks to prevent exposure to the community are not commonly recommended for asymptomatic persons. Social distancing is recommended, especially in places with a high transmission rate to the community. Strict cross-infection control at healthcare organizations is also essential to prevent further transmission of the epidemic. There is no question that further research is needed to establish better the exact human-to-human and animal-to-human transmission mechanism to accelerate the formulation of an effective virus-specific vaccine.

Within this reference, investment in epidemiological and economic modelling could become a substantive progression. There has been a recent demand for such an integrated epidemiological and economic modelling framework to be developed, which comes mainly from the COVID-19 outbreak. Moreover, there is a need to understand better and effectively manage the risks encircling outbreaks of infectious diseases.

References

1. J. Yang, Y. Zheng, X. Gou, K. Pu, Z. Chen, Q. Guo, R. Ji, H. Wang, Y. Wang, Y. Zhou, Prevalence of comorbidities in the novel Wuhan coronavirus (COVID-19) infection: A systematic review and meta-analysis. Int. J. Infect. Dis. **94**, 91–95 (2020)
2. A.R. Sahin, 2019 Novel coronavirus (COVID-19) outbreak: A review of the current literature. Eurasian J. Med. Investig. **4**, 1–7 (2020)
3. J.S. Guy, Turkey coronavirus is more closely related to avian infectious bronchitis virus than to mammalian coronaviruses: A review. Avian Pathol. **29**, 207–212 (2000)

4. F. Patrucco, F. Gavelli, R. Shi, N. De Vita, A. Pavot, L.M. Castello, P. Ravanini, P.E. Balbo, Coronavirus disease 2019 outbreak. Panminerva Med. **62**(2), 73–74 (2020)
5. H. Laude, K. Van Reeth, M. Pensaert, Porcine respiratory coronavirus: Molecular features and virus-host interactions. Vet. Res. **24**, 125–150 (1993)
6. S.L. Sawicki, S.G. Siddell, Comparative perception of COVID-19 transcript. J. Virol. **81**, 20–29 (2007)
7. D. Cavanagh, Coronavirus avian infectious bronchitis virus. Vet. Res. **38**, 281–297 (2007)
8. J. Pang, M.X. Wang, I.Y.H. Ang, et al., Potential rapid diagnostics, vaccine and therapeutics for 2019 novel coronavirus (2019-nCoV): A systematic review. J. Clin. Med. **9**, 623 (2020)
9. S.R. Weiss, S. Navas-Martin, Coronavirus pathogenesis and the emerging pathogen severe acute respiratory syndrome coronavirus. Microbiol. Mol. Biol. Rev. **69**, 635–664 (2005)
10. E.J. Snijder, M.C. Horzinek, Toroviruses: Replication, evolution and comparison with other members of the coronavirus-like superfamily. J. Gen. Virol. **74**, 2305–2316 (1993)
11. J.M.A. Van Den Brand, S.L. Smits, B.L. Haagmans, Pathogenesis of Middle East respiratory syndrome coronavirus. J. Pathol. **235**, 175–184 (2015)
12. C.C. Bergmann, T.E. Lane, S.A. Stohlman, Coronavirus infection of the central nervous system: Host-virus stand-off. Nat. Rev. Microbiol. **4**, 121–132 (2006)
13. L. Zhang, Y. Liu, Potential interventions for novel coronavirus in China: A systematic review. J. Med. Virol. **92**, 479–490 (2020)
14. M.M.C. Lai, Of genome. Policy Anal. **04**, 33–36 (2000)
15. S. Perlman, Review of pathological and immunological aspects. Adv. Exp. Med. Biol. **440**, 503–513 (1998)
16. P. Spychalski, A. Błażyńska-Spychalska, J. Kobiela, Estimating case fatality rates of COVID-19. Lancet Infect. Dis. **20**, 774–775 (2020)
17. J. Phua, L. Weng, L. Ling, M. Egi, C. Lim, J.V. Divatia, B.R. Shrestha, Y.M. Arabi, J. Ng, Review Intensive care management of coronavirus disease 2019 (COVID-19): Challenges and recommendations. Lancet Respir. **2019**, 1–12 (2020)
18. A. Cortegiani, G. Ingoglia, M. Ippolito, A. Giarratano, S. Einav, A systematic review on the efficacy and safety of chloroquine for the treatment of COVID-19. J. Crit. Care **57**, 279–283 (2020)
19. T. Singhal, A review of coronavirus disease-2019 (COVID-19). Indian J. Pediatr. **87**, 281–286 (2020)
20. D.M.G. Halpin, R. Faner, O. Sibila, J.R. Badia, A. Agusti, Do chronic respiratory diseases or their treatment affect the risk of SARS-CoV-2 infection? Lancet Respir. Med. **8**, 436–438 (2020)
21. J. Yazdany, A.H.J. Kim, Use of hydroxychloroquine and chloroquine during the COVID-19 pandemic: What every clinician should know. Ann. Intern. Med. **172**(11), 754–755 (2020)
22. A. Murphy, Z. Abdi, I. Harirchi, M. Mckee, E. Ahmadnezhad, Correspondence and Iran's capacity to. Lancet Public Health **2667**, 30083 (2020)
23. X.H. Jin, K.I. Zheng, K.H. Pan, Y.P. Xie, M.H. Zheng, COVID-19 in a patient with chronic lymphocytic leukaemia. The Lancet Haematology **7**(4), e351–e352 (2020)
24. B. Owens, Excitement around hydroxychloroquine for treating COVID-19 causes challenges for rheumatology. Lancet Rheumatol. **9913**, 30089 (2020)
25. X. Yao, F. Ye, M. Zhang, et al., In vitro antiviral activity and projection of optimized dosing design of hydroxychloroquine for the treatment of severe acute respiratory syndrome main point: Hydroxychloroquine was found to be more potent than chloroquine at inhibiting SARS-CoV-2 in vitro. Clin. Infect. Dis. **2**, 1–25 (2020)
26. C. Vardavas, K. Nikitara, COVID-19 and smoking: A systematic review of the evidence. Tob. Induc. Dis. **18**, 1–4 (2020)
27. D. Zhou, S.-M. Dai, Q. Tong, COVID-19: A recommendation to examine the effect of hydroxychloroquine in preventing infection and progression. J. Antimicrob. Chemother. **75**(7), 1667–1670 (2020)

28. C. Sohrabi, Z. Alsafi, N.O. Neill, M. Khan, A. Kerwan, Since January 2020 Elsevier has created a COVID-19 resource Centre with free information in English and Mandarin on the novel coronavirus COVID-19. The COVID-19 resource Centre is hosted on Elsevier Connect, the company's public news and information (2020)
29. J. Liu, R. Cao, M. Xu, X. Wang, H. Zhang, H. Hu, Y. Li, Z. Hu, W. Zhong, M. Wang, Hydroxychloroquine, a less toxic derivative of chloroquine, is effective in inhibiting SARS-CoV-2 infection in vitro. Cell Discov. **6**, 6–9 (2020)
30. S.A. Rasmussen, J.C. Smulian, J.A. Lednicky, T.S. Wen, D.J. Jamieson, Coronavirus disease 2019 (COVID-19) and pregnancy: What obstetricians need to know. Am. J. Obstet. Gynecol. (2020). https://doi.org/10.1016/j.ajog.2020.02.017
31. O. Mitjà, B. Clotet, Use of antiviral drugs to reduce COVID-19 transmission. Lancet Glob. Health **8**(5), e639–e640 (2020)
32. R. Viner, S. Russell, H. Croker, J. Packer, J. Ward, C. Stansfield, O. Mytton, R. Booy, School closure and management practices during coronavirus outbreaks including COVID-19: A rapid narrative systematic review. SSRN Electron. J. **2019**, 1–8 (2020)
33. H. Wang, T. Li, P. Barbarino, et al., Dementia care during COVID-19. Lancet **6736**, 19–20 (2020)
34. R. Verity, L.C. Okell, I. Dorigatti, et al., Estimates of the severity of coronavirus disease 2019: A model-based analysis. Lancet Infect. Dis. **3099**, 1–9 (2020)
35. P.M. De Salazar, A.R. Taylor, Article used experimental data to measure the bias of visitor-derived COVID-19 prevalence rate in Wuhan, China. Lancet Infect. Dis. **3099**, 1–6 (2020)
36. W. Zhang, Y. Zhao, F. Zhang, Q. Wang, T. Li, Z. Liu, The use of anti-inflammatory drugs in the treatment of people with severe coronavirus disease 2019 (COVID-19): The experience of clinical immunologists from China. Clin. Immunol. **214**, 108393 (2020)
37. H. Topic, Can Chinese medicine be used for prevention of Corona virus disease 2019 (COVID-19)? A review of historical classics, research evidence and current prevention programs. Chin. J. Integr. Med. **26**, 243–250 (2020)
38. Y. Yang, S. Islam, J. Wang, Y. Li, X. Chen, Traditional Chinese medicine in the treatment of patients infected with 2019-new coronavirus (SARS-CoV-2): A review and perspective. Int. J. Biol. Sci. (2020). https://doi.org/10.7150/ijbs.45538
39. Y. Yan, W.I. Shin, Y.X. Pang, Y. Meng, J. Lai, C. You, The first 75 days of novel coronavirus (SARS-CoV-2) outbreak: Recent advances. Prev. Treat **17**(7), 2323 (2020)
40. D.M. Roden, R.A. Harrington, Considerations for drug interactions on QTc in exploratory COVID-19 treatment. Circulation **141**(24), e906–e907 (2020)
41. H. Fan, L. Wang, W. Liu, X. An, Z. Liu, X. He, L. Song, Y. Tong, Repurposing of clinically approved drugs for treatment of coronavirus disease 2019 in a 2019-novel coronavirus-related coronavirus model. Chin. Med. J. **133**, 1051–1056 (2020)
42. H. Zhu, N. Sze, A. Mak, Y. Yan, Y. Zhu, Novel coronavirus treatment with ribavirin: Groundwork for an evaluation concerning COVID - 19. J. Med. Virol. **92**(7), 740–746 (2020)
43. T. Tian, Y. Doctor, J. Dan, Q. Doctor, W. Yan, Z. Doctor, Y. Wang, A. Gui, Q. Wang, A systematic review of lopinavir therapy for SARS coronavirus and MERS coronavirus—A possible reference for coronavirus disease-19 treatment option. J. Med. Virol. **92**, 556–563 (2020)
44. J. Storz, R. Rott, G. Kaluza, Enhancement of plaque formation and cell fusion of an enteropathogenic coronavirus by trypsin treatment. Infect. Immun. **31**, 1214–1222 (1981)
45. C. Sargiacomo, F. Sotgia, M.P. Lisanti, COVID-19 and chronological aging: Senolytics and other anti-aging drugs for the treatment or prevention of corona virus infection? Aging **12**, 6511–6517 (2020)
46. L. Yang, Y. Ren, Moral obligation, public leadership, and collective action for epidemic prevention and control: Evidence from the corona virus disease 2019 (COVID-19) emergency. Int. J. Environ. Res. Public Health **17**(8), 2731 (2020)
47. Z. Wang, X. Chen, Y. Lu, F. Chen, W. Zhang, Clinical characteristics and therapeutic procedure for four cases with 2019 novel coronavirus pneumonia receiving combined Chinese and Western medicine treatment. Biosci Trends **14**(1), 64–68 (2020)

48. X. Yao et al., In vitro antiviral activity and projection of optimized dosing design of hydroxychloroquine for the treatment of severe acute respiratory syndrome coronavirus. Clin. Infect. Dis. **71**, 732–739 (2020)
49. H.B. Harmful, Clinical infectious diseases, 2019–2020 (2020)
50. J. Wu, W. Li, X. Shi, et al., Early antiviral treatment contributes to alleviate the severity and improve the prognosis of patients with novel coronavirus disease (COVID-19). J. Intern. Med. **288**(1), 128–138 (2020)
51. A.H. De Wilde, V.S. Raj, D. Oudshoorn, et al., MERS-coronavirus replication induces severe in vitro cytopathology and is strongly inhibited by cyclosporin A or interferon-a treatment. J. Gen. Virol. **94**(Pt 8), 1749–1760 (2013)
52. Z. Min, C. Jun, F. Fu, et al., Diagnosis and treatment recommendations for pediatric respiratory infection caused by the 2019 novel coronavirus. World J. Pediatr. **16**, 240–246 (2020)
53. F. Violi, D. Pastori, R. Cangemi, P. Pignatelli, L. Loffredo, Hypercoagulation and antithrombotic treatment in coronavirus 2019: A new challenge. Thromb. Haemost. **120**(6), 949–956 (2020)
54. M.R. Basiri, Treatments and morbidity prevention of Covid-19. J. Pharm. Pharmacol. **8**, 89–90 (2020)
55. J. Dyall, C.M. Coleman, B.J. Hart, et al., Repurposing of clinically developed drugs for treatment of Middle East respiratory syndrome coronavirus infection. Antimicrob. Agents Chemother. **58**, 4885–4893 (2014)
56. B.S. Chhikara, B. Rathi, J. Singh, Corona virus SARS-CoV-2 disease COVID-19: Infection, prevention and clinical advances of the prospective chemical drug therapeutics. Chem. Biol. Lett. **7**, 63–72 (2020)
57. A.K. Panda, S. Kar, A.K. Dixit, Ayurveda consensus develop strategies for prevention of COVID-19. J. Ayurveda Integr. Med. Sci. **5**(1), 96–107 (2020)
58. S. White, M. Omer, G.N. Mohamma, International knowledge, attitude and practice on prevention of airborne and droplet infections during the outbreak of corona virus among the college students in University of Bisha, Saudi Arabia, Reviewed By Introduction. Med. Sci. **11**, 20773–20776 (2020)
59. J.F. Burke, Letter: The coronavirus disease 2019 global pandemic: A neurosurgical treatment algorithm. Neurosurgery **87**, E50–E57 (2020)
60. H. Lu, Drug treatment options for the 2019-new coronavirus (2019-nCoV). Biosci. Trends **14**, 69–71 (2020)
61. Z. Yang, J. Liu, Y. Zhou, X. Zhao, Q. Zhao, J. Liu, The effect of corticosteroid treatment on patients with coronavirus infection: A systematic review and meta-analysis. J. Infect. **81**, 13–20 (2020)
62. B.D. Vakser, O.P. Pishchulina, Prevention of marginal corona discharges in the insulation of high-voltage electric machines. Russ. Electr. Eng. **80**, 136–138 (2009)
63. L. Zha, S. Li, L. Pan, B. Tefsen, Y. Li, N. French, L. Chen, G. Yang, E.V. Villanueva, Corticosteroid treatment of patients with coronavirus disease 2019 (COVID-19). Med. J. Aust. (2020). https://doi.org/10.5694/mja2.50577
64. D. Vauzour, A. Rodriguez-mateos, G. Corona, M.J. Oruna-concha, J.P.E. Spencer, Mechanisms of action. Nutrients **2**(11), 1106–1131 (2010)
65. K.L. Shen, Y.H. Yang, Diagnosis and treatment of 2019 novel coronavirus infection in children: A pressing issue. World J. Pediatr. **16**, 219–221 (2020)
66. S.A. Baron, C. Devaux, P. Colson, Teicoplanin: An alternative drug for the treatment of coronavirus COVID-19? Int. J. Antimicrob. Agents **55**, 105944 (2020)
67. End-winding CING, Jf/ ‘fa/$77 5. 106273017, 16–18 (1948)
68. H. Liang, G. Acharya, Novel corona virus disease (COVID-19) in pregnancy: What clinical recommendations to follow? Acta. Obstet. Gynecol. Scand. **99**, 439–442 (2020)
69. N. Tang, H. Bai, X. Chen, J. Gong, D. Li, Z. Sun, Anticoagulant treatment is associated with decreased mortality in severe coronavirus disease 2019 patients with coagulopathy. J. Thromb. Haemost. **18**, 1094–1099 (2020)

70. K. Shen, Y. Yang, T. Wang, D. Zhao, Y. Jiang, R. Jin, Y. Zheng, Diagnosis, treatment, and prevention of 2019 novel coronavirus infection in children: Experts' consensus statement. World J. Pediatr. **16**, 223–231 (2020)
71. M. Kawase, K. Shirato, L. Van Der Hoek, F. Taguchi, S. Matsuyama, Simultaneous treatment of human bronchial epithelial cells with serine and cysteine protease inhibitors prevents severe acute respiratory syndrome coronavirus entry. J. Virol. **86**, 6537–6545 (2012)
72. N. Lee, K.C.A. Chan, D.S. Hui, et al., Since January 2020 Elsevier has created a COVID-19 resource centre with free information in English and Mandarin on the novel coronavirus COVID-19. The COVID-19 resource centre is hosted on Elsevier Connect, the company's public news and information. (2020). https://doi.org/10.1016/j.jcv.2004.07.006

Chapter 5
Statistical Analysis of Novel COVID-19 Based on Real-Time Data and Future Epidemics

C. H. Sekhar, M. Srinivasa Rao, and Debnath Battacharyya

5.1 Introduction to Coronavirus

5.1.1 Worldwide COVID-19

The nCoV (novel coronavirus) infection is the most recent rising infection after the Ebola, Zika and Nipah infections and the previous crises presented by bird influenza and swine influenza infections. The decent variety of CoVs in the bat populace needs further examination in subtleties, just as the reconnaissance and checking of bats get essential to forestall future episodes in animals and the public. The ongoing nCoV event features the shrouded wild creature store of destructive viruses. The creating novel coronavirus (2019-nCoV) has become overall stress inside a constrained capacity to centre time. First reported in Wuhan, and is present throughout the world, the total confirmed cases have reached to 929,6202 and death tolls to 479,133.

- The number of infected individuals is a lot higher in China than in different places of the world.
- Apart from singular cases, fatalities happen just in China.
- The number of individuals who recovered from infection is developing at a quick, nonlinear rate.

C. H. Sekhar (✉) · M. Srinivasa Rao
Department of Computer Science and Engineering, Vignan's Institute of Information Technology, Visakhapatnam, India

D. Battacharyya
Department of Computer Science and Engineering, K L Deemed to be University, KLEF, Guntur, India
e-mail: debnathb@kluniversity.in

L. Garg et al. (eds.), *Healthcare Informatics for Fighting COVID-19 and Future Epidemics*, EAI/Springer Innovations in Communication and Computing,
https://doi.org/10.1007/978-3-030-72752-9_5

- Mortality is falling at a slow pace and never exceeded 5.15% in history.
- The number of individuals who recovered at first dropped; however, from January 27, it has been developing quickly.
- The quantity of relief is moderately expanding to the dead.

As the pandemic evolves, so do the actions required by each country as they face different transmission scenarios [1]. And on June 24, WHO updated the interim guidance on the critical preparedness, readiness and response actions for COVID-19.

WHO has outlined four transmission synopses for COVID-19:

1. *No cases*: Nations/territories/regions not affected or do not have confirmed cases.
2. *Sporadic cases*: Countries/territories/areas with one or more cases, imported or locally detected.
3. *Clusters of cases*: Countries/territories/areas experiencing cases, clustered in time, geographic location and by common exposure.
4. *Community transmission*: Countries/territories/areas experiencing larger outbreaks of local transmission, defined through an assessment of factors including, but not limited to [1]:

    (a) Large quantities of cases which can't be connected to transmission chains.
    (b) Vast quantities of tests from sentinel lab reconnaissance or expanding positive tests through sentinel tests.
    (c) Multiple disconnected groups in a few regions of the count-attempt/an area/region.

A few countries have shown that COVID-19 transmission starting from one individual to another can be controlled. The "no cases" transmission situation presently covers the two nations that have never had any COVID-19 cases and nations that recently had COVID-19 cases, however right now have no dynamic cases. The updated guidance document provides an overview of the key actions and links to WHO interim guidance documents according to each transmission scenario. This spreads crisis reaction systems, chance correspondence and network commitment, epidemiological observation, contact following, general wellbeing measures, contamination anticipation and control, lab testing, case the executive procedures, maintaining essential health services and societal responses [1].

5.1.2 COVID-19 in India

The buzzword in the health sector globally COVID-19 alias coronavirus. Present all over the world, the virus spread rapidly from one person to another. The outbreak was first reported in Wuhan, China, in December 2019, exponentially spreading to the entire China. In the past months, COVID-19 becomes an outbreak throughout the world. The impact of this new virus damage brought horror to several countries as cities are quarantined and hospitals are overcrowded. A high infectious ailment that compromises the worldwide world, part of things is not entirely comprehended. It is a great challenge for all crisis centres and clinical staff. As of now, controlling contamination and reducing the spread of the disease are the most significant issues. We believe that with everybody's cooperation, the possibility of overcoming this pandemic is clear. In this chapter, we will discuss causes and possible ways of detection and necessary remedy steps to control COVID-19. Here we also provide the analysis of the COVID-19 in India. The data have been collected from the Indian Council of Medical Research (ICMR) and the Ministry of Health and Family Welfare, Government of India.

5.2 Human Family of Coronavirus

5.2.1 History of Coronavirus

Like any other family of infections, coronavirus is also named a family of similarly related viruses that create potentially dangerous diseases in mammals and birds. There are many different types of coronaviruses. Some of the significant illnesses occurred in human, as shown in Fig. 5.1—they usually spread through respiratory droplets produced by infected individuals.

Figure 5.1 shows the family of coronavirus and its sub-families. Presentation of COVID-19 comes under the betacoronavirus.

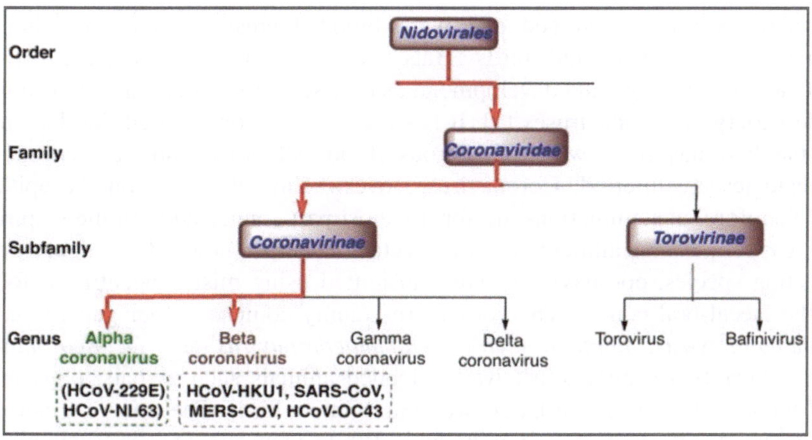

Fig. 5.1 Coronavirus family

5.2.1.1 When Did It Start?

A novel infection identified by Tyrrell and Bynoe in 1965, the common symptom of virus infection in humans is a common cold. In the 1970s, many scientists and researchers declared some morphologically comparable strains. They were clubbed together into this new gathering of infections, named coronavirus. The name came from the Latin word 'corona'. The shape of the virus looks like a crown, which alludes to the trademark appearance suggestive of a crown of sweet proteins. The ventures begin from the envelope encompassing the molecule [2].

With a distance across around 120 nm, the infection shows up as a sizeable, pleomorphic round molecule with bulbous surface projections. The morphology of the disease incorporates four fundamental basic proteins: the viral envelope (E); the spike (S), which frames the club-moulded bulges; the layer proteins (M); and the nucleocapsid (N), which is bounded to positive-sense single-abandoned RNA genome in a constant dot on a string-type compliance. Utilizing the essential proteins, the infection enters the host cells. It sets up contamination, reproduces, gathers its genome and discharges its offspring out of the host cell by exocytosis [3]. The encoding of coronavirus is the longest genome of any RNA-based virus, as a single strand of nucleic acid is approximately 26,000–32,000 bases in length.

The coronavirus has the most elevated known recurrence of recombination of any positive-strand RNA infection, indiscriminately joining genetic data from various sources when a host is tainted with different coronaviruses. These can transform/change at a lot quicker rate along these lines, and this property has made them a danger for the virology network.

5.2.1.2 Biological Properties

Coronaviruses infect winged and warm-blooded creatures, including humans, domesticated animals and birds. Bats are assumed to be a critical job in coronaviruses biology and development, as they seem to harbour an extraordinarily wide variety of coronaviruses [2]. It has even been recommended that bats might be the first has from which numerous if not all alpha and beta coronavirus genealogies are inferred. Coronaviruses overwhelmingly focus on the epithelial and therefore, contaminations are for the most part connected with the respiratory and gastrointestinal ailment. Natural vectors are not known. Contingent on the infection species, coronaviruses are transmitted using mist concentrates, fomites or the faecal-oral course. The coronavirus family comprises four genera, namely *Alphacoronavirus*, *Betacoronavirus*, *Gammacoronavirus* and *Deltacoronavirus*. The former two genera infect warm-blooded animals such as bats, pigs, felines and humans. However, the latter two genera infect birds. The infection can cause different side effects in among individuals. While a few strains cause flu in pigs and bovines, other strains can cause upper respiratory tract disorder in chickens [2].

In humans, coronavirus shifts fundamentally as far as pathogenicity. Some can kill over 30% of those contaminated (e.g. MERS-CoV), while some are generally innocuous, causing only common virus infection. As referenced, there are seven known strains of human coronavirus with the recent one found causing the COVID-19 pandemic.

SARS-CoV-2, MERS-CoV and SARS-CoV are the three highly pathogenic and deadly coronaviruses that spread rapidly and cause a significant number of deaths globally.

5.2.1.3 First Outbreak of SARS-CoV

During the year 2002–2003, SARS-CoV was identified in the southern part of China. The outbreak was first reported in Guangdong, China, in 2002. Human-to-human transmission of SARS-CoV is rapidly spreading at an alarming rate. The disease was declared a pandemic with an estimated confirmed case of 8000 around the world. SARS-CoV is viewed as increasingly pathogenic among coronaviruses as it can infect both the upper and the lower respiratory tract.

MERS-CoV

The Middle East respiratory syndrome coronavirus was first identified in Jordan and Saudi Arabia in 2012 when individuals showed symptoms of infection such as fever, cough and shortness of breath. In a few nations, it was speculated that the virus is transferred to humans from dromedary camels. However, the mode of transmission from dromedary camels to humans is still not yet clear. According to the WHO data, there are around 2500 confirmed cases of infection in 27 nations and 860 deaths reported since its outbreak.

SARS-CoV-2 (COVID-19)

At the end of the year 2019, the first outbreak of SARS-CoV-2 was recorded in Wuhan, China, and has since widely spread to different parts of the world. The WHO has declared SARS-CoV-2 also called COVID-19 a pandemic in March 2020. This infection was initially named 2019-nCoV and was later renamed to SARS-CoV2 after it was discovered to have the same characteristics as SARS-CoV. The infection is suspected to have originated from bats as it is fundamentally the same as the bat coronavirus.

5.2.2 Coronavirus Infection on Human

A coronavirus infection is an infection commonly found in animals and is seldom transmitted from animals to humans. Therefore, it can be spread from individual to individual. 2019-nCoV (COVID-19) disease is one of the diseases caused by one of the large family of coronaviruses infecting humans which is first reported in Wuhan, China, at the end of December 2019. The disease rapidly spreads, including over 31,000 confirmed cases with 638 deaths in just 1 month. The molecular analysis suggests that 2019-nCoV could have been originated from bats after passing on intermediate hosts, highlighting the high zoonotic potential of this coronavirus. As a highly contagious epidemic disease that threatens the human population globally, bunches of things about the virus are not completely comprehended. It is a great challenge for all emergency clinics and clinical staff. Right now, controlling and reducing the disease spread are the most significant issues. With everyone's cooperation and the endeavours made by many research centres around the world that started discovering vaccines for COVID-19, overcoming this disease is possible. Notwithstanding COVID-19, other human coronavirus infections have been included [5–8], such as the MERS infection or Middle East respiratory syndrome and the SARS (severe acute respiratory syndrome) infection, first reported in Guangdong, China.

5.2.2.1 Symptoms of COVID-19

COVID-19 symptoms range from mild to severe. It takes 2–14 days after being acquainted with an infected person for symptoms to appear. Common symptoms may include fever (the Centers for Disease Control and Prevention considers an individual to have a fever when he/she has a measured temperature of 100.4 °F or 38 °C), cough and shortness of breath. Those with weak immune systems may develop severe reactions, like pneumonia or bronchitis. Up until recently, adults are mostly the infected ones, but a couple of youths have also been infected. However, this finding is still under study by many research centres around the world and even how new symptoms can be seen about this epidemic's new wave. As far as it is very smart like a robot and can make changes in itself in new environmental conditions the same as HIV virus can have different behaviours and that is why virologists have confronted with an ill-posed virus that can be cured easily in different types of people throughout the world.

5.2.2.2 What Causes a Coronavirus Infection?

An individual at first is infected if he/she comes in contact with an infected individual. By then, it can be spread from one individual to another. Thriving experts don't have the haziest considered what creature caused COVID-19. COVID-19 can be spread through direct contact with infected people through nose and mouth secretions when sneezing or coughing. Moreover, it can also be spread through indirect contact through contaminated objects or surfaces and then touching their eyes, nose and mouth without washing their hands.

The coronavirus (CoV) influences the wellbeing of animals and people. Respiratory and gastrointestinal diseases often appear. For people, the CoV infection affects the upper respiratory tract and gastrointestinal tract, ranging from mild infections, for example, common cold, to severe infections like bronchitis and pneumonia. Since its discovery in the mid-1970s, a variety of neurotic conditions in animals was ascribed to CoV contaminations such as canine respiratory coronavirus, ox-like coronavirus and cat coronavirus, to name a few examples. The flexibility of CoVs varies in the two creatures and people. A portion of the CoVs is as of now adjusted in people (i.e. 229E, OC43, NL63 and HKU1 human coronaviruses), causing gentle ailments in people with powerless invulnerable frameworks. Be that as it may, on account of the tremendous deep MERS-CoV (i.e. Middle East respiratory syndrome coronavirus) and SARS-CoV (severe acute respiratory syndrome coronavirus), these CoVs are not adjusted in people and are found primarily in creature stores [4, 9, 10].

The transmission of illness from an animal to a human is known as a zoonotic overflow. Overflow occasions concern infection environmentalists, researchers and general well-being authorities because these are profoundly imperceptible. Right when it occurs, when it happens, the zoonotic illness hatches into the new host for a few days before it shows and spreads to the new host's populace with a wide scope of deadly diseases. All the more critically, overflow occasions present worldwide general well-being trouble. The gravity of overflows is lined up with environmental, epidemiological, and socio-social determinants [11, 12].

Figure 5.2 shows how the virus is transmitted from animal to human and human to human [13]. When transmission happens, the infected human being suffers from health issues. The kind of health issues only can be identified by the symptoms.

Nowadays, real-time image processing involves various sectors like security, healthcare, banking and face recognition. While capturing an image, there is more

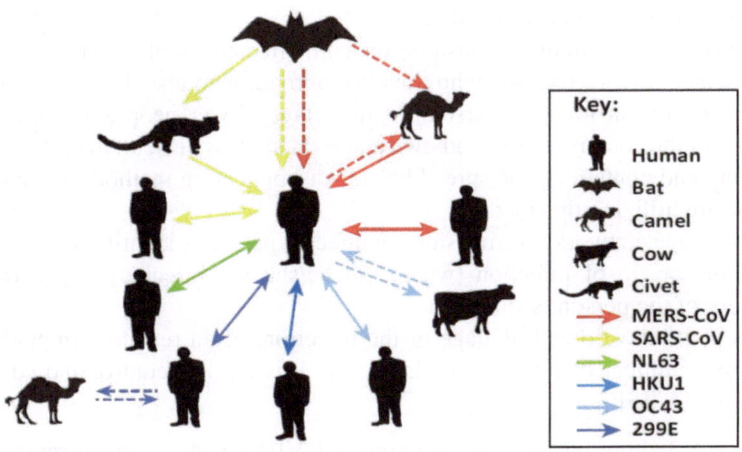

Fig. 5.2 Transmission of the virus from human to human and animal to human

chance of noise being engaged with multiple aspects of the surroundings. To improve the image's quality and get better classification results, we need to clean the picture, which is called pre-processing of the image. For the past 30 years, there is tremendous research happening on image processing by many researchers. Deep learning-based autoencoders are producing better results with minimum loss. Image denoising can be achieved with autoencoder architecture. The denoised image is taken as the input and then processed to the next level to improve the resolution. This paper has considered the popular dataset fashion mnist to denoise the image, which includes the noise. We used back-to-back autoencoders to perform both image denoising and resolution enhancement. This approach can do the pre-processing stage once on the dataset for both image denoising and enhancement of image resolution. We have used binary cross-entropy as loss function to evaluate the model's performance, and later we have focussed on improving the resolution of the image. Denoising of an image followed by resolution enhancements in the same process minimizes the time and pre-processing steps separately.

5.3 Life Cycle of COVID-19

5.3.1 Stages of COVID-19

Novel coronavirus infection occurs due to the transmission from one person to another person. It happened rapidly in China, Italy, South Korea and the rest of the world. Here, we will mention the various stages and how the mechanism of transmission of COVID-19 is done. The stages are as follows:

1. When infections are just imported from affected nations, only the individuals who have moved abroad are identified by the positive test. At this phase, there is no spread of the sickness locally.
2. When there is community transmission from infected people usually, from family or friends of work location who travelled abroad, who tested positive after close contact with an infected person. At this stage, fewer people are infected; the origin of the contamination is known and is thusly less difficult to perform contact tracing and containing the spread by self-disconnecting methods. Countries like India are utilizing this method.
3. In this stage, network transmission, an infected person is identified, but we cannot find the origin of infection (where did he/she get infected). Thus, the travel history of the person is validated.
4. This is the most dreadful stage of the infection, often resulting in epidemic. A colossal number of infection is rising, and it is hard to control and contain the spread [14, 15].

Figure 5.3 shows significant symptoms COVID-19. A graphical representation of significant parts of the body being infected is shown [13].

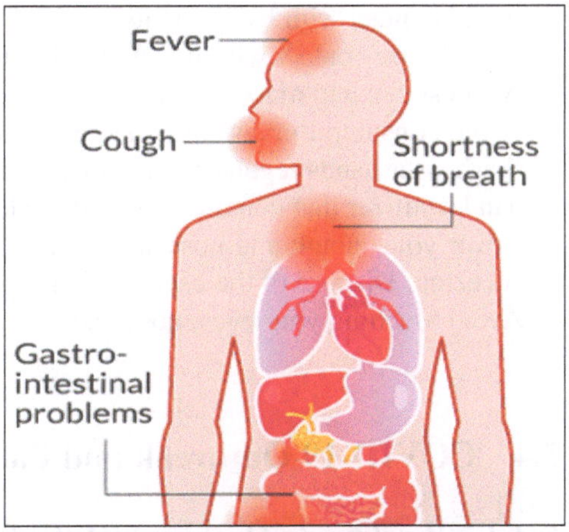

Fig. 5.3 Symptoms of COVID-19

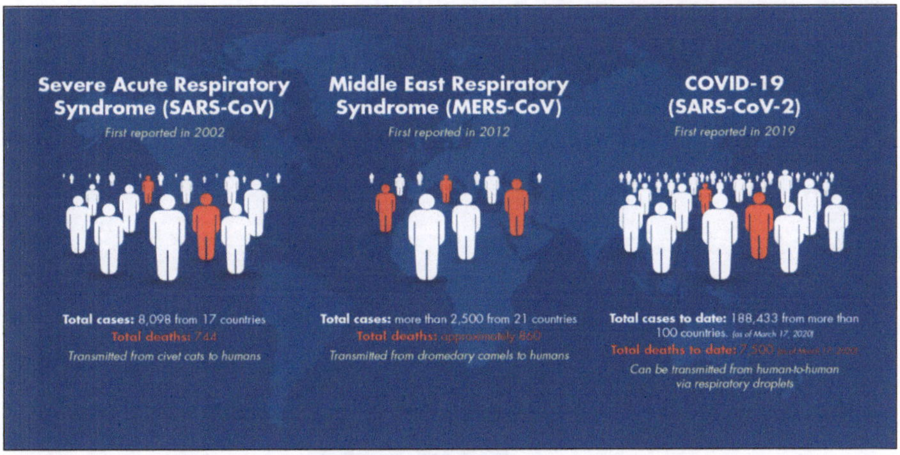

Fig. 5.4 Spread of coronavirus family infections [2]

5.3.2 Prevention and Control

Till date, there has been no specific medication prescribed for the treatment of coronavirus diseases like MERS, SARS and COVID-19. In that case, such diseases can be treated by frequently observing symptomatic patients and treating them with suitable existing drugs available. For the safe transportation of the viral sample, the CDC suggests gathering the speculated tests in the Viral Transport Medium and afterwards performing RT-PCR to affirm sickness. Hence, today, cleanliness has become a fundamental consideration.

Figure 5.4 shows the number of cases and number of countries affected with coronavirus family infections. And the following necessary preventive measures are needed to avoid transmission of infection:

- Avoid contact with live animals.
- Avoid close contact with infected individuals.
- Avoid social and mass gatherings.
- Avoid consumption raw and uncooked meats.
- Wash your hands regularly with soap and water for 20 s, or use an alcohol-based hand sanitizer that contains 70% ethyl alcohol.
- Cover your mouth and nose with your elbow or a tissue when you coughing or sneezing. Dispose of the used tissue properly.
- Avoid touching your eyes, nose and mouth when touching objects or surfaces.

5.4 COVID-19 Outbreak and Pandemic

5.4.1 Worldwide Outbreak Data Analysis

Figure 5.5 shows the worldwide outbreak of COVID-19 as regards confirmed cases, number of deaths, recovered cases and infected cases to date. With the help of this data, in the future, we can analyse the death rate and infected rate as were explained in the next sections.

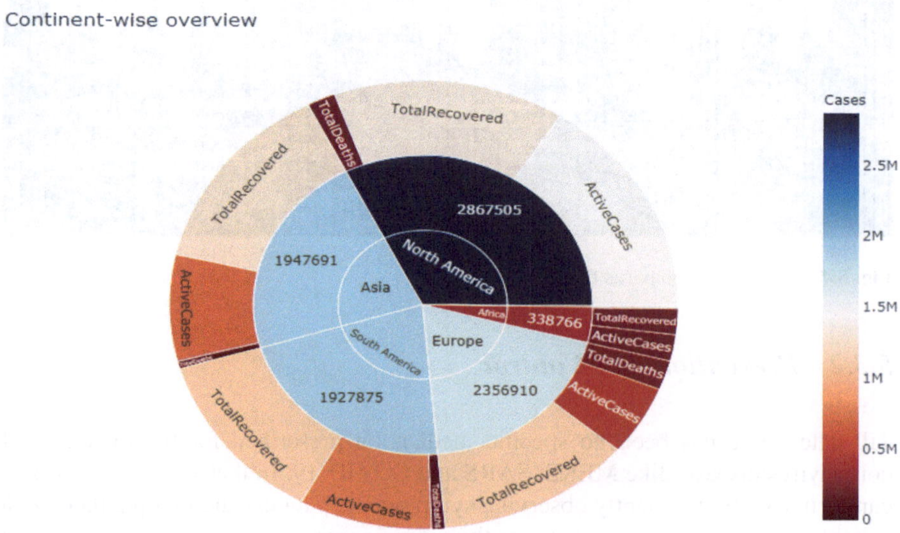

Fig. 5.5 Worldwide COVID-19 cases [2]

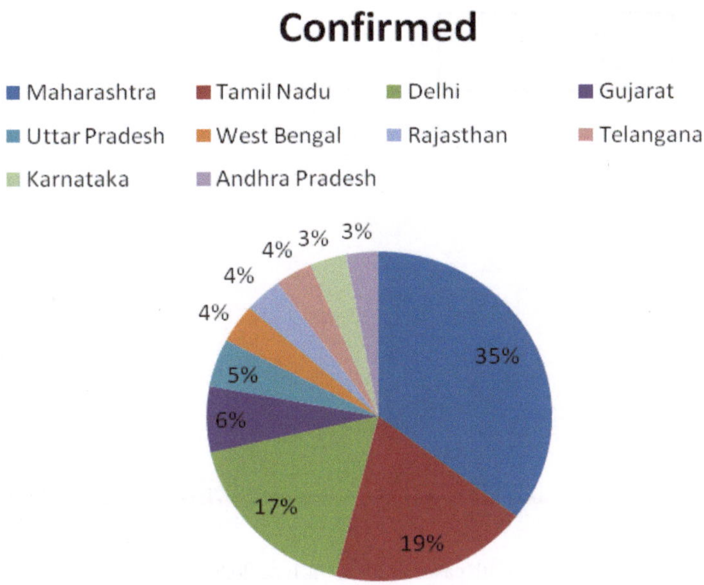

Fig. 5.6 Statewise COVID-19 analysis

5.4.2 Indian Outbreak Data Analysis

Figure 5.6 shows the statewise confirmed, recovered and death cases due to COVID-19. The red colour bar graph shows the confirmed cases, the green colour bar graph shows the recovered cases after treatment, and yellow colour bar graph shows the number of deaths up to April 26, 2020. All the data we have taken from the ICMR and states of India up to date make customized information.

India is a country in South Asia having a population of 1.3 billion. It consists of 30 states and 8 union territories. It is the second most populous country and the seventh largest country in terms of land area in the world. The first COVID-19 case was identified in the state of Kerala at the end of January 2020, and later in March 2020, new cases are identified. From March onwards, infections are increasing slowly. Based on the severity of infections on March 22, 2020, a 24-h lockdown was initiated. After 2 days, a 21-day lockdown was imposed throughout the country. The clear picture of confirmed cases was shown in Fig. 5.6 and recovered and death cases in Fig. 5.7 [16, 17].

5.5 Case Study in India

On January 30, 2020, the first case of COVID-19 in India was reported in the state of Kerala, which rose to three cases by February 3; all were students who returned

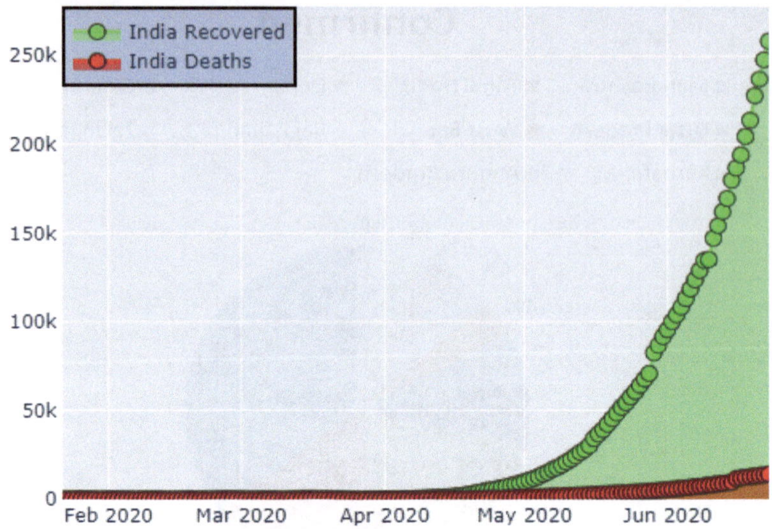

Fig. 5.7 Recovered cases vs. death cases in India till June 2020

from Wuhan, China [18]. And no rise in cases was recorded in the remainder of February. On March 22, 2020, India launched a 14-h curfew on Sunday initiated by Prime Minister Narendra Modi to lessen the spread of the virus. Seventy-five districts in India were put on lockdown with confirmed COVID cases. Further, on March 24, the officials announced a 21-day lockdown, affecting India's 1.3 billion people.

Transmission of infection rose in March after a couple of cases were reported throughout the country. On March 12, a 76-year-old individual returned from Saudi Arabia experiencing a difficulty in breathing. On March 4, 22 new cases became evident, including an Italian vacationer who contaminated 14 individuals.

Since then, the number of cases began to rise drastically after March 19; however, the pinnacle of infection was in April.

Authorities recommend that contamination could be a lot higher as India's troublesome rates are among the least on the planet. The contamination rate of COVID-19 in India is said to be 1.7, essentially lower than in the most conspicuously terrible affected nations.

5.5.1 Statewise Analysis in India

2019-nCoV is a contagious coronavirus that originated from Wuhan, China. This new strain of virus has posed fear in many countries as cities are quarantined and hospitals are overcrowded. We have taken the dataset to analyse the number of confirmed, recovered and death cases. This dataset will help us understand how

2019-nCoV is spread around the world. Moreover, this dataset is transformed into a format that is easier for kaggle to handle [19], 2019-nCoV_data.csv: daily level information on the number of 2019-nCoV confirmed cases across the globe. It contains five major parameters: country, daily level information, registered cases, recovered cases and death cases across the globe.

As of April 24, 2020, over 3.15 million cases have been confirmed in 200 countries and territories worldwide with 200,000 deaths. In addition to major outbreaks in the past 2 weeks were reported in the USA, Spain, Italy, France, the UK, China and Iran, and emerging outbreaks are currently being observed in Russia, Brazil, European countries and Asian countries.

In India, the COVID-19 cases are slowly increasing day by day. Compared to advanced countries, the spread is under control. Here we customized dataset prepared based on the government of India's data provided by ICMR. Tables 5.1 and 5.2 show the COVID-19 tests and COVID-19 cases, respectively [16, 17], based on the recent updated and implemented analysis of data. The numbers of COVID-19 tests and the contagious cases are increasing day by day. In India, initially, a limited number of the clinical laboratories were available, but after 1 month, the government gave permission and established 100 laboratories to hasten the testing process.

In Tables 5.3 and 5.4, statistical values of confirmed, recovered and death cases from the start of COVID-19 to June 25, 2020, have been demonstrated. Figure 5.6 shows the number of cases based on the tests conducted up to 790,000 above tests. Based on the tests, the top pie charts below show that number of confirmed cases and below the pie chart showing the active cases, cured cases and number deaths.

Table 5.1 Coronavirus family [4]

S. no	Name	Short name	Year of identification
1	Human coronavirus 229E	HCoV-229E	1960
2	Human coronavirus OC43	HCoV-OC43	1960
3	Severe acute respiratory syndrome coronavirus	SARS-CoV	2003
4	Human coronavirus NL63	HCoV-NL63	2004
5	Human coronavirus HKU1		2004
6	Middle East respiratory syndrome-related coronavirus (MERS-CoV)	HCoV-EMC	2012
7	Severe acute respiratory syndrome coronavirus 2 (SARS-CoV-2)	2019-nCoV	2019

Table 5.2 Covid-19 tests

S. no.	Feature	Remarks
1	S. no.	Unique number for the country/province
2	Name of state/union territory (UT)	Name of state or union territory in India
3	Total tested	Total COVID-19 tests conducted by each state
4	Positive	No. of positive cases based on tests
5	Negative	No. of positive cases based on tests
6	Active	No. of active cases present doing the treatment

Table 5.3 COVID-19 cases

S. no.	Feature	Remarks
1	S. no.	Unique number for the country/province
2	Name of state/UT	Name of state or union territory in India
3	Confirmed	No. of confirmed cases
4	Recovered	No. of recovered patients after treatment
5	Deaths	No. of deaths
6	Active	No. of active cases present under treatment

Table 5.4 shows the statewise confirmed, recovered and death cases due to COVID-19. All the data we have taken from the ICMR and states of India up to date make customized information.

5.5.2 *Age Group and Gender Analysis*

Unfortunately, in India, deaths were higher among younger individuals, i.e. 30–40 years old. A small percentage of COVID-19 deaths was recorded among patients 60 years of age and above. The extent of COVID-19 deaths among youngsters and patients 45 years of age and more in India is fundamentally higher than those recorded in the USA or China. The number of COVID-19 cases based on age was shown in Fig. 5.8, while the number of COVID-19 cases based on age vs. gender was shown in Fig. 5.9.

5.5.3 *COVID-19 Impact on Indian Economy*

The worldwide spread of COVID-19, across outskirts and geologies, has seriously affected and threatens the economy of nearly the entire world, including India. Because of the lockdown, the Indian economy was constrained by falling revenues. Most of the organizations, the stoppage could be as flexibly interruptions, fall in utilization request, and weight on the banking and budgetary segments.

The three economic scenario models of Indian GDP estimates during this pandemic situation were shown in Fig. 5.10. Those scenarios are as follows:

Scenario 1

- Nationwide lockdown lifted on April 15, 2020.
- Back to work in "spare lives and vocations" mode with solid security conventions.
- Support to family units, partnerships and banking framework with financial and money-related boosts.

Table 5.4 Statewise COVID-19 case details

S. no.	State	Confirmed	Active	Deaths	Mortality rate	Recovered	Recovery rate
1	Maharashtra	186,626	77,260	8178	4.38	101,172	54.21
2	Tamil Nadu	98,392	41,050	1321	1.34	56,021	56.94
3	Delhi	92,175	26,304	2864	3.11	63,007	68.36
4	Gujarat	33,999	7511	1887	5.55	24,601	72.36
5	Uttar Pradesh	24,825	6869	735	2.96	17,221	69.37
6	West Bengal	19,819	6083	699	3.53	13,037	65.78
7	Rajasthan	18,785	3307	435	2.32	15,043	80.08
8	Telangana	18,570	9226	275	1.48	9069	48.84
9	Karnataka	18,016	9404	272	1.51	8336	46.27
10	Andhra Pradesh	16,097	8586	198	1.23	7313	45.43
11	Haryana	15,509	4239	251	1.62	11,019	71.05
12	Madhya Pradesh	14,106	2702	589	4.18	10,815	76.67
13	Bihar	10,682	2610	78	0.73	7994	74.84
14	Assam	9435	3311	14	0.15	6107	64.73
15	Odisha	8106	2567	37	0.46	5502	67.88
16	Jammu and Kashmir	7849	2760	115	1.47	4974	63.37
17	Punjab	5784	1488	152	2.63	4144	71.65
18	Kerala	4754	2088	26	0.55	2638	55.49
19	Chhattisgarh	3013	637	14	0.46	2362	78.39
20	Uttarakhand	2984	510	42	1.41	2405	80.6
21	Jharkhand	2634	631	15	0.57	1988	75.47
22	Goa	1482	744	4	0.27	734	49.53
23	Tripura	1440	293	1	0.07	1146	79.58
24	Manipur	1279	663	0	0	616	48.16
25	Himachal Pradesh	1014	360	9	0.89	632	62.33
26	Ladakh	991	261	1	0.1	729	73.56
27	Puducherry	802	459	12	1.5	331	41.27
28	Nagaland	539	342	0	0	197	36.55
29	Chandigarh	450	55	6	1.33	389	86.44
30	Dadra and Nagar Haveli and Daman and Diu	254	141	0	0	112	44.09
31	Arunachal Pradesh	232	160	1	0.43	71	30.6
32	Mizoram	162	36	0	0	126	77.78
33	Andaman and Nicobar Islands	116	65	0	0	51	43.97
34	Sikkim	101	49	0	0	52	51.49
35	Meghalaya	59	15	1	1.69	43	72.88
36	Lakshadweep	0	0	0	0	0	0
	Total	621,081	222,786	18,232	47.92	379,997	60.7225

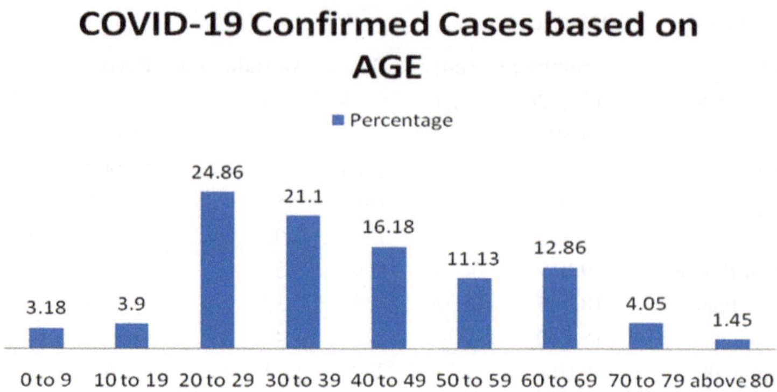

Fig. 5.8 No. of COVID cases based on age

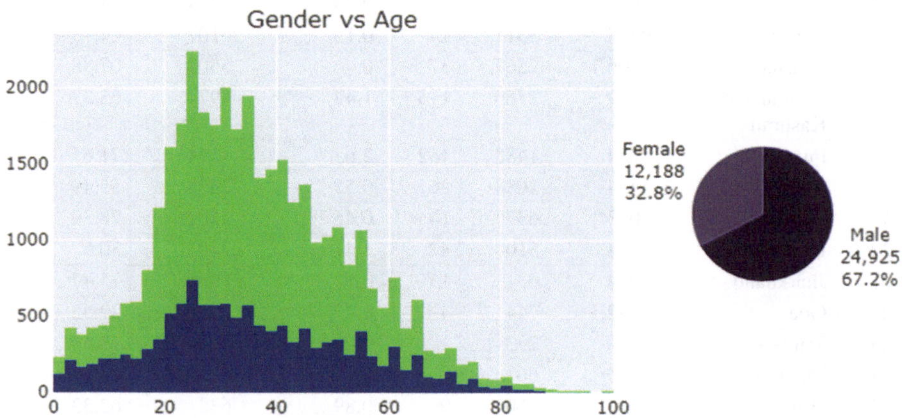

Fig. 5.9 No. of COVID-19 cases based on gender vs. age

Scenario 2

- Lockdown proceeds until mid-May 2020, moderate unwinding after April 15, 2020. Restarting chains gracefully and normalizing creation and utilization takes 3–5 months.
- Stabilization and improvement bundle more extensive than in scenario 1.

Scenario 3

- Lockdown as in situation 2 with extra 2-multi-week lockdowns in Q2 and Q4 FY 2021 due to infection resurgence.
- Low work accessibility as a result of constrained opposite relocation.
- Stabilization and upgrade bundle significantly more extensive than in scenario 2.

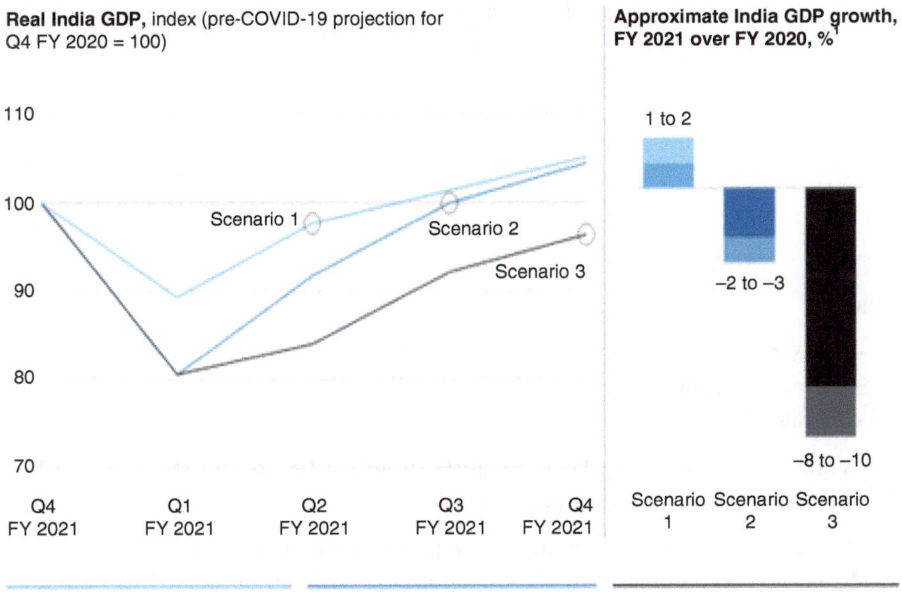

Fig. 5.10 Economic scenario models of Indian GDP estimates

5.6 Prediction of COVID-19

5.6.1 SEIR Model

COVID-19 disease spread drastically throughout the world, and the number of infected individuals increased day by day. When we want to identify infected individuals, one of the popular used models for is the SEIR model [20]. SEIR model consists of compartmental models in epidemiology. Compartmental models are a system used to streamline the scientific approach of infectious disease to predict how a disease spreads. The total population is split into compartments, with the suspicion that each person in a similar compartment has similar qualities [20].

The infectious rate, β, controls the pace of spread which is the likelihood of transmitting a virus between a helpless and an infectious person. The incubation rate, σ, is the pace of inert people getting irresistible (mean time of incubation is $1/\sigma$). Recuperation rate, $Y = 1/D$, is dictated by the normal length, D, of disease. For the SEIRS model, is the rate which recouped people come back to the helpless sculpture because of loss of immunity [9, 11]

$$\frac{dS}{dt} = \mu N - vS - \frac{\beta SI}{N} \tag{5.1}$$

$$\frac{dE}{dt} = \frac{\beta SI}{N} - vE - \sigma E \tag{5.2}$$

$$\frac{dI}{dt} = \sigma E - \gamma I - vI \tag{5.3}$$

$$\frac{dR}{dt} = \gamma I - vR \tag{5.4}$$

where

$N = \sum(S,E,I,R)$
μ is the rate of births
v is the rate of death

While solving the differential equation shown above to find the *S*, *E*, *I*, *R*, we have considered the following parameters [10, 16]:

- *R*_0 & *R*_t: Reproduction number; it tells about whether it is infected or not.
- *T*_inf: Average duration of the infection; 1/*T*_inf can be treated as individual experiences one recovery in *D* units of time [14].
- *T*_inc: Average incubation period.

Figure 5.11 shows the SEIR model prediction versus historical data of COVID-19 cases. Straight lines indicate the SEIR model predictions and dotted lines indicate the historical data. As of June 22, 2020, the COVID-19 cases rose to 459,626 based on the SEIR model, whereas it was 440,215 based on historical data.

Based on application, the SEIR model is fit for analysing the historical data of the spread of COVID-19 in India. We got results showing that we are experiencing the peak in these days and that for the next 30 days an increment is to be expected in

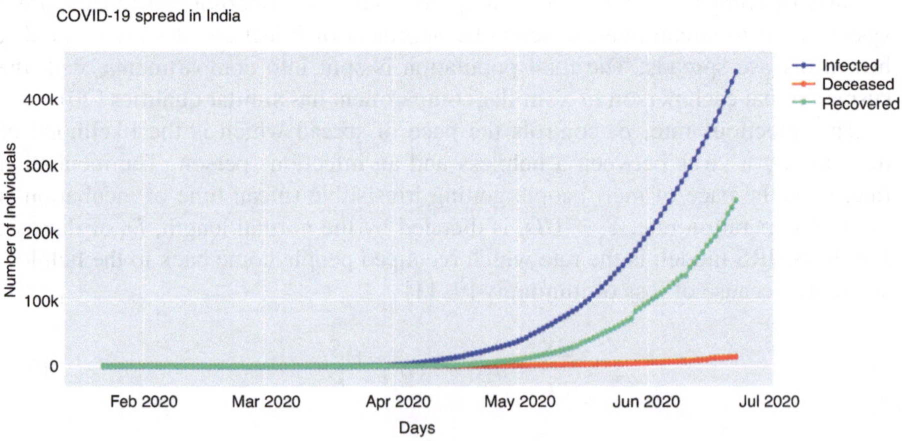

Fig. 5.11 Month-wise analysis using the SEIR model

the number of infected, deceased and recovered individuals. A proof of the model is given by the estimates of both the reproductive number and mean incubation period obtained, which are similar to the values present in literature. A more solid study should be done, estimating the confidence interval by considering the effect of bias introduced in historical data with the Indian testing policy.

5.6.2 ARIMA Model

ARIMA models stands for autoregressive integrated moving average models. Univariate (single vector) ARIMA is an estimating procedure that extends the future estimations of an arrangement dependent on its own inactivity. Its principal application is in the zone of momentary gauging requiring at any rate 40 recorded information focuses. It works best when your information displays a steady or predictable example after some time with a base measure of exceptions. ARIMA technique endeavours to depict the developments in a fixed time arrangement as a component of what is designated 'autoregressive and moving normal' boundaries. These are alluded to as AR boundaries (autoregressive) and MA boundaries (moving midpoints). An AR model with just a single boundary might be composed of the following (Fig. 5.12):

$$X(t) = A(1) \times X(t-1) + E(t)$$

where

$X(t)$ = time series under investigation
$A(1)$ = the autoregressive parameter of order 1

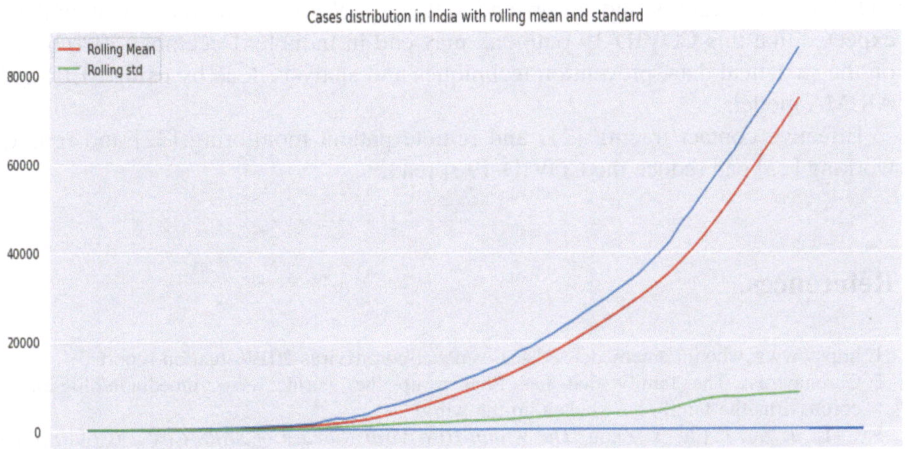

Fig. 5.12 ARIMA forecast

$X(t-1)$ = the time series lagged 1 period
$E(t)$ = the error term of the model

Based on application, the ARIMA model is fit for analysing the historical data of the spread of COVID-19 in India. We got results showing that we are experiencing the peak in these days, and that for the next 30 days, an increment is to be expected in the number of infected, deceased and recovered individuals. A proof of the model is given by the estimates of both the reproductive number and mean incubation period obtained, which are similar to the literature's values. A more solid study should be done.

5.7 Conclusion

Present circumstance, not having any prompt acting adversary of viral administrator and vaccinations, dangerous utilization of high caution for 2019-nCoV and fitting shirking and control measures are of most extreme significance to check the further spread and control of this contamination. Researchers and government authorities globally are making efforts to fight this pandemic. They are also perceiving the possible foundation of this novel disease and trying to structure and make incredible antibodies and therapeutics. It includes mulling over the contamination in nuances, its sub-nuclear science and immunology, adaptable innate changes, changes and recombination occasions, explaining clinical pathology and pathogenesis, perceiving the course of starting point, work of any blending vessels (like fowls, pigs, and all-around cutting edge creatures), ricocheting as far as possible, zoonotic potential and human-to-human transmission occasions which totally would clear the ways to organize convincing evasion and they control measures to counter 2019-nCoV.

This chapter gives a detailed knowledge about COVID-19 and the outbreak of COVID-19 in India and around the world. It provides a statistical analysis of COVID-19 as regards age group and statewise. With this prediction, it will be expected that this COVID-19 outbreak may end in India by December 2020 based on the statistical data, prevention techniques and analysis done by using SEIR and ARIMA models.

Effective contact tracing [21] and remote patient monitoring [22] and remote working [23] can reduce the COVID-19 spread.

References

1. https://www.who.int/emergencies/diseases/novel-coronavirus-2019/situation-reports
2. Coronavirus: The family that has Shaken up the world, www.tmmedia.in/blog-entry/coronavirus-the-family-has-shaken-up-the-world
3. C. Li, J. Xu, J. Liu, Y. Zhou, *The Within-Host Viral Kinetics of SARS-CoV-2* (Cold Spring Harbor Laboratory, Cold Springer Harbor, 2020)

4. Y.G. Sánchez, Z. Sabir, J.L.G. Guirao, Design of a nonlinear SITR fractal model based on the dynamics of a novel coronavirus (COVID-19). Fractals **28**(32) (2020)
5. C. Salata et al., Coronaviruses: A paradigm of new emerging zoonotic diseases. Pathogens Dis **77**(9) (2019). https://doi.org/10.1093/femspd/ftaa006
6. L. Pan, L. Wang, X. Huang, How to face the novel coronavirus infection during the 2019–2020 epidemic: The experience of Sichuan Provincial People's Hospital. Intensive Care Med **46**(4), 573–575. https://doi.org/10.1007/s00134-020-05964-0
7. L. Hui, T. Qiao-Ling, et al., *Can Chinese Medicine Be Used for Prevention of Corona Virus Disease 2019 (COVID-19)? A Review of Historical Classics, Research Evidence and Current Prevention Programs* (The Chinese Journal of Integrated Traditional and Western Medicine Press and Springer-Verlag GmbH Germany, part of Springer Nature, New York, 2020)
8. Y.S. Malik, S. Sircar, S. Bhat, K. Sharun, D. Kuldeep, M. Dadar, R. Tiwari, W. Chaicumpa, Emerging novel Coronavirus (2019-nCoV) - Current scenario, evolutionary perspective based on genome analysis and recent developments. Vet. Q. (2020). https://doi.org/10.1080/01652176.2020.1727993
9. A.N. Alagaili, T. Briese, N. Mishra, V. Kapoor, S.C. Sameroff, P.D. Burbelo, E. de Wit, V.J. Munster, L.E. Hensley, I.S. Zalmout, et al., Middle East respiratory syndrome coronavirus infection in dromedary camels in Saudi Arabia. mBio **5**(2), e00884–e00814 (2014)
10. A. Lin, H.W. Lee, J.Y. Choi, J. Zhang, M.S. Lee, Herbal medicine and pattern identification for treating COVID-19: A rapid review of guidelines. Integr Med Res **9**(2), 100407
11. S.K. Dey, M.M. Rahman, U.R. Siddiqi, A. Howlader, Analyzing the epidemiological outbreak of COVID-19: A visual exploratory data analysis approach. J. Med. Virol. (2020)
12. A. Thapa, Nepal and COVID-19: A strange case and the dilemma. Nepal J. Neurosci. **17**(1), 1–4 (2020)
13. The Novel Coronavirus Pneumonia Emergency Response Epidemiology Team, The epidemiological characteristics of an outbreak of 2019 novel coronavirus diseases (COVID-19)—China, 2020. China CDC Weekly **2**(8), 113–122 (2020)
14. Stage of COVID19, Article by C to I News, https://www.connectedtoindia.com/the-four-stages-of-covid-19-explained-7280.html
15. S. Tomar, S. Mahajan, R. Kumar, *Advances in Structure-Assisted Antiviral Discovery for Animal Viral Diseases* (Elsevier BV, Amsterdam, 2020)
16. Data set from ICMR, https://www.icmr.nic.in/content/covid-19
17. Data Set for India case study, https://api.covid19india.org/
18. China virus death toll rises to 41, more than 1300 infected worldwide, CNBC, 24 Jan 2020. Archived from the original on Jan 2020
19. COVID19 Dataset Analysis, https://www.kaggle.com/sekhar1203/covid-19-analysis-viz-prediction-comparisons
20. Compartmental models in epidemiology, https://idmod.org/docs/hiv/model-seir.html
21. L. Garg, E. Chukwu, N. Nidal, C. Chakraborty, G. Garg, Anonymity preserving IoT-based COVID-19 and other infectious disease contact tracing model. IEEE Access **8**, 159402–159414 (2020). https://doi.org/10.1109/ACCESS.2020.3020513
22. M. Jayalakshmi, L. Garg, K. Maharajan, K. Srinivasan, K. Jayakumar, A.K. Bashir, K. Ramesh, Fuzzy logic-based health monitoring system for COVID'19 patients. Comput. Mater. Continua (2022)
23. A.K. Bhardwaj, L. Garg, A. Garg, Y. Gajpal, E-Learning during COVID-19 outbreak: Cloud computing adoption in Indian Public Universities. Comput. Mater. Continua **66**(3), 2471–2492 (2022). https://doi.org/10.32604/cmc.2021.014099

Chapter 6
A Real-Time Approach with Deep Learning for Pandemic Management

A. Raghavendra Rao and Debabrata Samanta

6.1 Impact of Artificial Intelligence (AI) on Medicine

As per the proposal from authors of [1], artificial intelligence systems have made a mark in the medical fields of pathology, radiology, ophthalmology, and cardiology. This has led to collaborative efforts from physicians and the AI in the field. Though the concept of general AI is being explored deeply, today's reality is the narrow AI specializing in specific tasks. These specific tasks would be image recognition, speech recognition, and so on. Among many influencing factors for AI's role in medicine and healthcare is the availability of a large amount of medical data and data generated from medical wearables that have become highly popular. Prominent contribution of AI comes in the role of a decision-making layer on top of the current system. This is considerably improving the accuracy of treatment and cost involved. It also raises concerns about the possibility of AI replacing physicians. Electronic medical records (EMR) make this domain a data-rich endeavour that makes it more appropriate for AI to work on it and derive practical information. With quite a bit of progress in technology around scanners like magnetic resonance imaging (MRI), the next leg of the progress will be for AI to utilize the imaging data generated by imaging technologies [2]. Deep learning techniques like convolutional neural networks (CNNs) have been making useful contributions in imaging for object recognition and localization. Patients diagnosing the capability of AI are closely

A. Raghavendra Rao
Data Science Department, CHRIST (Deemed to be) University and Specialist-QMS, First American India Private Ltd., Bengaluru, India
e-mail: raghavendra.a@res.christuniversity.in

D. Samanta (✉)
Department of Computer Science, CHRIST (Deemed to be University), Bangalore, India
e-mail: debabrata.samanta369@gmail.com

L. Garg et al. (eds.), *Healthcare Informatics for Fighting COVID-19 and Future Epidemics*, EAI/Springer Innovations in Communication and Computing,
https://doi.org/10.1007/978-3-030-72752-9_6

competing with that of doctors. Works of Norman [3] emphasize that the AI's involvement is not about replacing the physician but complements and improvises their ways of work. A significant focus is also on cutting down on the administrative work that medical fraternity end up doing, which can be automated with machine learning. It is critical as the error that can creep into these documentations may be costly.

A more in-depth focus of AI in the medical field understands the pattern within the domain to assess the behaviour and derive appropriate logic for current scenarios. The key aspect that needs to be considered is the literal adoption of the AI algorithms to the objectives provided to them, rather than adapting to the unseen scenarios. Also, the algorithms' black box natures make it tough to dive deep and derive useful interpretation; this needs attention.

6.1.1 Ensemble Models for Pandemic Management

Possible architecture that can add value to pandemic situations like that of COVID-19 would involve ensembling of various machine learning and deep learning models. Since the idea is to organize and put all the available data in a meaningful way, ensemble models are the right approach. Since works are happening around the utilization of radiology images associated with the patients, the convolutional neural network (CNN) is one component. Work is done by Tulin et al. [4], banks on the radiology images of the patient's chest to identify the COVID-19. Here the author's banks on utilizing salient information are hidden in these radiology images. This work's advantages are also highlighted to help in remote areas where the doctors' availability is a concern. Here, the approach highlights the usage of chest X-rays as a means for COVID-19 detection. The proposed model focuses on binary classification between presence and absence of COVID-19 and multi-class classification to differentiate between the presence of COVID-19, pneumonia, and none of these. In the case of the YOLO (You Only Look Once) model for object detection, the darknet model was used as a classifier. Series of convolution layers was the architecture component with intermittent filters.

Artificial neural network (ANN) is another critical component of the ensemble model. Due to the complexity of the diagnosis involved, it is imperative to study various features' influence. The information on how each of the features influences each other can be handy in refining these systems and improving their performance. It would be an appropriate fit to use ANN with explainable features to address this concept. Since there is quite a bit of work on explainable AI, that thought process will be helpful. Recurrent neural network (RNN), with its specialization in managing time-series data, will play a key role in studying the evolution of the virus behaviour across the timeline, particularly on the characteristics of the virus and the possibility of its mutations. This characteristic of the virus will be significant to understand and device the mechanism for studying viruses and the possibility of the cure. In work [5], the author studies the spread of COVID-19 in India and the effect of the remedial measures taken to control the pandemic. With the largest economies struggling due to the virus's impact and its spreading nature, resources employed are turning out ineffective. Considering the growing pressure on the health system and administration, there is a need to build a prediction system that provides heads-up. Authors have employed long short-term memory (LSTM) data-driven estimation methods and try to fit the curve to predict future cases of COVID-19 and also assess the effectiveness of preventive measures like social distancing and lockdown. This proposal seems to provide useful insights into the administration of health officials.

Potential information is available from social media, which can also be plugged into the ensemble model. Social data is mainly about the information that people share about themselves in the media, such as Facebook and Twitter. Crunching this information will play a significant role as an early indicator of the potential impact such a pandemic situation can bring in. This would be leveraged to the plugin as one of the sources in pandemic management. Natural language processing (NLP) is an obvious choice to model these data and plug it into its ensemble model. NLP will also put together the learned knowledge in the literature and building the solution on top of it. Work done in [6] stresses the scientific literature being searched for answers on COVID-19 questions. The novel neural ranking approach is proposed to ensure that all the new information that comes in is put together and analysed and learned in all the information's overall context. Transfer learning, being a recent advancement in AI, can fit well on top of the ensemble model, bringing in the knowledge from various other domains and customizing the ensemble's architecture to fit the learning needed for specific situations of COVID-19. Work done in [7] emphasizes leveraging deep transfer learning with the rapidly increasing rate of COVID-19 and challenges associated with the testing kits. It becomes paramount to look at all possible knowledge being plugged in for the detection of the virus. The development of COVID-19 testing methods is a significant area of exploration. CT (computed tomography) of the chest is seen as an excellent potential source for COVID-19 detection. However, it is not a straightforward method and involves some challenges. Authors in this work propose deep transfer learning to classify COVID-19 infections. Authors also employ top two smooth loss functions to handle noisy and imbalanced datasets of this problem. This approach seems to provide better performance in comparison to other supervised learning models. Transfer learning can also be leveraged to study the individual's physiological and health state in the context of other pandemics, which can be extended into the context of COVID-19 infection. This provides a platform to build on top of learning from other pandemics (Fig. 6.1).

Convolutional neural network (CNN) in this architecture will have the primary role of managing the image data, particularly chest X-rays that are found to be one of the top sources of data of the virus infection. This module's critical outcome is to identify the virus's existence and retrieve the virus's critical characteristics as much as possible from this source of data (Fig. 6.2).

CNN specializes in picking the image data's essential features, such as the chest X-ray using the convolutional filters. These filters need to be architected effectively based on expected features to be learned from the X-ray. The max-pooling layer

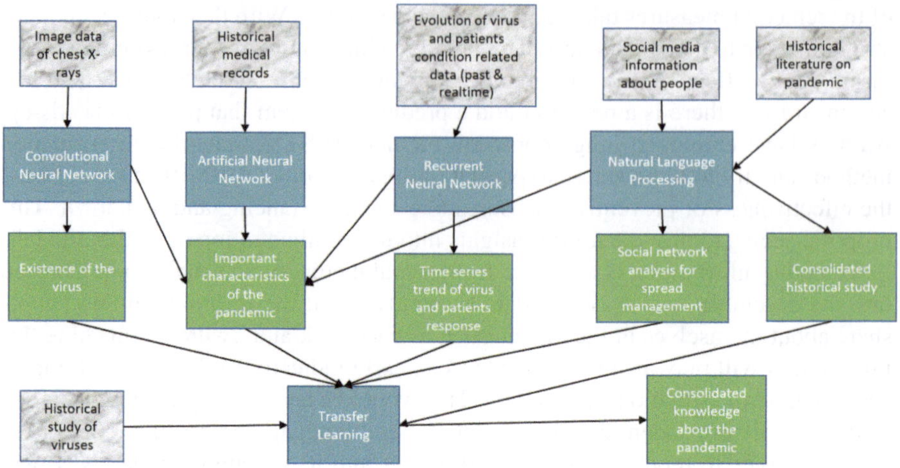

Fig. 6.1 Architecture of ensemble model proposed for pandemic management

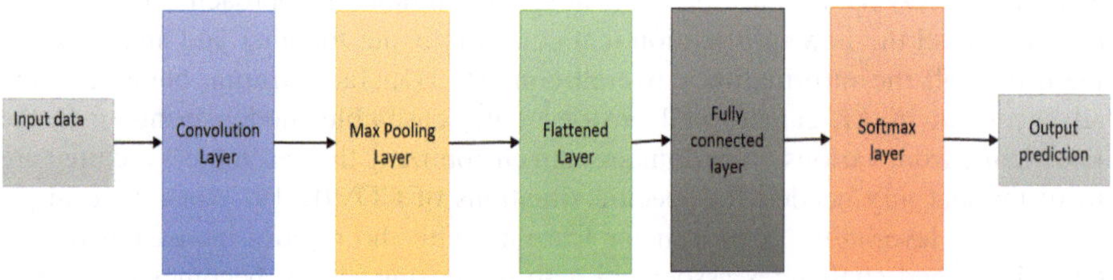

Fig. 6.2 Basic structure of convolutional neural network for image analysis

next in line will help comprehend the image's critical characteristics into significant knowledge. A further layer of fully connected one will formulate the summarized knowledge for the final prediction of the virus's existence in the subject. Apart from figuring out the existence of the virus, CNN's architecture can also be customized to learn enough critical characteristics from the virus that can be plugged in the ANN module that stands next in line with the framework. Convolution layer and pooling layer structure also need a study based on the target domain to customize its effective operation to generate expected output.

In this architecture, ANN will specialize in identifying the critical parameters from the study of the virus. Feature importance is the expected outcome. Historical medical information will be the critical inputs consumed by this model to generate important feature information. With a wide variety of historical information being fed in as input for the ANN part of the framework, layers of ANN and their neuron configuration must be customized to study the critical features for the study effectively. Backpropagation and gradient descent concepts can be leveraged to enhance ANN architecture to make it a focused study to generate useful output from this part.

Recurrent neural network (RNN) in this architecture will specialize in the study of time-series data. The time trend of the virus behaviour and the patients' responses on the medications are the critical input data. RNN architecture specializes in capturing the knowledge across the time from input data. Some of the variations of RNN like long short-term memory (LSTM) are of specific interest here as they overcome the problem of RNN, where they were tending to miss out on the vital information as the time passed by. LSTM bridges that gap by carrying forward crucial information in time and helping consolidate the knowledge over time. This pipeline in the architecture can also play the role of active plugging in data as it is gathered so that the outcomes can be kept refined over the period. RNN is critical here, as it is significantly vital to focus only on the characteristics that matter. This becomes crucial as the fight against time is a situation in handling this pandemic when it hits.

Natural language processing (NLP) pipeline of this architecture will specialize in plugging data from the social platforms. That information generates from people in real time some critical insights into the possibility of spreading the pandemic and also assesses the social network influence on the pandemic and other related information. The second part of the NLP pipeline task would be to effectively consolidate the historical literature to make it a meaningful data for present situations. With a lot of literature that sits from history and tons for further study getting added, specializations from the NLP domain will be crucial in this framework. NLP pipelines will also specialize in working on natural language data, from text and audio. As this part of the architecture is built, it will be crucial to study the landscape from where the data is plugged in and devise the NLP pipeline accordingly. As part of the NLP pipeline, social network study is involved. Graph theory can be banked on to make this objective of study more robust. Graph theory is about the entire network that can be represented as vertices and nodes. Here, the relation between the nodes is established by the vertices. This thought process came out of the travelling salesmen problem that looked at a situation where the salesman was expected to travel all the cities without revisiting the same city. It was about visiting all the cities once and picking the shortest distance to accomplish this. Here, in graph theory, the social network can be established with these graphs and plug in the input's knowledge.

Work in [8] studies the social network model of COVID-19. Here, the dynamic social network model of COVID-19 is built, where epidemiological models are used with person-to-person interaction graphs. Graphs are the thought process of establishing the mathematical relation between the objects and their entities. The consolidator role in this framework is taken by transfer learning (TL), which takes as its input all the key learnings from CNN, ANN, RNN, and NLP pipelines. Also, it will be fed with historical data of the pandemic. The TL pipeline's primary focus would be making the effective transfer of knowledge from the source domain, which is the historical data with the current situation of COVID-19.

6.1.2 *Transfer Learning (TL) and Its Capabilities for Pandemic Management*

The capability of transfer learning is an ability that is leveraged from the way the human brain operates. We learn from the tasks that we carry out and develop the intuition for performing similar tasks. Transfer learning builds on the limited ability of conventional machine learning, where learning of pattern happens with the focus of solving specific tasks in hand. There is a need to revalidate the pattern studied when the data feature space distributions change in these cases. Article [9] provides comprehensive coverage of transfer learning and its real-world applications. We look for leveraging the TL approach's critical characteristics to build into the ensemble architecture discussed here. Transfer learning is also a good leap towards the thought process of artificial general intelligence (Fig. 6.3).

In the case of traditional machine learning, it boils down to learned weights to capture patterns. However, in the case of TL, features and knowledge from previous learning will be leveraged into new scenarios and domain. This will be of interest to encapsulate all the learnings gathered in other pandemic experiences in COVID-19. TL also enables faster learning without dependencies on a large amount of data for learning. This will be a great advantage to use every learning that we add on as we go forwards in handling the virus. This also fits in well in the proposed ensemble architecture, as the proposal is to integrate the models from various specialities that work with a variety of data. In work [10], the author focuses on categorizing and reviewing TL's progress for clustering, regression, and classification problems. They also provide a comparison of multi-task learning and domain adaptation. TL's potential issues are also highlighted, which will provide useful insights into improvements that can enhance TL architecture's performance.

In work [10], the definition of transfer learning is defined as follows: for a domain, '*D*,' defined as two-element-base tuples 'χ', and P(*X*), which is a marginal

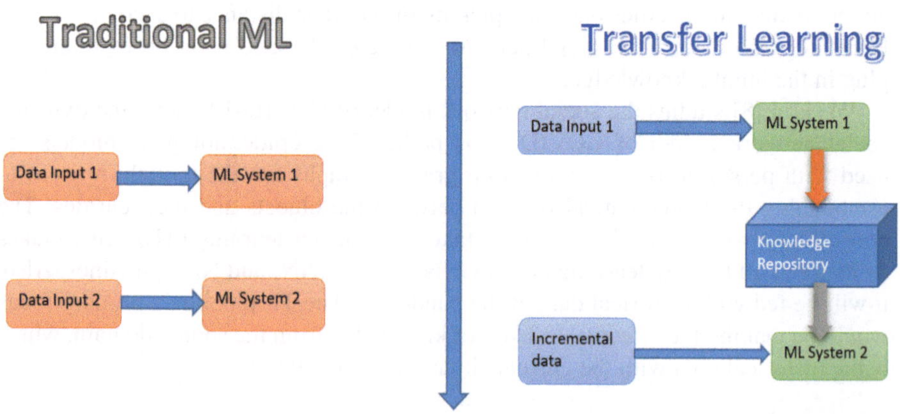

Fig. 6.3 Traditional learning and transfer learning

probability, with 'X' as sample data, the domain can be represented as $D = \{\chi, \mathrm{P}(X)\}$.

Domain will have two components, feature space 'χ' and marginal distribution $\mathrm{P}(X)$, $X = \{x_1, \ldots, x_n\}, x_i - \chi$.

'X_i', is the specific vector, task 'T' will be the two-element tuple for 'γ' label space, and 'η' is objective function. From the probabilistic view, the objective function can be depicted as $\mathrm{P}(\gamma|X)$.

For a domain D, task T is defined as

$$T = \{\gamma, \mathrm{P}(Y|X)\} = \{\gamma, \eta\}$$

$$Y = \{y_1, \ldots, y_n\}, y_i - \gamma$$

A predictive function 'η', learned from feature vector $(x_i, y_i), x_i - \chi, y_i - \gamma$. For each feature vector for the domain, 'η' predicts a label for each, $\eta(x_i) = y_i$.

One of TL's essential aspects is to decide upon which part of the knowledge from the previous domain must be taken forwards in the new domain. Similarly, there is a need to study the historical pandemics, more so with viruses that belong to the same family, and figure out what aspects of this historical information are relevant to be carried forwards to the context of COVID-19. This is important to ensure that the performance of the model is at its best. All available historical knowledge may not be of significance for the latest context, and just plugging in all available knowledge may lead to negative learning and will not help. Correlation needs to be established with the new virus and earlier ones and then pick a crucial part of authentic learning to be plugged into the latest studies (Fig. 6.4).

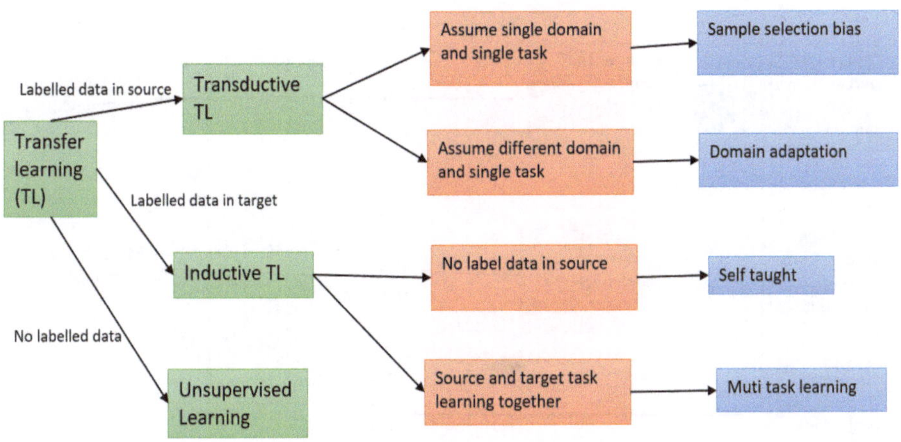

Fig. 6.4 Transfer learning formats

In the case of inductive learning, there is the possibility of extending the learning between the same family classes. Viruses of the corona family can be considered here. Through inductive learning, the source-target task of COVID-19 can be improved. In the case of the historical class of virus which does not have the required classification of information, the knowledge of that class can be extended to the study of the target class which is present, through unsupervised TL. Transductive TL can be leveraged to use the knowledge from other unrelated classes of the virus, where useful labelled data is available. With these three focus areas, layers of knowledge can be built between historical data and current scenarios (Fig. 6.5).

In the selective transfer for critical aspects of the source domain, which is historical knowledge with the target domain, COVID-19, TL's inductive learning aspect is adopted. AdaBoost is an approach that fits well here. Both target and source domains can be learned to balance the missing aspects in both and balance one another in a combination of supervised, semi-supervised, and unsupervised learning.

6.1.3 Deep Transfer Learning for Pandemic

In work [11], authors propose the detection of COVID-19-associated pneumonia with generative adversarial network (GAN) and fine-tuning the deep TL model with chest X-ray data as the virus leads to pneumonia that infects the lungs of humans. So, an X-ray of the chests is subject to study with GAN with deep TL. In this study, solution robustness with GAN helps avoid overfitting problem and generating images from available datasets. Standard and pneumonia X-rays form the dataset. GoogLeNet, AlexNet, SqueezeNet, and ResNet-18 are employed as deep TL architecture in this study. Careful attention is put in to balance the architecture's

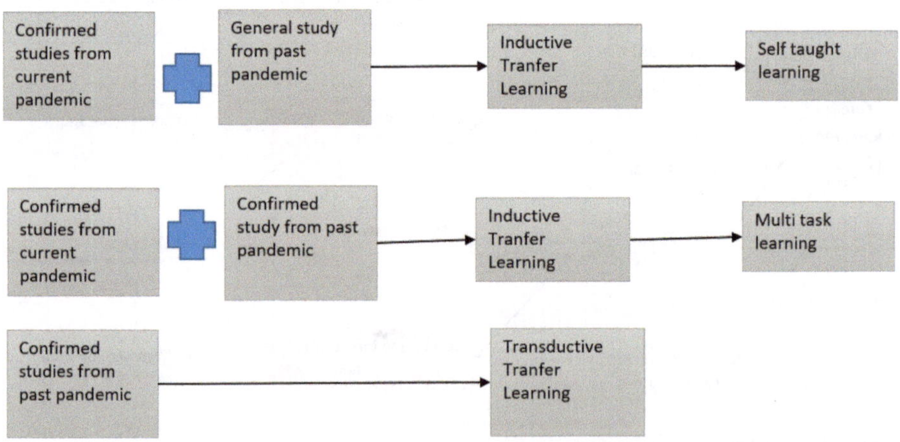

Fig. 6.5 Transfer learning methods in the context of COVID-19

complexity and make it optimal in consumed memory. Authors propose ResNet-18 to be the optimal deep TL model based on testing accuracy and performance on precision, recall, and F1 score, where GAN played the role of image augmenter (Fig. 6.6).

Pre-trained data models can work as feature extractors for source domain, and customized networks can be built on top of this to adapt to the need of the target domain, in this case COVID-19 (Fig. 6.7).

The critical thought process is to use the source domain weights learned to extract features from the target domain and not modify the source domain's weights. It is essential to do white-box modelling where the focus is to see the influence of various characteristics of the other viruses historically from the source domain. It will become essential to pay attention to every step in the architecture and see how the prediction evolves. Deep learning architectures offer high flexibility in terms of

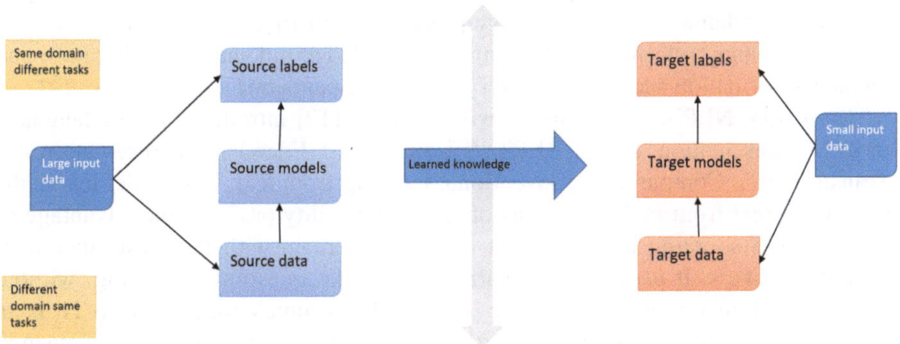

Fig. 6.6 Deep transfer learning

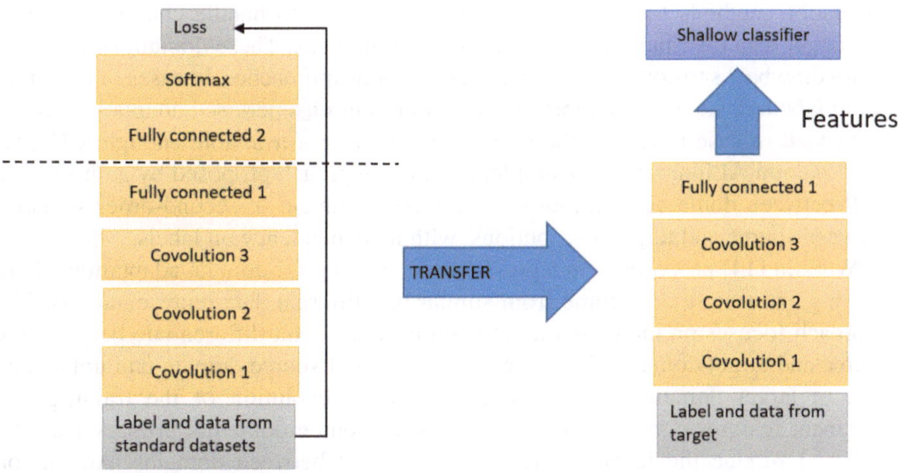

Fig. 6.7 Pre-trained deep transfer learning acting as a feature extractor

the layers and hyper-parameters that can be tuned to customize them. It becomes possible to fine-tune these architectures. As per the characteristics of the deep learning architectures, they tend to learn simpler patterns in the data as they begin to dig deeper into the architectures' layers, and patterns identified to become more domain-specific of task-specific. This helps to visualize the importance of various aspects of the source domain and customize the target domain. These capabilities also will contribute to strengthening the effort towards research on vaccines, and the source domain knowledge can be dug deep for further study. Another prominent aspect of deep TL uses parameters like freezing and fine-tuning the network based on the need. Based on the extent to which the labels are available in the target domain, we may more freely fine-tune the layers where the weights get updated in the backpropagation. However, if the target domain labels are limited, we will freeze the layers so that their weights do not get updated in the backpropagation. Computer vision and NLP being the top focus areas for deep learning find multiple pre-trained models that are open-sourced by the community and can be leveraged to study a pandemic. Natural language processing (NLP)-based pre-trained models can play a handy role in consolidating the knowledge hidden in the literature and the new information accumulated every day on the pandemic.

To explore NLP's advancement, work done in [12] introduces a new language model representation called BERT (Bi-directional Encoder Representation for Transformers). Compared to conventional learning from text, this model learns the unlabelled text from both directions of text. This ability provides the advantage of utilizing and adopting this model in the target domain with the least amount of change in layers. It uses them in various tasks like question answering, without major re-architecting needed specific to tasks. The primary focus in deep TL is an adaptation of the domains between the source and target domains. Work on pushing the architecture to learn what is essential is a critical differentiating fact that can add much value which is expedited learning on target. In work [13], the author's domain adaptation methods focus on the machines' inability to handle change in source and target data distribution compared to that of humans. These domain shifts cause major drawbacks to conventional machine learning approaches. In cases of the target being labelled, supervised approaches do well, but unsupervised adaptation would be needed in case labels on the target domain are not available enough. CORAL (CORelation ALignment) is a simple, practical approach proposed by authors. The shift between domains is minimized with the alignment of second-order statistics between source and target distributions, with no dependency on labels.

Work in [14] proposes new representation learning for domain adaptation where training and testing data come from similar but different data representations. The approach focuses on the bank on the features that do not differentiate between the source and target domains. Here the labelled data of source domain and unlabelled data of target domain are considered. With the evolution of the training, the dominant features come to the forefront as the source domain's primary learning task and subdue the facts that represent the shift between domains. Adaptation characteristics are achieved with a feedforward model that is combined with gradient reversal layers. Standard backpropagation and stochastic gradient methods are used to train this setup. Image classification and document sentiment analysis tasks are chosen here for demonstration (Fig. 6.8).

Deep learning has always faced data availability challenges; in that light, one-shot learning is a great approach. In work [15], authors propose one-shot learning for object categories. With the challenge of learning from a visual-based domain needing hundreds of data points in the form of images, this approach demonstrates the possibility of using a few images to learn. The idea is to avoid work from scratch but leverage the knowledge from past occurrences. Object categories are represented as probabilistic models to represent the Bayesian implementation. Using prior knowledge of the subject, the probability density function is established on these parameters. Multiple observations prior are updated to obtain the posterior model for the object category. Models learned from maximum a posterior (MAP) and maximum likelihood (ML) methods are compared with Bayesian models learned from this approach proposed by authors. With few data samples, the Bayesian approach seems to exceedingly well recognize hundreds of categories compared to other approaches which are struggling. Zero-shot learning takes it to the next level, which will have on top of the standard input '*X*' and output '*y*', a random variable that explains the task and makes necessary training adjustments itself when it looks at unseen data. Machine translation is an appropriate scenario where zero-shot learning can fair well. This is of interest to expedite the learning in situations of a critical pandemic, where every bit of knowledge gathered daily has to be conceived to build the knowledge on an ongoing basis.

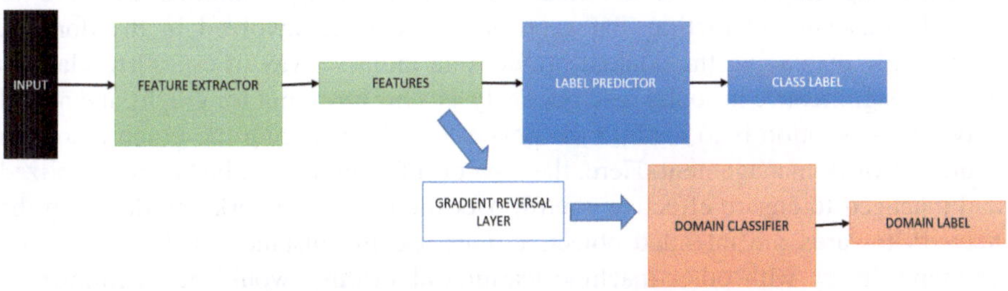

Fig. 6.8 Architecture proposed in work [14]. An in-depth feature extractor and profound label predictor compose the forward feed network of the architecture. The domain classifier provides the unsupervised adaptation to the domain. Backpropagation-based training is done with a feature extractor connected to a gradient reversal layer, multiplying with some negative constant in the process. The rest of the training process is standard, with domain classification loss optimized in all samples and prediction loss optimized in source examples. Domain-invariant features are ensured with domain classifier by gradient reversal, where feature distribution of the two domains involved is maintained similarly. Multi-task learning makes learning between source and targets a random learning approach, where there is no segregation or sequence involved in learning. All the tasks involved between the source and target are exposed for the learners

6.1.3.1 Challenges to Tackle in Transfer Learning (TL) from a Pandemic Management Perspective

Managing the organization of when to transfer the knowledge is a key focus area that can play a significant role in deciding the success of the approach. Negative transfer is another critical focus area which leads to the degradation of the performance if the knowledge transferred is not appropriate. This may lead to degradation of the performance, instead of improvement. These can occur because relevant connections between the source and target are not established, or relevant tasks between the source and target are not connected. Bayesian approaches are explored to tackle some of these issues. Another critical aspect of TL is to make sure that quantification is possible in case of transfer learning. This gives an excellent opportunity to explore in-depth the relationship between source and target domains.

6.1.4 Graph Theory for Social Network Analysis for COVID-19

Graph theory finds its applications in airline networks, physician networks, and supply chain networks. In a physician network, doctors would be the vertices, with specialities, demographics, and patient volumes being some of the vertex attributes. Patients will be the edges in the graph connecting the physicians, and edges carry the history of the diagnosis, visit frequencies, and other information related to patients. The graph plays a significant role in providing a summarized view of the relations and interactions between various entities involved in the domain. Graphically displaying the content provides an intuitive way to establish relations and is of significance in social network analysis. One key input for graphs and neural network association is to explore the possibility of leveraging the graph theory in neural network management. Here, the flow of information can be better visualized and managed to ensure effective control over the neural network and directing the network towards the intended objective. One specific instance of the application of graph theory with other machine learning algorithms would be as follows. If there are scenarios of grouping the data in this pandemic management effort, then algorithms like K-means and graph theory can go hand in hand.

In case if any scenarios involved the optimization of the paths, then graphs are well suited. In general, there is an advantage associated with memory consumption as the data space is represented by graphs which are more efficient. In work [16], authors recognize the graph theory importance in science and technology. They highlight the possibility of depicting any situation with a graph. With the pandemic situation of COVID-19 and precautions, graph theory seems to play a significant role. The virus growth is mapped in different types of graphs, and the number of infected people over a period is accounted for. Some of the concepts in graph representation that can be handy for the pandemic study are as follows. Among all the possible node pairs, the shortest path length represents the average path length. This can help to understand the pace of movement in the network. This will be of interest in the case of virus spread. Graph traversal where a search is happening from node to node involves searching across breadth or depth, where breadth search focuses on being close to the primary node. In contrast, depth search intends to remain away, as much as possible, from the root node. These concepts will help track the infected individuals and extend secondary and tertiary contacts of the primary infected individual [17].

Centrality concepts of the graph assist in the identification of the most critical node in the graph. In the identification of centrality, there is a classification aspect involved. Centrality may be decided based on the number of edges connected to the node. Based on the shortest distance to another node, centrality may be decided. These centrality measures play a prominent role in pandemic management to assess the network's essential entities while we trace the pandemic contacts. Graph density is measured concerning the number of edges. These graph density measures will assist in planning the medical facilities, including the reservations of the beds, ICUs, ambulances, and other facilities. Graph randomization is another useful concept that will be handy. Here, metrics for the graphs are generated by building hypothetical graphs based on the graph that we have in hand. The similarity between the target graph and the source one that we generate for reference would be based on the number of nodes, density, or other metrics. Here, the reference graphs can be created, making use of the historical knowledge of the pandemic. This provides the opportunity to use the historical learnings of the pandemic in current scenarios. This will provide a good benchmark for the latest study of the pandemic as well. Some graph analysis tools that are available for graph computation and visualization make the inferencing process more effective.

6.1.5 Importance of Transparent AI for Effective Pandemic Management

The importance of the machine learning approaches to be transparent relates to traceability that can be established from the study of pandemics to derive differentiating facts when a new virus-like COVID-19 hits hard. As the algorithms bring in their sophisticated architecture for solving problems, understanding the prediction process gets affected. To ensure knowledge accumulation can be ensured in a pandemic situation, this aspect of AI becomes key. This becomes extremely critical as the domain that is dealt with here is that of healthcare. To explore the interpretability of AI systems, one technical aspect to consider that will play a vital role in the system's success is to assess all data aspects' influence on the AI system's decision. For example, suppose we pick up an image recognition problem. It is significant to assess if the trivial aspects in an image like the background of the image influence decision-making. This is important because scenarios where the training data may come from the same set of backgrounds lead to systems assuming that this image may always have the same setting, which may not hold good.

This aspect points to one of the essential considerations of accounting the distribution of the data in the ecosystem that they are coming from. Training data need to be carefully curated to ensure that the data represents all possible distribution in the ecosystem. That does more vigorous training to be possible, resulting in a robust AI system. With the challenge in pandemic management in handling the knowledge coming from unrelated domains of the virus, this becomes a significant part. Feature importance identification is another substantial part of a robust AI system in the pandemic management domain that we are talking about. Some of the techniques that help build interpretability into the AI systems are as follows (Fig. 6.9).

In the global surrogate model, simple, intermediate models are built to interpret the complex models' predictions. In case the random forest algorithms are involved in a complex multi-class decision-making process, a simple decision tree can be used as an intermediate model to interpret the random forest model's predictions to interpret the results. This provides a rough map to get a sense of what is happening in the process of complex model predictions.

LIME (local interpretable model-agnostic explanations) is a framework that helps determine the need for interpreting at the granular level of input data. In this approach, the data point of interest in the input domain is marked, and then fake data is generated around the target data point using standard data distributions. More weights are assigned for data points that are closer to the target data point. Now prediction model is built for these new data distributions. This model is used as a surrogate model for interpretation (Fig. 6.10).

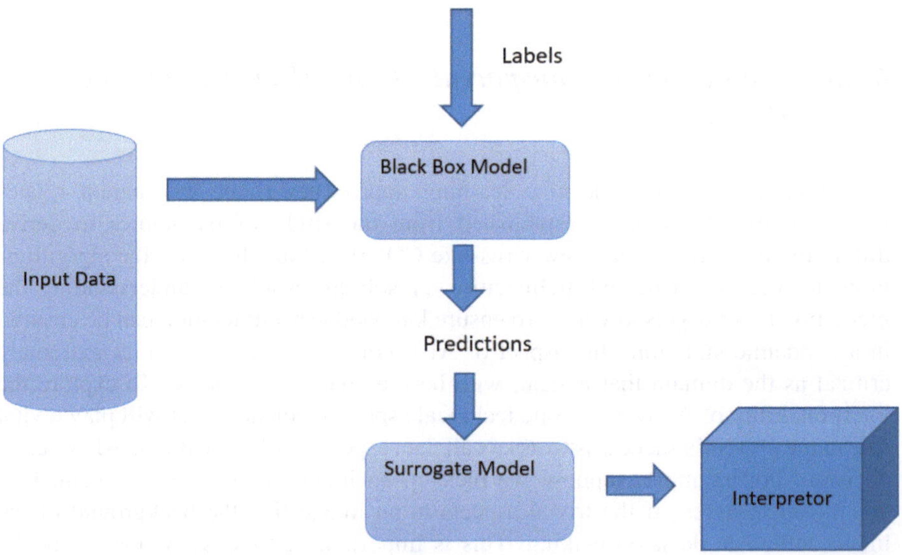

Fig. 6.9 Global surrogate model

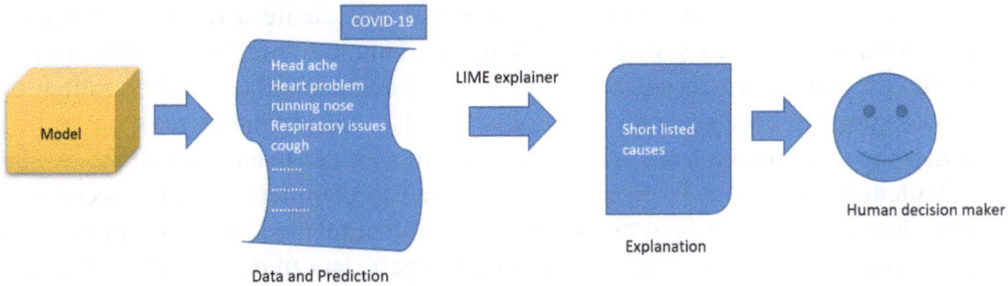

Fig. 6.10 LIME interpretation demonstration in case of virus identification. LIME explains individual prediction. The model predicts the outcome of the COVID-19 positive; the LIME model assists in shortlisting the key factors causing it. This provides interpretable outcomes of the model for the physician to make informed decisions

LIME models will help to work as intermediate to complex AI systems and humans to better interpretation. Complex AI system would identify the virus's characteristics by studying the symptoms of the virus in the affected individual and creating the library of characteristics of the symptoms by learning from the source domain. At the same time, the LIME interpretation model that fits in between will highlight the key characteristics of the library that are significant in the study. This scenario will be of prime importance to determine the plan for early identification of the symptoms so that the physician gets enough time to treat the affected person. Asymptotically affected cases have been a massive challenge in handling this pandemic, making this improvement scenario explored.

6.1.6 Building an Active Data Pipeline for Pandemic Management

As much as the algorithm itself, it becomes crucial to building an active data management pipeline for the effective modelling of the virus. Since multiple nations are involved, they needed to strike collaborative efforts between nations. Another challenging task would be to make sure the doctors and medical community are engaged in this effort. Since they are in mid-term action, saving lives and paying attention to the data pipeline would not be easy. Doctors cannot end up spending hours to get the documentation right. There is a need to think about effective systems that can facilitate this. This process is crucial to understand in real time what is the essential features in the data and make sure they are tracked effectively. As part of the data pipeline building, the data privacy part must be counted as well. However, sophisticated data protection systems are built; there are counter-approaches to deriving the patient's related information from the data by leveraging the people's available social data. This makes it a key challenge in building an active data pipeline for the study. Since the hospital end's data collection mechanism is a traditional system, leveraging those data for research purposes is challenging.

Though there is an effort to put them together and create a database, ensuring the information's accuracy will be challenging. This may need more commitment between the data research team and the medical team to strike good coordination to make sure the data accuracy is improved. Also added challenge is on putting together the information from across the globe in an inconsistent manner.

Challenges in these data pipelines also extend to complete traceable records of patient history and their final health state being documented. To ease out the data management part, it is not easy to get in an expert data management corporation due to many challenges involved concerning data privacy. All possible approaches to ease this data pipeline should explore smart natural language processing (NLP)-based system where doctors can record and upload to the database, possibly real-time data validation with the doctors to help improve data quality. Exploring the possibilities of engaging student doctors for managing the documentation part would be the right approach. The importance of these data is also in tracking essential medicines that are tried on patients and their evolution.

6.1.7 Deep Learning Models for Integrating Social Media and Epidemic Data

Infectious disease management across the globe is a critical aspect that needs focused attention. In these situations, understanding the virus and studying its evolution becomes a critical need. These are computational frameworks under epidemiology that provide the required framework, but they lack real-time monitoring abilities. On the other hand, the right amount of information is available on social media but will not provide a complete picture of how the network of virus spans out. In work [18], the author proposes a deep learning semi-supervised approach to bring social media mining techniques and epidemiology information together. The approach focuses on studying social media information for health and how they interact with each other. This information is modelled, taking into reference models associated with the disease and network of the contact. The approach has also attempted to feed in social media knowledge to an epidemic model built on computation to improve the model's efficiency built on controlling the disease. To achieve consistent integration of both aspects of the data, an optimization algorithm is proposed to ensure an interactive learning process and consistency in the integration. The approach has been said to demonstrate the ability to characterize, time-based, and space-based diffusion of the disease better than other models. One of the highlighting factors of this epidemic is its spread resulting from the increased local and global travelling. The rapid spread of the virus in a short period also adds to the concern. The root action to this situation lies in understanding the characteristics of the virus and studying its evolutionary pattern. Recent trends have said to contribute to both social data mining and computational epidemiology. The individual-based epidemiology network is proposed in computational epidemiology where time and space influence are epidemic spread is accounted for. The study starts with the personal impact of the epidemic and then extends up to how various actions have influenced the epidemic's control. Network-based models are simulated with high-performance simulation abilities related to epidemics. These simulation results help forecast the evolution of epidemic that can also help forecast the spread of disease, peak time associated with the spread, and how practical the prevention measures are. Some of the limitations of computational epidemiology are lack of spatial data that is fine-grained and eligible for surveillance and model tuning.

There is a dependency on the data received from the Centers for Disease Control and Prevention (CDC) to estimate model parameters [19]. However, there is no granularity of the CDC's data at the state level, and the data is not enough for disease diffusion within a state. Real-time detection of dynamic networking of the contact is another challenge. There is a significant influence of actions such as closing the school, medications given on the infection level, and spreading viruses that change the network structure. Real-time updating of the network with the ongoing changes is a critical challenge that needs attention. The cost of real-time training with real-time data is high. Mostly, the existing approach relies on batch training with the CDC data. The limitation of CDC data is updated once a week, making it tough for real-time updates. Social media data provides a better supply of data and a timely one from the socially located sensors [20]. Data based on social media provide detailed health information and disease surveillance at the aggregate level. Social media users are reporting the disease's self-symptoms to help in aggregating the trend and looking at possible outbreaks. There will be a twofold focus: one trying to highlight the current spread and the other forecasting the possible breakout in the future. Another part of the focus is to model social media data to assess health behaviour and disease informatics.

Social media data would suffer from a granular view of real-time contact information to establish a network that will facilitate diffusion of the disease based on its pattern. Just depending on the user location to assess the social contact network would not be enough. Visualizing the complete demography would not be possible as the restriction is towards social users' health information. Limitation continues in terms of data used which is restrictive to the disease level and not to the extent of deriving knowledge from the disease model. With limitations of their own in computational epidemiology data and social media data, in work [18], the author put the approach to make use of both sources of data with a deep learning framework called SocIal Media Nested Epidemic SimulaTion (SimNest) (Fig. 6.11).

The framework focuses on deriving insights from social media based on interventions utilizing deep learning. In the case of unsupervised learning, it facilitates disease model understanding from computational epidemiology. So, the disease model from epidemiology will in case be fed with granular data from social media feed that optimizes the disease parameters. This establishes the iteration between both sources of data to build an integrated model. A semi-supervised multilayer perceptron is involved in the framework, which focuses on mining epidemic features. Epidemic disease progress model is used to derive the unsupervised pattern

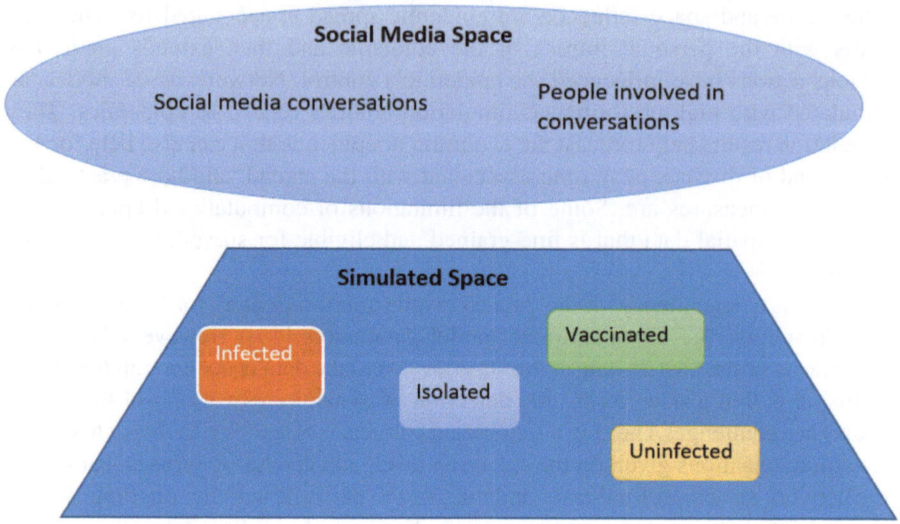

Fig. 6.11 SimNest framework from work [18]. Simulated space is the mirror of social media conversations among people. Based on the conversations, infection, isolation, and vaccination are mapped. Demography-based contact information is used to establish network connections in the simulated world

from epidemic disease and later subjected to supervised classification. The sparsity of labelled data is managed with a semi-supervised approach. Online learning is employed to ensure the gap between the social media world and the simulated world is minimized—the algorithm focuses on injecting real-time data into the model and reduces the cost of retraining.

Historically, computational epidemiology has been utilized to study the clustered data of population based on the health state of people and demography. Differential equations have been used to model these data [21, 22]. In terms of supporting network epidemiology, an individual computational model is used to study stochastic propagation of the epidemic in people's network. Random models of people interactions are a common approach in network epidemiology [23, 24]. Network epidemiology has also attempted to represent people networks and attempt to simulate individual-based data to assess the epidemic spread network. Individual-based attributes are built into this model, like social, geographical, and other attributes that create a population's synthetic simulation model close to the real population. This model is regularly updated based on daily activities and its location to build a social contact network for the population [25]. This individual-based epidemic spread model helps in assessing the spread of who infected who and time of the same [26]. Apart from this disease model and synthetic network, individual-based epidemic models are also composed of individual intervention and public health information like vaccination and medication and other aspects like social distancing. Network node or edge properties are modified by this intervention that's done as precautions. Epidemic knowledge mining approaches have considered social media sources of data like focusing on disease surveillance data that is rolled up. Approaches in [27] have highlighted the reliability of social media feed data regarding how people feel about their help. Generally, the disease information is not explicit from people unless diagnosed by experts. Health information semantic analysis is another source of reference. Here, the social message's intent is used to assess public health scenarios, interventions that are tried out, and other health behaviour. The topic model proposed by Biswas et al. [28] considered the symptoms of the ailment and possible treatments and then assessed the geographical patterns of such health issues. Classification of social tweets was proposed by Barrett et al. [29], where user behaviour is accounted for. In work [30], accurate geographical locations were explored for the outbreak. The health condition of Twitter users was assessed based on user interaction by the work of Krieck et al. [31]. Individuals' disease progression tracking was a different dimension of exploration in the work of [20].

6.1.8 Importance of Secured E-Health in a Pandemic Situation

E-health systems will play a prominent role in the pandemic situation like that of COVID-19. It will be essential to make sure that the information is disseminated quickly and all the knowledge is plugged in for better management. It is essential to ensure that E-health's entire ecosystem is built with patients as the focus centre. E-health systems need to consider data collection mechanisms, data transfer mechanisms, and decision-making systems. With all these, as focus security of the E-health systems is a vital one that needs attention. The primary driver for the E-health systems is to optimize the cost of healthcare services. With the associated benefits, E-health suffers the security concern of the data handled. The security concerns' primary theme revolves around data privacy, authentication of the right user, and integrity. Biometric has been the solution to account for security and works better than traditional approaches. Work in this focuses on addressing privacy and security issues with the biometric technology-enabled E-health. Biometrics provides a reliable solution if other aspects, like patient privacy of using biometrics, processing time, and complexity of the process, are taken care of. Singh et al. [32] focuses on building an encryption technique that is lighter but is strong to manage large data transferred on the network.

E-health facilitates easy access to patient's information where efficiency and cost are improved. With limited time between patients and physicians, an efficient information system would be an excellent facilitator. Securing E-health application and their components is the key focus, focusing on user authentication and authorization. Traditional authorization methods are not user friendly from various perspectives, including managing the credentials. Fingerprint, face, voice, and signature are explored to strengthen biometric capabilities. Deep learning techniques can be employed to make biometric more efficient, to make sure that the system does not depend on the database being created for the user. One-shot learning kind of advanced techniques is explored to perform on the fly learning. Voice and face authentication are done as a comprehensive solution. Biometric features are difficult to be reproduced and make it a healthy control. Health data encryption is an important area to be considered as E-health systems are built. Biometric systems have enrolment and recognition as their key phrases. As a system, it will comprise pattern identification with sensors, extracting the feature, creating a database, and running the comparison. Based on the scenario in which the application fits in, there is a need to decide on an identification and authentication approach.

Unimodal or multimodal features of the users are used to figure out the right users. Evaluation of identifying approach is based on the parameters like trait chosen to be constant over time, uniqueness of the feature, quantification possibility of the feature, people accepting the system, the strength of the system to face hacking, and so on. A similarity score is generated to identify the identity. False non-match rate (FNMR) and false match rate (FMR) are necessary biometric system accuracy measures. These are sources of error from the system where FNMR is the wrong declaration of the correct user as the wrong one. FMR is the wrong identification of the identity resulting in fake identities getting access to the system. Failure to capture, failure to acquire, and failure to enrol are the other possibilities of system failure. Failure to acquire is the deficiency of the biometric system to capture the input.

There would be cases where there are difficulties in enrolling the user. Receiver Operating Characteristic (ROC) curve helps to depict the trade-off between FMR and FNMR. Detection error tradeoff (DET) is also a mechanism for measurement [33]. ROC is the accuracy of the system in the test environment. Equal error rate (EER), which is the point in the curve of DET where FMR and FNMR are equal, provides a measure for the biometric system's performance. The lowest value of EER is expected for an effective biometric system. E-health has expanded as telemedicine, which is about providing healthcare delivery systems using information technology and telecommunication. Electronic health record systems storing patient's information are an E-health system. Customer medical needs are assessed based on consumer health information. The health knowledge management system also has a significant role to play. Medical decision-making systems play a vital role and assist the physician—M-health with mobiles involved in various healthcare support. Digitization of the data is a common theme for all these systems, so E-health stands for digital health management systems in place of a paper-based system (Fig. 6.12).

In this biometric technology-based E-health system architecture, level 1 has all devices that assist in data transmission across various parties involved in the transaction. Sensors, mobile devices, and computers form part of this. In level 2, primary communication architecture is hosted that establishes a connection between level 1 and level 2. Telemedicine, healthcare information storage, and healthcare provision are involved in level 3. Levels 1 and 3 are devised to be authenticated with biometrics of physicians or patients. Enhancing the knowledge of the consumers and medical care individuals is one of the critical objectives. This objective also facilitates consumers to develop their knowledge to manage primary

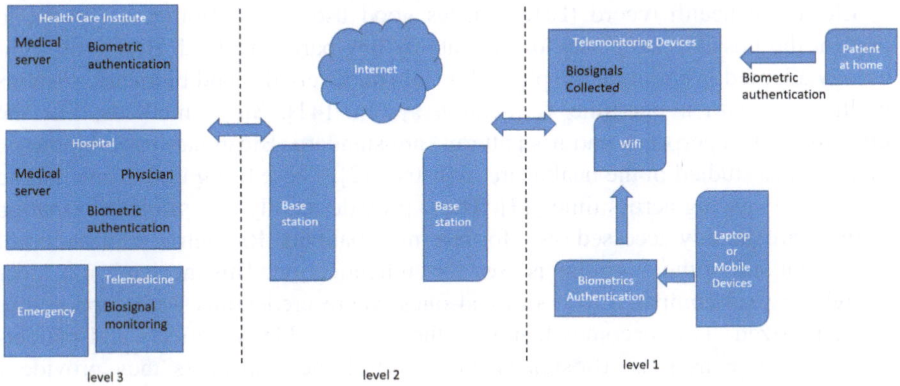

Fig. 6.12 Biometric technology-based E-health system architecture

health conditions. There is a broader focus on moving from a provider-driven system to a patient-centric system. This is a significant change in mindset that will increase people's confidence in the healthcare system and play a significant role, particularly during a pandemic like COVID-19 [14]. With tremendous pressure on both consumers and providers during this pandemic, such a robust system stronger from all dimensions will make a significant difference. Studies taken on various E-health systems have provided knowledge on the system architecture of the system. The most common theme is the three-layer architecture presented [34, 35]: the first layer for devices to collect the information, the second layer of the network that transfers data from patients to the interested parties' databases, and the third layer about the systems for intelligent decision-making. Network layer architecture is presented in the work by Samanta et al. and Brennan et al. [36, 37].

6.1.8.1 Security Challenges

Since the information is stored and moved in digital format, it attracts security vulnerabilities. Information is seen in storage, transmit, and processing stages. The data's confidentiality is impacted as the data gets moved by medical fraternity with the information network systems' confidence. Any instance of the confidentiality breach will impact the patient's privacy. That calls for effective access control for the data processing systems. Password-based smart cards are a traditional method that is vulnerable and not user friendly [38, 39]. Wireless sensor network (WSN) strives to protect the patient's data from securing communication across biosensors. Within this network, there is a need for more robust controls for ensuring the security of confidentiality, integrity, and privacy of the data. Encryption has a prominent role in protecting transmitted data. However, key generation and key distribution requirements make it hard as resources constrain the biosensors [40].

Electronic health record (EHR) makes good use of the biometric system, to prevent the possible tampering of the data by any party involved. Biometric technology adopted is based on the physiological characteristics and biometric systems multimodal with a one-time verification system [41]. Static methods, like the utilization of fingerprints and iris patterns, are standard. Biosignal-based biometric modules are studied in the healthcare industry [42]. These bring in dynamic nature as they are varying across time [43]. These provide readily accessible information as these are already accessed once for returning patients. Biometric information of the patient and of the physician is used for authentication. This mechanism is more straightforward compared to traditional ones where credentials were supposed to be memorized. This becomes handy in the case of elderly patients and patients who are not conscious. Biosignals are a useful mechanism as they provide a seamless experience to the user without intervening in the user's regular activity [44–46]. Systems like photoplethysmography (PPG), electrocardiogram (ECG), and electroencephalography (EEG) are the popular biosignal systems. Wireless secure communication with biometric encryption on the sensors is seen in wireless body sensor networks (BSNs). BSN specializes with the sensors that are worn on the human body. BSN helps monitor health conditions, enhance memory, access medical data, and communicate in case of emergencies [47].

Health information is protected with encrypted access to sensitive information. The generation of cryptographic keys is the crucial aspect of biometric cryptography. Authentication key generation and wireless communication of the data are ensured by biometrics. With randomness and time variation characteristics, key generation makes sense in biometrics where dynamic traits are considered [48]. In work], authors propose encryption and authentication combined biometric solutions for wireless communication in BSNs. Secure communication is ensured in case of work for BSN; here ECG or PPG kinds of physiological features are employed to generate the cryptographic keys that get communication within the network. Fast Fourier Transform (FFT) is employed for feature extraction like interpulse interval (IPI) from PPG and ECG, frequency domain, or time domain. The quality of keys that are generated is essential to ensure cryptosystems are secure [49].

Distinctiveness and randomness decide the quality of the keys generated. The distinction between the people is covered by distinctiveness, measured with FAR, hamming distance (HD), and FRR. Making unique keys unpredictable is the role of randomness. The entropy of the generated keys decides the randomness [50].

6.1.8.2 Future Vision

E-health security issues are tackled well by the biometric system. Besides providing identity management, encryption is provided to ensure the secure transfer of the information across the pipeline of exchange [51, 52]. Data modification and eavesdropping kind of attack can be managed by protecting health information with biometric encryption. Biometrics promises to tackle several issues faced by the healthcare industry in the midst of technological evolution. Efficiency and robustness of the biometric system are crucial features. Even with these possibilities, there are potential areas that must be improved around authentication, attracting security attacks. Biometric templates can be compromised, leading to security attackers manipulating the templates and replaying the attacks. Since the biometric templates are linked to an individual, it will not be possible to reverse the manipulation. This will need a biometric system that can be cancelled. Time taken for identification and verification needs a closer focus for further improvement [53]. Multiple biometric processes like noise removal, feature extraction, feature matching, enhancement, and classification are managed in a time-optimal way.

Data encryption plays a significant role in transforming institution-based healthcare into home healthcare with telemedicine and mobile health, with a wireless communication approach leveraged. Biometric systems' speciality in encryption and decryption of the information plays a significant role, with crucial generation playing a vital role in cryptographic systems. Wireless communication networks have challenges in the generation and distribution of keys [54]. These needs focused attention and research. Keeping older adults in mind while devising these biometric systems is a scope of further exploration. In work, authors have focused upon the importance of E-health in the healthcare industry and exploring the challenges that need focused research. Focus is drawn upon patient privacy data security in E-health. All the drawbacks in the conventional system are focused on being addressed. Unimodal to multimodal biometric range of systems is proposed as part of E-health applications [55]. Biometric technology is explored to secure wireless sensor networks with continuous and unobtrusive authentication methods. ECG, EEG [56], and PPG biosignals that gather unconventional biometrics provide a new direction for technological adoption in the E-health domain. Specific areas like biometric database protection and processing time involved should be focused on.

6.2 Conclusion

With the technology evolving rapidly, so is the situation of a pandemic caused by a deadly virus. Based on the experience gained over the last few decades, it is essential to invest regularly in a well-planned effort to learn these pandemics and tackle them effectively in a short period. Exploration of artificial intelligence (AI) in the field of medicine was presented in this chapter. There is greater collaboration between the healthcare industry and the technology industry. Exploring the possibility of bringing critical concepts of deep learning together in an ensemble model approach to utilize these models' best aspects is proposed. With revolutions taking place in transfer learning, it finds its place as a good fit for making use of all the knowledge gathered every time a pandemic hits the world. Social network analysis plays a significant role in the pandemic management situation; graph theory highlights its significance. AI solutions have been striving to make themselves more explicit and transparent; this thought process can be handy when struggling with a complex domain like that of the COVID-19. The ability to break into the data analysis patterns helps to device the solutions faster and effectively.

With a large amount of data that is spread across the globe, it is essential to build a robust data pipeline that can put all the useful information together and conduct a relevant exploration to build intelligence against the pandemic. The discussion is extended to put together the past knowledge of the pandemic and real-time data generated on social media. Putting social media data into meaningful use can be achieved with this thought process. E-health system's role in these uncertain times is highlighted from building confidence among the people. The demand for healthcare exponentially growing in these pandemic times builds tremendous pressure to respond to the need. Automating all possible elements of the healthcare system can play a prominent role in this demand management need. As the demand is addressed, healthcare systems cannot compromise people's data security and privacy. So, this is a tricky scenario to balance all dimensions of the people's needs.

References

1. A.S. Ahuja, C.E. Schmidt, The impact of artificial intelligence in medicine on the future role of the physician, Ahuja, Distributed under Creative Commons CC-BY 4.0 (2019)
2. B. King Jr., Artificial intelligence and radiology: What will the future hold? J. Am. Coll. Radiol. **15**(3 Part B), 501503 (2018). https://doi.org/10.1016/j.jacr.2017.11.017
3. A. Norman, Your future doctor may not be human. This is the rise of AI in medicine (2018), https://futurism.com/ai-medicine-doctor. Accessed Jan 2018
4. T. Ozturk, M. Talo, E.A. Yildirim, U.B. Baloglu, O. Yildirim, U.R. Acharya, Automated detection of COVID-19 cases using deep neural networks with X-ray images. Comput Biol Med **121**, 103792 (2020). https://doi.org/10.1016/j.compbiomed.2020.103792
5. A. Tomar, N. Gupta, Prediction for the spread of COVID-19 in India and effectiveness of preventive measures. Sci. Total Environ. **728**, 138762 (2020)
6. V. Nguyen, M. Rybinski, S. Karimi, Z. Xing, *Searching Scientific Literature for Answers on COVID-19 Questions, 1CSIRO Data, Sydney, Australia* (The Australian National University, Canberra, Australia)
7. Y. Pathaka, P.K. Shukla, A. Tiwari, S. Stalin, S. Singhe, K. Shukla, Deep transfer learning based classification model for COVID-19 disease. Ing. Rech. Biomed. (2020). https://doi.org/10.1016/j.irbm.2020.05.003
8. A. Karaivanov, A social network model of COVID-19. PLoS One **15**(10), e0240878 (2020). https://doi.org/10.1371/journal.pone.0240878
9. Dipanjan (DJ) Sarkar, A comprehensive hands-on guide to transfer learning with real-world applications in deep learning; Deep learning on steroids with the power of knowledge transfer!, https://towardsdatascience.com/a-comprehensive-hands-on-guide-to-transfer-learning-with-real-world-applications-in-deep-learning-212bf3b2f27a
10. S.J. Pan, Q. Yang, A survey on transfer learning, IEEE Transactions on Knowledge and Data Engineering, https://www.cse.ust.hk/~qyang/Docs/2009/tkde_transfer_learning.pdf
11. N.E.M. Khalifa, M.H.N. Taha, A.E. Hassanien, S. Elghamrawy, Detection of coronavirus (COVID-19) associated pneumonia based on generative adversarial networks and a fine-tuned deep transfer learning model using chest X-ray dataset, https://arxiv.org/abs/2004.01184
12. J. Devlin, M.-W. Chang, K. Lee, K. Toutanova, BERT: Pre-training of deep bidirectional transformers for language understanding
13. B. Sun, J. Feng, K. Saenko, Return of Frustratingly Easy Domain Adaptation, AAAI

14. S. Roy, M.M. Kanti, D. Samanta, Venkatanagaraju, Awareness with informatics on hypertension and effects on hemoglobin. Int. J. Adv. Sci. Technol. **29**(4), 423–433 (2020)
15. F.-F. Li, R. Fergus, P. Perona, One-shot learning of object categories. IEEE Trans. Pattern Anal. Mach. Intell. **28**(4), 594–611 (2006). https://doi.org/10.1109/TPAMI.2006.79
16. H.R. Bhapkar, P. Mahalle, P.S. Dhotre, Virus graph, and COVID-19 pandemic: A graph theory approach. Preprints **2020040507** (2020). https://doi.org/10.20944/preprints202004.0507.v1
17. L. Garg, E. Chukwu, N. Nidal, C. Chakraborty, G. Garg, Anonymity preserving IoT-based COVID-19 and other infectious disease contact tracing model. IEEE Access **8**, 159402–159414 (2020)
18. S.L. Zhao, J. Chen, F. Chen, W. Wang, C.-T. Lu, N. Ramakrishnan, SimNest: Social media nested epidemic simulation via online semi-supervised deep learning, in *2015 IEEE International Conference on Data Mining*, (IEEE, New York)
19. CDC, Fluview interactive. Accessed 31 May 2015
20. L. Chen, K.T. Hossain, P. Butler, N. Ramakrishnan, B.A. Prakash, Flu gone viral: Syndromic surveillance of flu on Twitter using temporal topic models, in *ICDM*, (IEEE, New York, 2014), pp. 2783–2789
21. J. D. Murray. Mathematical Biology I: An Introduction, vol. 17 of Interdisciplinary Applied Mathematics, 2002
22. E. Vynnycky, R.G. White, *An Introduction to Infectious Disease Modelling* (Oxford University Press, Oxford, 2010)
23. M.E. Craft, E. Volz, C. Packer, L.A. Meyers, Disease transmission in territorial populations: The small-world network of Serengeti lions. J. R. Soc. Interface **8**(59), 776–786 (2011)
24. C. Groendyke, D. Welch, D.R. Hunter, A network-based analysis of the 1861 hagelloch measles data. Biometrics **68**(3), 755–765 (2012)
25. R.R. Althar, D. Samanta, Building intelligent integrated development environment for IoT in the context of statistical modeling for software source code, in *Multimedia Technologies in the Internet of Things Environment*, Studies in Big Data, ed. by R. Kumar, R. Sharma, P. K. Pattnaik, vol. 79, (Springer, Singapore, 2022). https://doi.org/10.1007/978-981-15-7965-3_7
26. A. Guha, D. Samanta, Real-time application of document classification based on machine learning, in *Proceedings of the 1st International Conference on Information, Communication and Computing Technology*, (Springer, Istanbul, Turkey, 2020), pp. 366–379. https://doi.org/10.1007/978-3-030-38501-9_37
27. A. Guha, D. Samanta, Hybrid approach to document anomaly detection: An application to facilitate RPA in title insurance. Int. J. Autom. Comput. (2020). https://doi.org/10.1007/s11633-020-1247-y
28. J. Biswas, J.V. Kureethara, D. Samanta, M. Sandhya, Efficient algorithm for people management in an elevator, TEST Engineering & Management, 83 (2020) ISSN: 0193-4120
29. C. Barrett, R. Beckman, M. Khan, V. Kumar, M. Marathe, P. Stretz, T. Dutta, B. Lewis, Generation and analysis of large synthetic social contact networks, in *WSC*, (2009), pp. 1003–1014
30. K. Bisset, J. Chen, X. Feng, V.S.A. Kumar, M. Marathe, Epifast: A fast algorithm for large scale realistic epidemic simulations on distributed memory systems, in *ICS*, (2009), pp. 430–439
31. M. Krieck, J. Dreesman, L. Otrusina, K. Denecke, A new age of public health: Identifying disease outbreaks by analyzing tweets, in *WebSci*, (2011)
32. R.K. Singh, T. Begum, L. Borah, D. Samanta, Text encryption: Character jumbling, in *Proc. of IEEE International Conference on Inventive Systems and Control, 19–20 Jan 2017, Coimbatore*, (IEEE, New York, 2017) 978-1-5090-4715-4
33. N. Collier, N.T. Son, N.M. Nguyen, Omg u got flu? Analysis of shared health messages for bio-surveillance. J. Biomed. Semant. **2**(S-5), S9 (2011)
34. M. Dredze, M.J. Paul, S. Bergsma, H. Tran, Carmen: A Twitter geolocation system with applications to public health, in *AAAI Workshop on Expanding the Boundaries of HIAI*, (Citeseer, 2013), pp. 20–24

35. B. Thomas, P. Shwetha, P. Dey, J. Biswas, D. Samanta, An efficient and holistic approach to reduce output and dependent parameters for multi-output learning. Int. J. Adv. Sci. Technol. **29**(4), 25–33 (2020)
36. D. Samanta, M.G. Galety, M. Shivamurthaiah, S. Kariyappala. A hybridization approach based semantic approach to the software engineering, TEST Engineering & Management, 83 (2020). ISSN: 0193-4120
37. S. Brennan, A. Sadilek, H. Kautz, Towards understanding global spread of disease from everyday interpersonal interactions, in *IJCAI*, (AAAI Press, Palo Alto, CA, 2013), pp. 2783–2789
38. E. Okoh, A.I. Awad, Biometrics applications in e-Health security: A preliminary survey, in *Health Information Science. HIS 2015*, Lecture Notes in Computer Science, ed. by X. Yin, K. Ho, D. Zeng, U. Aickelin, R. Zhou, H. Wang, vol. 9085, (Springer, Cham, 2015). https://doi.org/10.1007/978-3-319-19156-0_10
39. A. Jain, L. Hong, S. Pankanti, Biometric identification. Commun. ACM **43**(2), 90–98 (2000)
40. S. Ahmed, M. Raja, Integration of wireless sensor network with medical service provider for ubiquitous e-healthcare, in *9th International Conference on High Capacity Optical Networks and Enabling Technologies (HONET)*, (2012), pp. 120–126
41. G. Bai, Y. Guo, A general architecture for developing a sustainable elderly care e-health system, in *8th International Conference on Service Systems and Service Management (ICSSSM)*, (IEEE, New York, 2011), pp. 1–6
42. K. Chatterjee, D. Samanta, J. Biswas, Enhancement of education with wearable computing device. CSI Commun. **43**(10) (2020) ISSN 0970-647X
43. Z. Anwar, S. Banerjee, N.G. Eapen, D. Samanta, A clinical study of hepatitis B. J. Crit. Rev. **6**(5), 81–84. https://doi.org/10.22159/jcr.06.05.13. E-ISSN: 2394-5125
44. S. Manral, D. Samanta, S.K. Podder, Effective classroom activities on accounting using double entry system: The productive consequences, TEST Engineering & Management, 83 (2020). ISSN: 0193-4120
45. A. Khamparia, P.K. Singh, P. Rani, D. Samanta, A. Khanna, B. Bhushan, An internet of health things driven deep learning framework for detection and classification of skin cancer using transfer learning. Trans. Emerg. Telecommun. Technol. (2020, 2020) ISSN: 2161-3915
46. R. Gurunath, D. Samanta, Studies on encrypted secret data storage techniques analogous to steganography. Int. J. Adv. Sci. Technol. **29**(2), 3705–3711 (2020)
47. V. Kureethara, J. Biswas, D. Samanta, N.G. Eapen, Balanced constrained partitioning of distinct objects. Int. J. Innov. Technol. Explor. Eng.. ISSN: 2278-3075 (Online)
48. D. Samanta, S.K. Podder, Level of green computing based management practices for digital revolution and new India. Int. J. Recent Technol. Eng. **8**(2) (2019) ISSN: 2277-3878
49. B. Mahua, S.K. Podder, R. Shalini, D. Samanta, Factors that influence sustainable education with respect to innovation and statistical science. Int. J. Recent Technol. Eng. **7**(5S2) (2019) ISSN: 2277-3878
50. B. Praveen, N. Umarani, T. Anand, D. Samanta, Cardinal digital image data fortification expending steganography. Int. J. Recent Technol. Eng. **7**(5S2) (2019) ISSN: 2277-3878
51. M.K. Manu, S. Roy, D. Samanta, Effects of liver cancer drugs on cellular energy metabolism in hepatocellular carcinoma cells. Int. J. Pharm. Res. **10**(3) (2018) ISSN: 0975-2366
52. H. Silva, A. Loureno, A. Fred, J. Filipe, Clinical data privacy and customization via biometrics based on ECG signals, in *Information Quality in e-Health*, Lecture Notes in Computer Science, ed. by A. Holzinger, K. M. Simonic, vol. 7058, (Springer, Berlin, 2011), pp. 121–132
53. G. Zhang, C.C.Y. Poon, Y. Zhang, A biometrics based security solution for encryption and authentication in tele-healthcare systems, in *2nd International Symposium on Applied Sciences in Biomedical and Communication Technologies ISABEL, 2009*, (2009), pp. 1–4
54. G. Zhang, C.C.Y. Poon, Y. Zhang, A fast critical generation method based on dynamic biometrics to secure wireless body sensor networks for p-health, in *2010 Annual International Conference of the IEEE Engineering in Medicine and Biology Society (EMBC)*, (2010), pp. 2034–2036

55. Y. Ganin et al., Domain-adversarial training of neural networks. J. Mach. Learn. Res. **17**(1), 2096–2030 (2016)
56. M.P. Orenda, L. Garg, G. Garg, Exploring the feasibility to authenticate users of Web and Cloud Services using a brain-computer Interface (BCI), in *ICIAP 2017 International Workshops*, Lecture Notes in Computer Science (LNCS), ed. by S. Battiato et al., vol. 10590, (2017), pp. 353–363. https://doi.org/10.1007/978-3-319-70742-6_33

Chapter 7
Personal Protective Equipment for COVID-19: A Comprehensive Review

Debangana Das, Shreya Nag, Hemanta Naskar, Srikanta Acharya, Sourav Bakchi, Sheikh Saharuk Ali, Runu Banerjee Roy, Bipan Tudu, and Rajib Bandyopadhyay

7.1 Introduction

Coronaviruses encompass a broad spectrum of virions that can permeate into host cells implicating pathogenesis. They are so named because of their appearance (akin to Sun's corona; in Latin, "corona" meaning crown or halo) under the electron microscope. Wuhan in Hubei province of China reported the first outbreak of COVID-19 pandemic in mid-December 2019. The outbreak of coronavirus disease, across various topographical regions, has influenced the structure of healthcare and administrative settings throughout the world. This has led to the undertaking of sincere obligation towards public health measures. As per Yu et al. [1], the virus responsible for the disease is SARS-CoV-2, named so because of its similarity to the severe acute respiratory syndrome (SARS) epidemic in China in 2002–2003. The reference diagnosis method used for COVID-19 is reverse transcription-polymerase chain reaction (RT-PCR). COVID-19 pandemic engulfed the mind of millions of people with stress and difficulties. The rumours and misinformation stimulate more stress and can disrupt our fight against COVID-19. The novel coronavirus has been unprecedented because it has affected more than 180 countries worldwide within a span of a few months. This can be primarily attributed to its transmission mode, primarily respiratory droplets (generally more than 5 μm in diameter) and sputum from infected persons. According to [2, 3], wheezing and coughing oust a haze of respiratory particles of a wide range of sizes between <1 and >500 μm or even up

D. Das (✉) · S. Nag · H. Naskar · S. Acharya · S. Bakchi · S. S. Ali · R. Banerjee Roy · B. Tudu
Department of Instrumentation and Electronics Engineering, Jadavpur University, Kolkata, West Bengal, India

R. Bandyopadhyay
Department of Instrumentation and Electronics Engineering, Jadavpur University, Kolkata, West Bengal, India

L. Garg et al. (eds.), *Healthcare Informatics for Fighting COVID-19 and Future Epidemics*, EAI/Springer Innovations in Communication and Computing,
https://doi.org/10.1007/978-3-030-72752-9_7

to 2000 μm. A wheeze or sneeze contains a larger number of particles than a cough, and for both cases, the level of dispersal is drastically diminished by the patient wearing a surgical face mask as per Nicas et al. [3]. Thus, the danger of this disease transmission from coughing or sneezing is decided either from droplet or contact transmission.

All these have necessitated the usage of personal protective equipment (PPE) as a mitigative measure to diminish, if not completely eliminate, the viral load that is transmitted. As such, face masks and protective clothing like face goggles, face shields, protective coveralls, head covers and shoe covers are the need of the hour as these create a barrier between the human body and the virus. When coming in contact with an infected person or for medical personnel attending to infected patients, two types of masks are recommended for use: three-layered medical masks and N95 respirator masks. While three-layered masks offer adequate protection in an infected environment, N95 masks (prepared through advanced filtration techniques) provide a higher protection level. Additionally, when a person touches an infected surface and uses the same hand to touch his eyes, nose or mouth, he may advertently be exposed to the virus. This transmission mode may not be the most predominant one; however, it is advised that protection should address the same issue. As such, hand gloves prevent virus transmission from the contaminated surfaces when used in conjunction with face shields or face goggles. Face shields and goggles prevent the infection of the eyes and nose in cases of proximity with viral load. Body coveralls and head covers offer similar kind of protection to a person in an infected environment and are mostly recommended for use by healthcare workers. Aprons and gowns also offer 360° protection for the persons using them and are a must for healthcare staff working near symptomatic people. Shoe covers made of an impermeable fabric are necessary for effective protection and decontamination in a limited environment. The use of hand sanitizers made up of alcohol has also been known to deactivate the virus. Therefore, the use of sanitizers or even soap-water is being recommended increasingly as an effective way of combatting the threat.

7.2 Different Types of PPE

The transmission of SARS-CoV-2 either by direct or indirect contact from one person to another is the current pandemic's primary cause. Recent studies by Esposito et al. [4] also reflected the possibilities of aerial transmission of this virus, with probabilities of infection even from an asymptomatic patient. Rothe et al. [5] reported that the adoption of different infection-preventive actions can impact the reduction of community transmission rates. Exercise of good respiratory and hand hygiene has become essential. The use of PPE can provide primary protection to the global population and the health workers and their patients. Formerly, the exercise of PPE use was prevalent in selective hazardous working environments to protect workers from physical injuries. However, the COVID-

19 pandemic has disclosed the potential of PPE to condense infection hazards in contaminated environments effectively. Different types of PPE can be classified based on the physical organ to be protected, the type of risks and the type of clothing and equipment required. PPE comprises the following elements: filtration masks, preemptive clothes (gowns), hand covers (gloves), face shields (helmets), eye gears (goggles) and hand sanitizers. These fabricated protective accessories must abide the standards of the Food and Drug Administration (FDA). Product quality control and maintenance are significant for customer care and satisfaction. On the contrary, high demand in the PPE supply chain is causing an upsurge of plastic usage. The abundant use of polyester, polyamide, polyethylene and other polymers in the manufacture of medical devices like face masks, face shields, suits and sanitizer bottles have been observed, thus producing a large mass of the unusable solid waste. The sustainability of PPE materials can be preserved with the use of natural fibres. The various types of PPE elements are illustrated in details as follows.

7.2.1 Types of Face Masks

Respiratory tract infections generally occur via inhalation and exhalation of contaminated droplets (5–10 μm) or fine aerosol particles [6]. The World Health Organization (WHO) specified that SARS-CoV-2 virus transmission could take place via coarse droplets [7]. However, recent research article presented the aptitudes of airborne transmission as well by Eikenberry et al. [8]. The basic principle of face masks is the filtration of airborne particles. Generally, face masks are made of different filter material layers. Lynteris [9] has reported the use of cloth face masks became scientifically relevant during the plague epidemic period. Patients with COVID symptoms and other respiratory infections like pulmonary tuberculosis or influenza are strongly recommended to wear face masks [4]. A greater part of the population includes asymptomatic patients having the equal potential to transmit their viral loads to healthy people. Hence, the exercise of universal public masking should be sincerely endorsed at the earliest. There may be a shortage in supply relative to demand of the proactive masks and surgical masks in recent times. Masks should properly fit on one's nose and mouth and not cause any constraint in breathing. Hands should be properly washed using soap and water or cleaned using alcohol-based sanitizers before wearing a mask. One should never touch the mask on the front end while wearing it. Similarly, during removal, one should gently pull out the mask by holding the ear loops [10]. After removing the mask, once again, hands should be washed and sanitized. Masks should be regularly washed with care; if not washable, they should be replaced after short intervals of use. Apart from wearing a face mask, one should also continue social distancing and follow hand hygiene practices.

7.2.2 Body Coveralls

Body coveralls are protective apparels that cover most of the body parts from harmful contagions. Medical gown, an example of the kind, is mostly necessary for healthcare workers. These gowns prevent them from direct contact with infections from bodily fluids. This will also help protect the patients from contacting contagions. These gowns are further categorized according to the risk regulation as surgical, surgical isolation and non-surgical gowns. The isolation gowns are made of impermeable materials that prevent microorganisms' diffusion via fabrics [11]. The isolation gowns may also be disposable or reusable. The disposable gowns are manufactured from synthetic fibres like polyester, while reusable gowns are made of cotton [11]. The fibres are the smallest unit of fabrics, and depending on their physical structure, the viral trapping is possible by high absorbance fibres. The natural fibres are higher absorbing fibres over the synthetic fibres [11]. The protective gowns should be absolutely sterilized during manufacture. Reusable gowns must be washed with care after every use. Likewise, gloves are also an important element of the PPE kit providing hand safety. The healthcare staff commonly uses disposable gloves made of latex, vinyl or nitrile. Both gowns and gloves need to be a perfect fit for the wearer. While wearing a gown, it must be secured at the neck and waist. Gloves should be worn on the hands and extended over the gown cuff areas. While removing a gown, it should be pulled from the neck, securing the contaminated part inside, followed by immediate disposal. Disposal of PPE kits is of significant concern because they can add to a large mass of the non-biodegradable waste. Also, proper care should be taken while disposing to avoid unwanted contaminations. Appropriate sanitization of hands is always necessary before wearing and after removing the gowns or gloves.

7.2.3 Face Shields

Face shields serve as a defensive layer of the entire face protecting the eyes, nose and mouth from dispersed bodily fluids or contaminated aerosols. But face shields are not the sole protector and must always be used along with other PPE elements [12]. Severe communicable diseases from the past like severe acute respiratory syndrome (SARS), influenza and Ebola had influenced the face and eye protection technologies. The present-day COVID-19 pandemic has consequently increased this awareness. A face shield comprises of a visor, a frame and a suspension system. The visor is a type of transparent window mostly made of polyvinyl chloride, polycarbonate or polyethylene. Frames support adjustments of the visor. The suspension systems are usually of elastic material and assist to position the face shield. Although eye contamination can be limited by protective eye gears like safety glasses or goggles, face shields can be an alternative to goggles. However, face shields can also be used in addition to goggles if potential infections are anticipated.

The dressing up sequence of a PPE should be as follows: medical gown, face masks, face shield or eyewears and gloves; the reverse while undressing [12]. Necessary considerations should be concerned for correct care conducts.

7.2.4 Hand Sanitizers

Hands are the most common body part which is vulnerable to interaction with infected environments. Proper hand sanitization may reduce SARS-CoV-2 viral transmission according to [13]. The Centers for Disease Control and Prevention (CDC) recommends the use of hand sanitizers and handwashing for effective hand sanitation. Different types of commercial products like disinfectant soaps and water- or alcohol-based sanitizers are available in the market. Hands should be cleaned by soap or alcohol sanitizer for a minimum of 20 s. The WHO promoted the use of alcohol-based hand sanitizers due to their verified actions against virus and bacteria loadings. Dixit et al. [14] has reported usually sanitizer products with a minimum of 62% alcohol are suitable for virus inactivation. But risks of fire hazards and skin denaturation due to high alcohol quantity may cause concern [15]. The direct or indirect spread of the SARS-CoV-2 virus through hands can be restricted by proper sterilization. Health workers must perform hand hygiene before and after contact with patients or medical devices. Eventually, good hygiene and efficient dissemination of safety norms by medical professionals can help improve community health.

7.3 Types of Face Masks

To combat the spread of coronavirus, various health organizations have advised the human population to use face masks. A number of face masks have been recommended by international organizations like WHO and CDC. Some of the important types of masks have been elucidated below.

7.3.1 Telephone Mouthpiece Mask

The telephone mouthpiece mask has been designed by Turkevich et al. [16]. These masks are made up of a synthetic polymer (polyolefin fibre) and an electret treated non-woven web (meltdown web). It has been intended to work utilizing the standard of a telephone handset. The non-woven web is covered with a pressure-responsive glue and goes through the air into the mouthpiece and causes the layer to vibrate. That layer changes over the sound into power to make the external layer electret in order to destroy the approaching viral particle. The utilization of this face mask can relax the weaved threads used while designing, thereby reducing the propagation of sound waves.

7.3.2 Strapless Flexible Tribo-Charged Respiratory Face Mask

This type of face mask has been proposed by Weinberg [17], where the activated carbon layer is included within a multilayer flexible flat filter. The filtration depends on the actuation of the carbon layer dissimilar to triboelectricity. Reutilizing the mask is a requirement to refill the carbon in the mask. Additionally, working of such a face mask relies upon the skin type the user bears. The user may experience the ill effects due to the mask's non-suitability for his/her skin.

7.3.3 Electrically Charged Filter Mask

This type of electrically charged filter and the mask has been proposed by Turkevich et al. [18]. In this type, four layers are available wherein there are three-layered liquid charged non-woven fibres and one layer of tribo-charged non-woven fabric. The temperature induced because of fluid charge power is liable to be under 40 °C, which is deficient to battle novel coronavirus infection. Refilling of polar fluid in the fluid charged texture may be problematic as it requires apparatus for immersion which is the same as spraying in the form of droplets, fog, shower, etc.

7.3.4 Medical Protective Breathing Mask

Verpoort et al. [19] proposed a multilayer made of chitin or silk fibre and hydrophilic and chemical fibre fabrics. The active gas is moved to the earth through the adsorption-dispersion-desorption procedure of the hydrophilic gathering of the practical film. The epitome of the created cover is encouraging. However, the working system of such fibre, including the commitment of synthetics required here, is very vague.

7.3.5 Surgical Masks (Multilayer Composition)

A surgical mask is widely used in the medical field for protection against bacterial infection. It can be used for respiratory disease control. These are typically a three-layer (three-ply) mask. The innermost part is made of polypropylene spunbond non-woven fabric; its purpose is to soak water or droplets. The middle layer is made of PP melt-blown and active carbon non-woven fabric, whose purpose is to filter a minimum of 95% bacteria. The outer layer is made of hydrophobic non-woven fabric, which repels water or liquid. This mask can stain the user's droplets, so you can wear this mask to protect others if you have any respiratory disease or you are COVID-19 positive. All are advised to wear this type of mask in addition to maintaining social distance.

7.3.6 Respiratory Protection Masks (Respirator)

Respirators are used to protect from inhaling airborne virus, bacteria, dust or industrial pollution, hazardous gas, etc. There are mainly two types of respirators: air-purifying type and supplied air-type respirator (particulate respirator, gas and vapour respirators, etc.) Descriptions of the N95 mask and half-face respirator are given. The N95 mask is a disposable particulate filtering facepiece. These types of masks are made of polypropylene and comprise of four layers of the same cloth material. The significance of N95 mask is that it can filter at least 95% of airborne particles. The half-face mask is a reusable mask which gives respiratory protection from particulates, gas, vapour, etc. These are made of thermoplastic elastomer. The half-face respirator covers the nose and mouth. As a result, it gives better protection when compared to ordinary face masks. We can use it with an added particulate filter (N95) or cartridges (gas or vapour cartridges) for better filter efficiency. This comes with a respiratory valve. It provides better security, but according to WHO and CDC guidelines, only healthcare workers should use it as the supplies are limited. The materials that are used for the construction of such respiratory masks are explained by Konda et al. [20].

7.3.7 Self-Powered Smart Masks

This is the most recent type of face mask designed by Ghatak et al. [21]. The material used for the purpose of designing is nylon-polyester, cotton-polyester, PMMA-PVDF, nylon-PVDF and polypropylene-polyester. This mask affirms its capacity to work when the user is talking, singing or making any signals of the lips of the wearer without any challenges of external sources. The active layer is dynamic during breathing in and breathing out the mask's time, which the electronic converter's capacitance can accomplish. Any infection that is comprised amidst the layers gets deactivated under the tribo-field. These masks generate thermal power of 0.4 W per second, and as per literature, this amount of power is enough to destroy the virus-loaded aerosols.

7.3.8 Cloth Face Mask/Covering

If a person does not have any kind of specially designed face mask in an emergency, he can use a cloth as a face mask. Handkerchief, cotton tees, towels, etc. can be used to wrap it over the face ensuring that nose and mouth openings are covered. Though CDC recommends it, this will not protect a person from biohazardous and small particles but can save the person and prevent the large particles from spreading from coughing and sneezing from one person to another. Kids under 2 years of age can use this and the CDC has recommended this.

7.4 Types of Hand Gloves

Among the different PPE components, gloves are the most commonly used component for handling object or surface contamination caused by germs. CDC recommends some rules for wearing and removing a pair of gloves which can serve as a protective layer against a surface contaminated with germs. As is obvious and suggested by Nazarko [22] and the Ministry of Health and Family Welfare, the user should dispose off the gloves after each use to prevent contamination.

Medical gloves are made of latex or rubber; however, WHO recommends gloves that are powder-free, non-sterile and at least 230–280 mm long. The quality and ability of gloves depend on the absence of perforation and overall integrity. The strength of the barrier of the glove is defined by the acceptable quality level (AQL). A low value of AQL is preferred for a high level of protection. As the virus is extremely small in size, gloves' resistance power plays a major role in selecting the appropriate PPE for the healthcare industry and being tested against ISO 16604:2004 standards. Gloves should meet the following standards:

1. EU standard directive 89/686/EEC Category III, EN 374
2. EU standard directive 93/42/EEC Class I, EN 455
3. ASTM D6319-10
4. ANSI/SEA 105-2011

Gloves are categorized into two variants, namely, disposable gloves and reusable gloves. On the one hand, disposable gloves are also of different types like medical purpose gloves and the gloves used for any other purposes like in salons, for food handling and for automotive purposes. On the other hand, the types of medical purpose gloves include surgical gloves, examination gloves, chemotherapy gloves and other medical care gloves. Reusable gloves, which are also called industrial or heavy-duty gloves, offer good protection in hazardous situations. These types of gloves are thicker, less flexible and less sensitive than disposable gloves. Reusable gloves can be washed and dried after every use. Gloves used in the healthcare industry are regulated by the Food and Drug Administration (FDA) guidelines. The different types of disposable gloves are given below.

7.4.1 Latex Gloves

Latex gloves are stretchable and made of natural rubber with high-quality materials that are flexible, waterproof and resilient. These gloves are washable and oil resistant. Latex gloves are very tactile, hence preferred for sensitive application. Other advantages of latex gloves are that they are comfortable, flexible and durable. Like nitrile gloves, latex gloves can also cause skin allergy problem. However, latex gloves are expensive and hardy disposable gloves.

7.4.2 Nitrile Gloves

These gloves are made of synthetic material such as nitrile, created from monomers acrylonitrile and butadiene. These are used in tattoo parlour, food preparation unit and industrial and healthcare sector. They show a high level of chemical and puncture resistance. But their pathogen protection and temperature handling ability are moderate. These types of gloves are soft, comfortable and flexible but can be torn easily. However, they show some disadvantages like less sensitivity and more coarseness than latex gloves.

7.4.3 Vinyl Gloves

Vinyl gloves are latex-free, inexpensive, lightweight and soft, which provides average resistance to the chemicals. These are mainly used for food preparation and janitorial purposes. The main disadvantages are a lower degree of protection from pathogens and low tensile strength; thus, they can be torn easily.

7.4.4 Poly Gloves

Poly gloves are polymer-based, thin, latex-free and less expensive used mainly for food preparation purposes. These offer low protection against pathogens and should be used in normal room temperature (25 °C ± 2).

According to Cook [23], the activity or the distance between two persons, the level of risk and the recommended PPE have been tabulated in Table 7.1.

Table 7.1 Activities, risk and recommended PPE

Activity	Risk	Recommended PPE
Distance $\geq$1 m	Low risk	Triple-layer mask and gloves
Distance = 1 m	Moderate risk	Triple-layer mask and gloves
Contact with COVID patient	High risk	Full PPE

Table 7.2 Classification of hand disinfectant chemical compounds with their antimicrobial activities

Type of compounds	Chemicals	Type of antimicrobial actions
Alcohol	• Ethanol (C_2H_6O) • Isopropanol (C_3H_8O) or *n*-propanol	Rapid denaturation of protein by interfering metabolism and cell rupture
Chlorine	• Chlorine dioxide (ClO_2) • Chloramine-t trihydrate ($C_7H_7ClNNaO_2S$)	Oxidants that can destroy protein structures by disrupting cell activities
Iodine	• Povidone-iodine	Fast penetration into cell with subsequent hit on protein groups (cysteine, methionine), resulting in collapse of the cell
Peroxygens	• Hydrogen peroxide • Peracetic acid	An oxidant which releases free radical to destroy cellular lipids and proteins
(Bis)phenols	• Triclosan	Adversely affects the cytoplasmic membranes
Biguanide	• Chlorhexidine	Ion interactions cause cell wall lysis

7.5 Suitable Hand Sanitizer Against COVID-19

Hand sanitizer is one of the essential antiseptic ammunition to combat the COVID-19 disease. Commercial hand disinfectant products are available in different forms like antiseptic soaps and water- or alcohol-based sanitizers with dispense systems such as gel, foam or wipes. Hand sanitizers are broadly classified into two categories: alcohol-based and alcohol-free. Alcohol-based sanitizers primarily contain different types of alcohol with necessary additives like glycerine or fragrance. These types of sanitizers can effectively deactivate a wide range of microorganisms without water. However, the antimicrobial effects are temporary and may be weak to counter some specific protozoa and non-enveloped viruses. On the contrary, alcohol-free sanitizers are based on antiseptic chemical solutions to deliver sterilization. These sanitizers are incombustible and hence are comparatively safe for children. Classifications of hand disinfectants with their antimicrobial activities are listed in Table 7.2 [13].

COVID-19 viruses can be disinfected using sterile solvents like ethanol,ether, chlorine compounds and chloroform [13]. Ethanol (60–80%) is a potent disinfectant that can deactivate any lipophilic viruses like influenza, herpes and hydrophilic viruses like rhinovirus and rotavirus. WHO in 2015 recognized ethanol (80%) and isopropanol (75%) as potent disinfectant hand rubs [13]. Nevertheless, further studies by WHO estimated ethanol as the most efficient viricidal agent against ZIKV, EBOV, SARS-CoV and MERS-CoV [13]. Studies conducted have reported the efficacy of ethanol (minimum 60%) rub for 30 s to deactivate SARS-CoV [13].

7.6 Advantages and Disadvantages of PPE

PPE is the final frontier against disease, injury or death. Using the control hierarchy, controls are considered if the risks of injury or exposure are medium or high. Unmitigable hazards require further administrative and engineering control for their elimination. Thus, understanding the limitations and failure becomes imperative.

- PPE does not attenuate the health hazards of the chemical or pathogen.
- PPE can imbibe a false sense of security.
- PPE are effective only when basic safety principles like engineering controls, housekeeping, etc. are already applied.
- PPE may not match the risk of changing risks, if any, of the prevalent hazards.
- PPE might hinder comfort and locomotion.
- PPE can restrict vision, normal breathing and communication.
- Using PPE for hours of work can cause anxiety attacks and claustrophobia.
- PPE might aggravate the risk of dehydration and heat stress-related problems.

PPE get contaminated by pathogens or chemicals and need to be duly removed before entering home, failing to infect healthy people. Some of the common advantages and disadvantages have been tabulated in Table 7.3. PPE can assure safety within a hazardous working place for the workers, as they do not fear short-/long-term health issues from exposure. Also, PPE can reduce the likelihood of workplace injury caused by working in such an environment.

Table 7.3 Types of PPE: advantages and disadvantages

Types of PPE	Advantages	Disadvantages
Face mask	Protection from pathogen-containing aerosols, masks are disposable	No indication of pathogen contact unless electric masks are used
Gown/coverall/lab coats	Gowns do not generate heat, covers large surface area of body	Coveralls cause heat production and gowns contain more openings
Face shield	Fairly simple to put on, covers the whole face and fogging is rare	No disadvantages as such. Protection at high risk not evidenced yet
Gloves	Ensures no direct contact with affected surfaces; hence pathogen transmission is reduced	Hands may become uncomfortable and slippery

7.7 Covid-19 and Health Informatics

Advances in technology framework and its applications have established a milestone to recover the catastrophe in healthcare management systems worldwide during the COVID-19 pandemic. Development of remote electronic healthcare monitoring tools has fast-tracked treatment facilities for COVID-19 as well as other diseases. A collaboration of well-equipped medical experts and technology consultants is necessary to assist in patient health surveillance. There should be elaborate research and analysis of existing operations and healthcare informatics before process execution. Basics of health informatics must include a review of the standard protocols for pandemic regulation by WHO and CDC. The factors that drive these protocols are strategy blueprints, coordination, communication, observation, screening, evaluation and medication facilities. Moreover, several research articles provide abundant information about premeditated recommendations to be pursued by regional administrations. Extensive knowledge of remote health inspection technologies is mostly significant for informatics archive. Taiwan's national health insurance database was interfaced with migration data, and medical alerts were directly sent to patients if required. The basic screening was done by interaction with travellers; medical permits were sent to the ones with low health risks. The ones with high health risk were instructed home quarantine with continuous health supervision via healthcare applications over mobile [24]. A remote communication network was developed in Texas between medics and their patients for immediate assistance [24]. People with high threats were delivered remote window visits to monitor intensive care and avoid unnecessary infections. On the contrary, many countries have also adapted emergency telemedicine facilities to drive down remote window visits. Telemedicine services include video consultancies for patients, virtual health scrutinization and symptoms tracker applications over mobile or other electronic gadgets. Telemedicine can also provide emergency medication assistance and continuous monitoring, hence reducing contacts between suspected patients and healthcare persons. Thus, prudent control over possible contagious interactions can be established. Augmentation of health monitoring platforms and tools for symptoms tracker can lead to an early screening of symptomatic persons and drain the healthcare administrations' liabilities. However, several aspects like project strategies, financial resources, process management, electronic appliances with strong communication network and collaborations with healthcare setups must be encountered in the beginning. Moreover, proper training and guidelines must be followed by the volunteers. Technologies and tools associated with healthcare and informatics have developed proficiency against pandemic control and management, including contact tracing [25], remote monitoring [26] and remote working [27]. The experience and expertise would head to beneficial health management amenities for similar confront in the future.

7.8 Summary

In this chapter, the perks of PPE custom have been manifested in detail, along with why investing in protective clothing for staff in all hazardous environments should be paramount. PPE is used to reduce the risk of germ dissemination to the environment and minimize transmission from patient to health worker or vice versa. All types of PPE have significant advantages as well as shortcomings. Utmost care must be taken while handling these PPE. On the positive side, these help in preventing unwanted infection from pathogens and injury from chemicals. PPE can be considered one of the most effective control methods and applied only when all other control measures are not accessible. While in a hazardous environment, complete PPE must be worn from goggles to gloves. PPE act as protective barriers between the persons wearing them and the pathogens in an infectious environment, which might prove infectious or fatal to the skin. Therefore, it is imperative for people working in such a setting to wear protective clothing. Respirators are essential in the protection of lungs from temporary as well as chronic infection or inflammation. It should be kept in mind that PPE use must be strictly confined to a specific person and must be cleaned thoroughly before and after wearing them. This is done mainly to prevent cross-contamination. Thus, PPE should be used by medical staff, visitors to hazardous worksites involving harmful chemicals, naked flame or infection-ridden places like hospitals and nursing homes.

References

1. I.T.S. Yu, Y. Li, T.W. Wong, Evidence of airborne transmission of the severe acute respiratory syndrome virus. N. Engl. J. Med. **350**, 1731–1739 (2004)
2. J. Gralton, E. Tovey, M.L. McLaws, W.D. Rawlinson, The role of particle size in aerosolised pathogen transmission: A review. J. Infect. **62**, 1–13 (2011)
3. M. Nicas, W.W. Nazaroff, A. Hubbard, Toward understanding the risk of secondary airborne infection: Emission of respirable pathogens. J. Occup. Environ. Hyg. **2**, 143–154 (2005)
4. S. Esposito, N. Principi, C. Leung, G. Migliori, Universal use of face masks for success against COVID-19: Evidence and implications for prevention policies. Eur. Respir. J. (2020). https://doi.org/10.1183/13993003.01260-2020
5. C. Rothe, M. Schunk, P. Sothmann, G. Bretzel, G. Froeschl, C. Wallrauch, T. Zimmer, V. Thiel, C. Janke, Transmission of 2019-nCoV infection from an asymptomatic contact in Germany. N. Engl. J. Med. (2020). https://doi.org/10.1056/NEJMc2001468
6. N.H.L. Leung, D.K.W. Chu, E.Y.C. Shiu, K.H. Chan, J.J. McDevitt, B.J.P. Hau, H.L. Yen, Y. Li, D.K.M. Ip, J.S.M. Peiris, Respiratory virus shedding in exhaled breath and efficacy of face masks. Nat. Med. (2020). https://doi.org/10.1038/s41591-020-0843-2
7. World Health Organization, Modes of transmission of virus causing COVID-19: Implications for IPC precaution recommendations: Scientific brief, March 2020 (No. WHO/2019-nCoV/Sci_Brief/Transmission_modes/2020.1) (2020)
8. S. Eikenberry, M. Mancuso, E. Iboi, T. Phan, K. Eikenberry, Y. Kuang, E. Kostelich, A. Gumel, To mask or not to mask: Modeling the potential for face mask use by the general public to curtail the COVID-19 pandemic. Infect. Dis. Modell. (2020). https://doi.org/10.1016/j.idm.2020.04.001

9. C. Lynteris, Plague masks: The visual emergence of anti-epidemic personal protection equipment. Med. Anthropol. (2018). https://doi.org/10.1080/01459740.2017.1423072
10. A. Desai, D. Aronoff, Masks and coronavirus disease 2019 (COVID-19). JAMA (2020). https://doi.org/10.1001/jama.2020.6437
11. F. Kilinc, A review of isolation gowns in healthcare: Fabric and gown properties. J. Eng. Fiber Fabr. **10**(3), 180–190 (2015)
12. R.J. Roberge, Face shields for infection control: A review. J. Occup. Environ. Hyg. (2016). https://doi.org/10.1080/15459624.2015.1095302
13. J. Jing, T. Yi, R. Bose, J.R. McCarthy, N. Tharmalingam, T. Madheswaran, Hand sanitizers: A review on formulation aspects, adverse effects, and regulations. Int. J. Environ. Res. Public Health (2020). https://doi.org/10.3390/ijerph17093326
14. A. Dixit, P. Pandey, R. Mahajan, D.C. Dhasmana, Alcohol based hand sanitizers: Assurance and apprehensions revisited. Res. J. Pharm. Biol. Chem. Sci. **5**, 558–563 (2014)
15. V. Erasmus, T.J. Daha, H. Brug, J.H. Richardus, M.D. Behrendt, M.C. Vos, B.E.F. Van, Systematic review of studies on compliance with hand hygiene guidelines in hospital care. Infect. Control Hosp. Epidemiol. **31**, 283–294 (2010)
16. M.H. Turkevich, L.A. Turkevich, D.L. Myers, Telephone Mouthpiece Mask, CA2217784
17. S. Weinberg, Strapless flexible tribo-charged respiratory facial, Patent No. CA2596342
18. M. Takeuchi, Y. Takashima, Electrically charged filter and mask, Patent No. EP2567744
19. T. Verpoort, L. Delaeter, N. Deneuville, Respiratory protection mask e.g. FFP2 type mask, for use by children, has porous protection part including non-woven type electrostatically charged melt-blown layer and non-woven type tribo-electrically charged felt layer, FR2970845
20. A. Konda, A. Prakash, G.A. Moss, M. Schmoldt, G.D. Grant, S. Guha, Aerosol filtration efficiency of common fabrics used in respiratory cloth masks. ACS Nano (2020). https://doi.org/10.1021/acsnano.0c03252
21. B. Ghatak, S. Banerjee, Sk.B. Ali, R. Bandyopadhyay, N. Das, D. Mandal, B. Tudu, Design of a self-powered smart mask for COVID-19 (2020). arXiv:2005.08305
22. L. Nazarko, COVID-19 and gloves: When to wear and when not to wear. Br. J. Healthc. Assist. **14**(4) (2020)
23. T.M. Cook, Personal protective equipment during the COVID-19 pandemic – A narrative review. Anaesthesia **75**(7) (2020)
24. R.S. Abeles, M. Tai-Seale, A.C. Longhurst, Rapid response to COVID-19: Health informatics support for outbreak management in an academic health system. J. Am. Med. Inform. Assoc. (2020). https://doi.org/10.1093/jamia/ocaa037
25. L. Garg, E. Chukwu, N. Nidal, C. Chakraborty, G. Garg, Anonymity preserving IoT-based COVID-19 and other infectious disease contact tracing model. IEEE Access **8**, 159402–159414 (2020). https://doi.org/10.1109/ACCESS.2020.3020513
26. M. Jayalakshmi, L. Garg, K. Maharajan, K. Srinivasan, K. Jayakumar, A.K. Bashir, K. Ramesh, Fuzzy logic-based health monitoring system for COVID'19 patients. Comput. Mater. Continua (2022)
27. A.K. Bhardwaj, L. Garg, A. Garg, Y. Gajpal, E-Learning during COVID-19 outbreak: Cloud computing adoption in Indian Public Universities. Comput. Mater. Continua **66**(3), 2471–2492 (2022). https://doi.org/10.32604/cmc.2021.014099

Chapter 8
Extensive Statistical Analysis on Novel Coronavirus: Towards Worldwide Health Using Apache Spark

Eali Stephen Neal Joshua, Debnath Battacharyya, Bhanu Prakash Doppala, and Midhun Chakkravarthy

8.1 Introduction to Coronavirus

The disease was initially called SARS-CoV-2 and later named as COVID-19. Coronavirus disease 2019 (COVID-19) is a highly contagious disease caused by a new strain of coronavirus.

COVID-19 infection is transmitted through respiratory droplets expelled from the nose and mouth when a person is coughing or sneezing. As a result, it's critical that you also follow breathing device policies (for circumstances, through hacking right into an arched junction).

8.1.1 Indicators

COVID-19 affects individuals of all walks of life. Many infected individuals will experience mild symptoms or no symptoms at all and will recuperate without hospital treatment.

E. S. N. Joshua (✉) · B. P. Doppala · M. Chakkravarthy
Department of Computer Science and Multimedia, Lincoln University College, Petaling Jaya, Malaysia
e-mail: stephen_neal@lincoln.edu.my; bhanu.doppala@lincoln.edu.my; midhun@lincoln.edu.my

D. Battacharyya
Department of Computer Science and Engineering, K L Deemed to be University, KLEF, Guntur, India
e-mail: debnathb@kluniversity.in

L. Garg et al. (eds.), *Healthcare Informatics for Fighting COVID-19 and Future Epidemics*, EAI/Springer Innovations in Communication and Computing,
https://doi.org/10.1007/978-3-030-72752-9_8

8.1.1.1 Most Common and Less Common Symptoms

- Fever
- Dry cough
- Fatigue
- Pains as well as aches
- Sore throat
- Diarrhoea
- Conjunctivitis
- Headache
- Loss of taste or smell
- Skin rash or discolouration of toes or fingers

8.1.1.2 Serious Symptoms

- Shortness of breath or difficulty breathing
- Pressure or chest pain
- Loss of speech or even movement

A large number of folks tainted along with the COVID-19 infection are going to experience moderate to reasonable breathing body health and wellness trouble as effectively as recuperate without phoning for an entire procedure. Much older people and those with hidden clinical problems like heart health condition, diabetes mellitus, constant breathing illness, and cancer tissues are much more likely to develop considerable health and wellness trouble [1]. The absolute best procedure is to stay away from as properly as decline transmittal is effectively informed concerning the COVID-19 disease. It develops as effectively as just how it spreads out (Fig. 8.1).

If you are experiencing serious symptoms, seek immediate medical attention. Always call a medical professional or even a health facility before visiting. Individuals experiencing mild symptoms and are healthy are advised to manage their symptoms at home. Typically, it takes about 5–6 days after the infection for symptoms to show.

8.1.2 Deterrence

To avoid infection and also to minimise transmission of COVID-19, the following protective measures should be exercised:

- Avoid touching your mouth, eyes and nose.
- Wash your hands often with soap and water or always disinfect your hands with alcohol-based sanitiser when touching surfaces.
- Avoid cigarette smoking so as not to harm the bronchi.

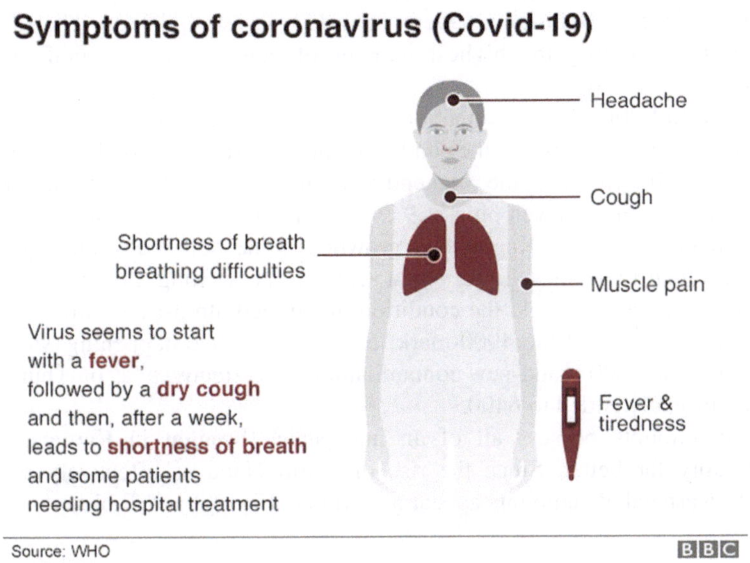

Fig. 8.1 Symptoms of person infected with COVID-19

- Maintain a minimum of 1 m distance from people to avoid contact with droplets from sneezing or coughing.
- Cover your mouth and nose when sneezing or coughing.
- Stay at home if you are sick.
- Avoid mass gatherings.

Forty-nine thousand four hundred and ten new circumstances were consisted of in the nation on Friday, along with Odisha, which has been incorporating over 2000 scenarios aimed at the final two times, however, to disclose its everyday varieties. COVID instances in South Africa have been decreasing day by day in recent days, whereas COVID cases in India have increased from 35,000 to 50,000.

COVID cases identified in Karnataka are very less when compared to Andhra Pradesh and Tamilnadu.

8.2 COVID-19 in India

In India there are 60,000 cases reporting daily. Where Andhra Pradesh is contributing with 10.7% cases and Karnataka with 6.68% cases per day.

Andhra Pradesh reported with high peak of COVID cases on Thursday with a total number of 9000 cases.

A total of 50000 instances were recorded across India on Thursday, with Maharashtra reporting the highest number of new cases compared to Andhra Pradesh.

The overall lot of contaminations in Andhra Pradesh came to 72,700 on Thursday, and also at this fee, the condition appears prepared to eclipse Karnataka's existing 81,000-figure over the weekend rest. The contamination varieties in Andhra Pradesh are presently developing at 9.7% per day (7-day compounded day-to-day development cost), while Karnataka's growth cost has boiled down to 6.68%.

For the final two times, Tamil Nadu seems to be seeking a brand-new amount. For higher than a full week, the condition mentioned almost the same selection of new situations, around the 4900-mark. It exposed a dive happening Monday and even more than 5600 brand-new contaminations, as effectively as on Thursday, this went additionally added to 6400.

These amounts possess all of an unexpected brought in Karnataka appear considerably far better. Since the rise of Tamil Nadu as effectively as Andhra Pradesh, Karnataka's amounts appear a lot tinier (Fig. 8.2 and Table 8.1).

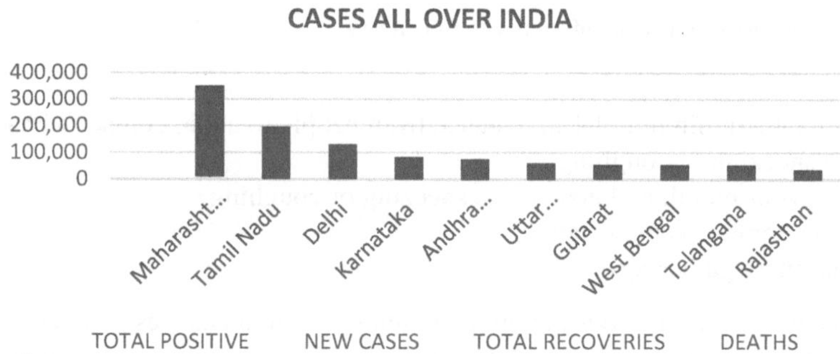

Fig. 8.2 COVID-19 cases recorded in India

Table 8.1 COVID-19 cases in India till July 2020

State's	Confirmed cases	New cases	Total recovered	Mortality
Maharashtra	347,501	9896	194,254	12,855
Tamil Nadu	192,965	6473	136,794	3235
Delhi	127,365	1042	109,066	3746
Karnataka	80,864	5031	29,311	1623
Andhra Pradesh	72,712	7999	37,556	885
Uttar Pradesh	58,105	2517	35,804	1299
Gujarat	52,564	1079	37,959	2258
West Bengal	51,758	2437	31,656	1256
Telangana	50,827	1568	39,328	448
Rajasthan	33,099	887	23,701	595

8.3 Coronavirus Family

Coronaviruses (CoVs) are single-stranded positive-sense RNA viruses. In patients with underlying illnesses, inflammatory and coagulation responses are lower than in patients without such disorders, and the need for vasopressors and mechanical breathing is more common. Initially named as severe acute respiratory syndrome (SARS-CoV-2) and later named COVID-19, the disease was quickly declared as a pandemic.

Coronaviruses are classified as zoonotic viruses (which imply that it is transmitted between animals and people). Fever, cough, respiratory symptoms, and breathing difficulty are some of the symptoms. Patients may get pneumonia, severe acute respiratory syndrome (SARS), kidney failure, and even death if the situation is not handled properly.

8.3.1 Severe Acute Respiratory Syndrome

Additionally, I also possess cardio problems. Rigorous coronary disorder was always kept in thoughts to take location after SARS. This low investigation study has undoubtedly not been validated in various other files [3].

In an additional investigation study of 121 individuals (indicate grow older of 37 years; 36a guys) along with a healthcare prognosis of SARS inhouse 12 people had covered cardiovascular disease, tachycardia was amongst the most popular (72%), in addition to various other concerns, including high blood pressure (50%), bradycardia (15%), short-term cardiomegaly (11%), and also temporary peroxyl little bit of atrial fibrillation in single detail [4]. A lot of these patients were asymptomatic and their disorders were actually mainly self-limiting.

A research study from Singapore disclosed post-mortem assessment in eight clients who passed away for SARS in which four people possessed bronchi apoplexy, as effectively as three individuals possessed deep-seated blood vessel apoplexy. One individual possessed marantic 5–12 mm vulvar vegetation resides, being made up of the mitral, tricuspid, and aortic regulators, along with infarction in centre, renal spleen. Still, the venerability of this measured analysis study is actually certainly not developed.

8.3.2 Middle East Respiratory Syndrome

The incredibly transmittable contamination broadcast comes from contaminated dromedary Beiges as the more advanced multitude to people and a shut telephone call. To get in right into the multitude tissue, it produces a serine peptidase as effectively as dipeptidyl peptidase as the receptor [5].

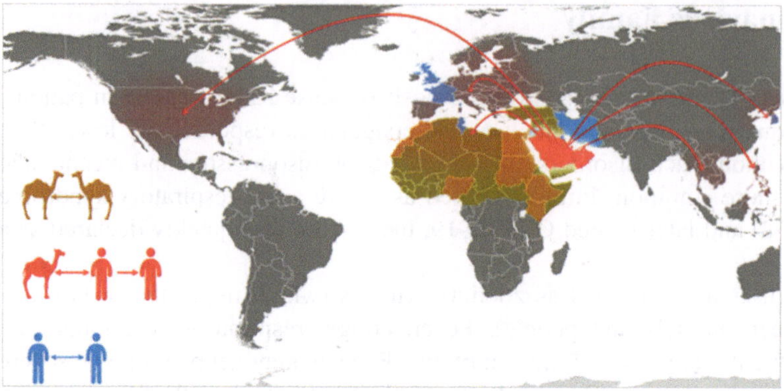

Fig. 8.3 The contagion of the Middle East respiratory syndrome

The study specifies that the MERS-CoV might possess been happened coming from baseball bats along with sent out to promissory beiges [6] (Fig. 8.3).

8.3.3 SARS-CoV-2

On 31 December 2019, an amount of neighbourhood health and wellness amenities uncovered that amounts of pneumonia of unknown ethology connected to giant fish, a lifestyle creature in Wuhan, Hubei Inception, China. In 10 January 2020, unfamiliar COVID 19, SARS-COVID, in the start phoned as 2019-nCoV, was officially identified as a description responsible for an appeal of virus-like pneumonia. Serious, excessive breathing health condition CoV-2 possesses an area along with the β-CoVs ton that possesses 89% nucleotide personality and baseball bat as effectively as 82% along with the individual SARS-COVID [7].

As of 29 November 2019, the downright amount of 2495 research workshop certified disease of MERS COVID had been actually accounted for, along with 858 hooked up casualties (occasion victim: 34%) in 26 Countries, along with a wonderful offer of instances coming from Saudi Arabia along with 2102 concerns along with an Occasion casualty of 37% [8].

As of Nov 30, 2019, the downright amount of 2494 research laboratory attested health problem of MERS-COVID had been accounted for, along with 858 linked casualties (occasion sufferer: 34%) in 26 Countries, along with a terrific bargain of situations coming from Saudi Arabia along with 2012 troubles along with a Case casualty of 39%. On 31 December 2019, various neighbourhood health and wellness centres showed that amounts of pneumonia of unfamiliar ethology connected to huge fish, a lifestyle pet in Wuhan, Hubei Inception, China. Intense, excessive breathing disorder CoV-2 possesses a location and the β-CoVs lot that possesses

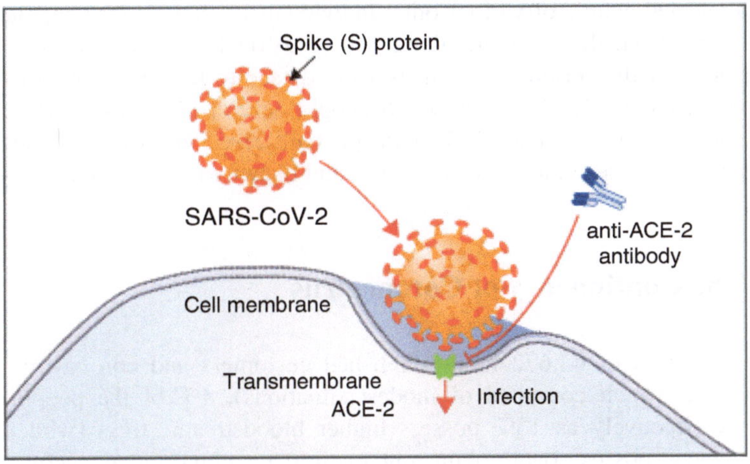

Fig. 8.4 ACE-2 is the host cell receptor responsible for mediating infection by SARS-COVID-2

88% nucleotide personality along by baseball bat as effectively as 82% along with the individual SARS-COVID (Fig. 8.4).

There are some stress and anxiety over the achievable faecal-oral system of transmission coming from SARS-CoV-2 considered that clients along with SARS and also MERS a considerable component of the minute possessed isolation of the gastrointestinal systems, along with SARS-COVID RNA pinpointed in chairs of individuals along with SARS [9]. The determined rate of infection of SARS-CoV-2 is actually in between 3 and also 3, which signifies that every person along with SARS-CoV-2 contaminants is traditional to corrupt a married couple of various other folks in an at threat populace. The three necessary evidence as well as likewise signs of COVID-19 are high-temperature hacking along with the conciseness of respiration. Much less general side results are muscular tissue mass discomfort, throbbing neck, nasal blockage, and frustration [4].

A bust figured out tomography examination made use of typically to even further evaluate individuals along with COVID-19 [10]. Hazardous documentation encourages that very first higher physical body determined tomography plans and also abnormality in a lowest of 85% of customers, along with 75% of individuals possessing an equivalent bronchi contamination that often turns up as Sab plural alongside outside areas of ground glass functionality as well as economic commitment loan consolidation [11]. First records coming from 4226 people along with COVID-19 in the USA reveal that the majority of serious difficulty is found face-to-faces 85 years similarly as additional widely known (10–27%), sticks to people developed 65–84 years (3–11%), people expanded 55–64 years (1–3%). People built 22–55 years (<1%), along with no mortalities amongst individuals 18 years and likewise a lot more much younger.

The predicted R0 of SARS-CoV-2 is actually between 3 and 4, which signifies that everybody along with SARS-CoV-2 contaminants is actually traditional to affect a married couple of various other individuals in an at danger populace. First files coming from 4226 people along with COVID-19 in the USA present that the majority of the serious problem is viewed face-to-face 85 years similarly as additional popular (10–27%), sticks to people developed 65–84 years (3–11%), people increased 55–64 years (1–3%). People built 22–55 years (<1.2%), along with no mortalities amongst individuals 20 years and likewise much more much younger.

8.4 The Contingency of Coronavirus

In a progression of 44,672 long-established customers and coronavirus coming from China (which consisted of modest situations), 4% of the people possess CVD, as effectively as 13% possess higher bloodstream stress (while 50% of circumstances possess overlooking out on info on comorbid concerns). In this populace, 81% mentioned possessing a mild ailment along with no fatality, 14% possessed severe ailment without death, and 5% possessed important ailment along with a case fatality fee of 49%. The COVID-19 death rows along with enhanced grow older, along with the scenario death price of 1.3% in customers expanded 50–58 years, 3.7% in individuals produced 61–68 years, 9% in individuals developed 71–80 years as properly as 14.9% in people 81 years or even above. People, along with CVD made up 4.2% of validated occasions but created up 2.7% of all harmful circumstances, along with the scenario death rate of 10.5%. The occasion fatality cost of individuals and high blood pressure was 6%, diabetic issues Mellitus was 7.3%, and the persistent respiratory system health condition was 6.3% [11].

In the growth of 44,672 confirmed customers and COVID-19 coming from China (which featured modest instances), 4% of the individuals possess CVD, as effectively as 13% possess higher bloodstream tension (while 50% of circumstances possess skipping out on info on comorbid complications). In this populace, 81% mentioned possessing a modest condition along with no fatality, 14% possessed severe problem without death, and 5% possessed crucial ailment along with a case victim cost of 49%. The COVID-19 death rows along with enhanced grow older, along with the instant death fee of 1.3% in customers expanded 50–58 years, 3.76% in individuals produced 61–68 years, 8% in people created 71–80 years as effectively as 14.88% in people 79 years or even above.

In one even more exam out of 138 laid up people along with COVID-19, 36 (26%) people relocated to EMERGENCY ROOM. Being obligated to pay to problems, comprising of ARDS (61%), arrhythmias (44%), as properly as a surprise (31%).

8.4.1 History Research Study

The SARS-COVID-19 outburst started in the Guangdong location in Southern China in November 2002, similarly as most likely affiliated along with a zoonotic celebration in the untamed pet screens in China, the gearbox of SARS-COVID near exclusive to particularly receive in contact along with and also through breathing grains, along with a gestation period of 22 eleven times after straight visibility. The whitewash of ACE2 articulation throughout SARS-CoV an ailment has actually been actually suggested to incorporate to the medical customisations in the bronchi in enhancement to incorporate to harsh pneumonia as effectively as additionally, extreme passion breakdown noted along with this contamination.

The SARS-CoV could be gone down right into the setting as well as furthermore specifying coming from environmental surface area places to palms of clients as properly as furthermore clinical treatment medical doctor [7].

There is no inoculation or even show antiviral tension versus SARS-CoV. For that cause therapy of SARS therapy allowed stimulating treatment and made use of broad-spectrum antimicrobial surveillance to work along with audio microbial contamination [12] (Fig. 8.5).

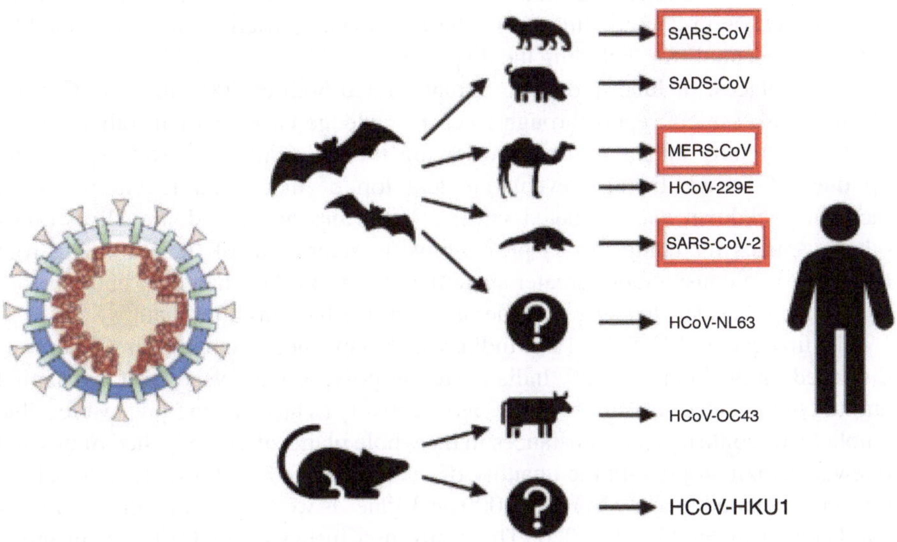

Fig. 8.5 Animal origins of human coronaviruses

8.5 Case Study on India

The COVID-19 pandemic in India enters into the world pandemic of coronavirus problem 2019 (COVID-19) caused by severe extreme respiratory system condition coronavirus (SARS-CoV-2). The first scenario of COVID-19 in India, which arose from China, was pointed out on 30 January 2020. India currently possesses the most significant choice of confirmed scenarios in Asia, and also likewise has the third ultimate feasible wide array of confirmed scenarios worldwide after the United States as well as Brazil in addition to the range of complete validated situations breaching the 100,000 outcomes on 19 May, 200,000 on 3 June, as well as 1,000,000 confirmed events on 17 July 2020.

India's occasion fatality cost is amongst the best economical on earth at 2.41% considering that 23 July and is steadily minimising. On 10 June, India's recoveries went over energised cases for the very first time.

On 22 March, India kept track of a 14-h volunteer social time frame at the prime pulpit Arian Narendra Modi scenario. Even more, on 24 March, the Prime Minister acquired a throughout the country lockdown for 21 opportunities, having an effect on the whole entire 1.3 billion-person people of India.

The United Nations (UN), as well as likewise the World Health Organization (WHO), possess commended India's response to the worldwide as 'likewise heavy duty as well as in-depth,' illustrating the lockdown restrictions as 'unfavourable, however, essential' for including the dispersing in addition to establishment critical treatment places. In June, India was actually rated 56th of 200 nations in COVID 19 safety assessment report through Deep Knowledge Group various other experts possess in reality enhanced issues worrying the financial end results specifying up due to the additional preventative and top of that usual requirements. In fact, the lockdown was validated via the authorities and ad-additionally various other agencies for being in fact pre-emptive to steer clear of India coming from obtaining in a considerably greater stage that might produce handling undoubtedly challenging, besides, to cause considerably extra reductions after that.

The first event of COVID-19 in India, which happened to come from China, was disclosed on 30 January 2020. India currently possesses the very most substantial amount of validated situations in Asia, as effectively as has the third greatest feasible whole lot of confirmed circumstances in the whole planet after the United States and likewise Brazil along with the quantity of overall verified circumstances breaching the 100,000 smudge on 19 May, 200,000 on 3 June, as well as additionally 1,000,000 validated cases on 17 July 2020. The really first instance of COVID-19 in India, which con-trolled coming from China, was disclosed on 30 January 2020 (Fig. 8.6).

Authorities advise the number of contaminations may be a whole lot higher as India's problematic percentages are actually amongst the minimum on the planet. The contaminants speed of COVID-19 in India is spoken with being 1.7, basically less than in one of the most conspicuously horrible affected nations.

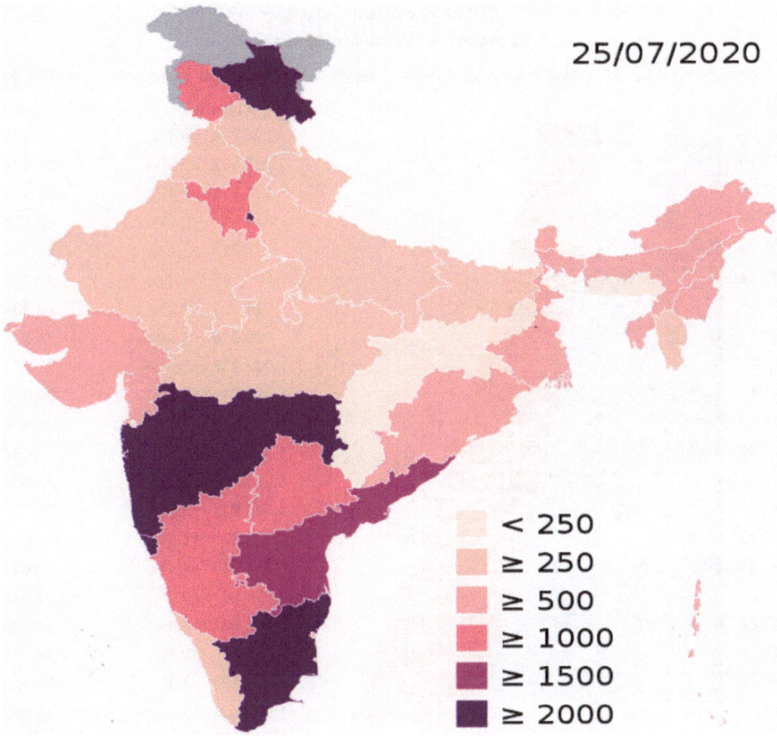

Fig. 8.6 Map of confirmed cases per million

8.5.1 Timeline

On 30 January, India stated its first case of COVID-19 in Kerala, which cheered three circumstances through 3 February; all were trainees coming back from Wuhan. Besides these, no massive increase in equipment cartons was actually observed in February. On 4 March 22 brand-new cases were mentioned, containing 14 afflicted individuals of an Italian tourist group. In March, the gearboxes grown after several people with excursion past to affected nations and their connection with checked beneficial. On 12 March, a 76-year-old fella, with a touring history to Saudi Arabia, became India's initial COVID-19 death.

Timeline of the global escalates throughout India (considering that 30 January 2020 and likewise till 3 April 2020).

A Sikh priest, that had a journeying record to Italy and additionally Germany, cultivated into a 'exceptionally spreader' with seeing a Sikh activity in Anandpur Sahib throughout 10–12 March. Twenty-seven COVID-19 circumstances were in fact summarised back to him. Over 40,000 people in 20 towns in Punjab were really sequestered on 27 March to contain the intensify.

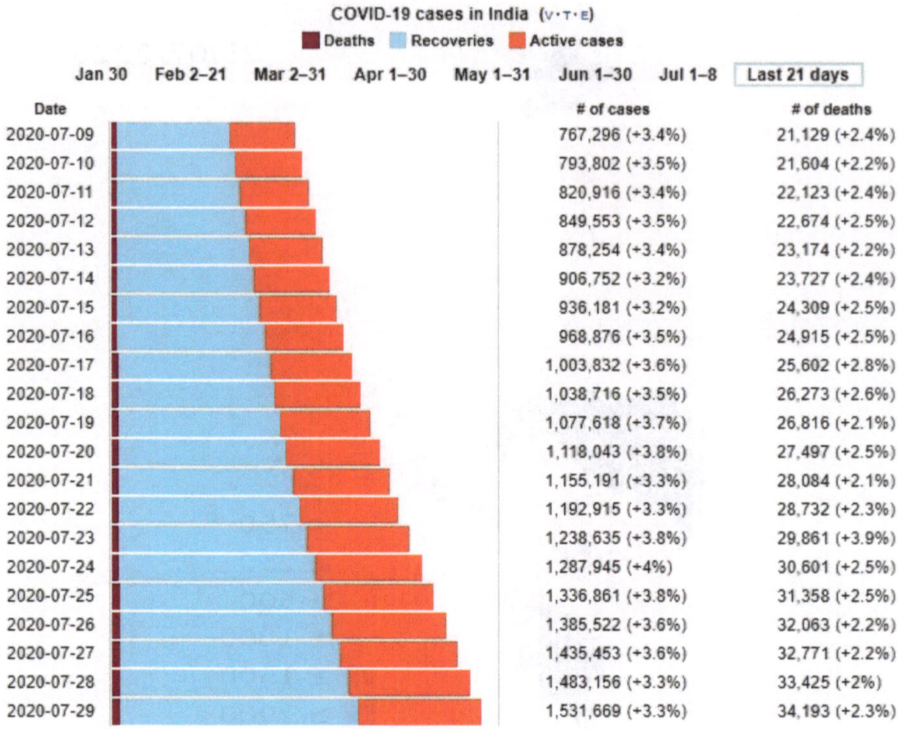

Fig. 8.7 Statistics of death, recovered and active cases

On 31 March, a Tablighi Jamaat supernatural theological goers' occasion in Delhi, which invited reality taken site previously in March, come up as a new contaminant tremendously spreader activity, after whole lots of cases throughout the country were outlined back to it. Countless of them had a look at pleasing, having 27 bus car vehicle drivers and conductors that had been an element of the transportation setup (Fig. 8.7).

8.5.2 Statewise Analysis in India

Utilise this graph to comprehend whether India or even one of its conditions or UT is flattening the curve or not. A higher arc shows that the infection is spreading quickly, and even more, people are finding therapy at any form of supplied time.

A gentler contour suggests that much fewer individuals are infected along with the infection, quitting a rise that will baffle the medical care unit. India has examined 14,381,303 samples, containing 333,395 samples in the last 24 h.

Utilise this graph to understand the assessment prices of every State/UT. Measurement of bubble signifies overall examination accomplished due to the condition. Colour signifies Status matched up to national standard: Test per thousand individuals/Percentage of beneficial instances, amongst example, examined. he rises in exams per million has really been obtained with a stable rise in the number of research laboratories and initiatives due to the Centre and State federal government authorities and likewise Union Territory administration to support in wide-spread screening.

For the third day right, many COVID-19 recoveries in 24 h viewed an extra document high, along with 34,602 patients having recovered pushing the healing price to 63.45%. The case death rate has more refused to 2.38%, it claimed. Depending on to information improved at 8 a.m., the general healings have reached 817,208, while there are 440,135 lively cases of coronavirus in the country presently. India similarly viewed a report single-day spike of 49,310 instances while the death-toll mounted to 30,601 along with 740 brand new disasters. Further, a progressing total of 15,428,170 instances have been actually checked out for COVID-19 around 23 July. On Thursday, 3, 52,801 examples were actually examined. The rise in TPM has actually been accomplished along with a regular rise in the assortment of laboratories (1290 so far) and efforts due to the Centre and State governments and Union Territory managements to promote wide-spread screening via a range of alternatives, it always remembered.

There are presently 897 labs in the federal government market as well as 393 personal labs. When it comes to the country registering an increasing variety of recuperations, the Ministry said that efforts of States and also Union Territories are bolstered due to the Central teams of pros sent to high caseload regions and likewise using planned conversations stored through Central federal government using video conferencing with State—as well as additionally district officials.

The dimension of blister works with total exam done due to the state. Colour denotes Status contrasted to nationwide standard: Test per thousand people/Percentage of positive circumstances, amongst instance, examined. The rise in TPM has been accomplished with a constant increase in the variety of labs (1290 until now) as well as efforts due to the Centre as well as likewise State governments and likewise Union Territory administrations to facilitate wide-spread testing along with a selection of substitutes, it noted.

Measurement of bubble means the overall exam carried out by the state. The boost in TPM has been attained with consistent growth in the range of labs (1290 thus far) and campaigns by the Centre as effectively as State governments and also Union Territory administrations to advertise wide-spread screening through a range of options, it always kept in thoughts. The rise in TPM has been obtained with a consistent rise in the number of laboratories (1290 so much) as effectively as initiatives through the Centre and State governments and Union Territory monitoring to assist in wide-spread screening with an assortment of choice (Figs. 8.8 and 8.9 and Table 8.2).

In Tables 8.3 and 8.4, statistical values of confirmed, recovered and deaths cases from the inception of COVID-19 to 25 June 2020, have been demonstrated. Figure

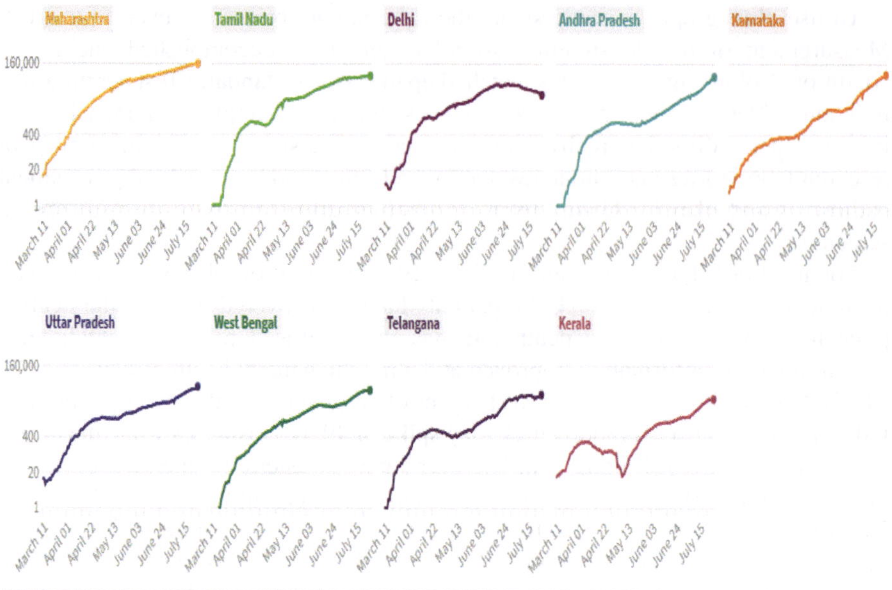

Fig. 8.8 Statewise active cases

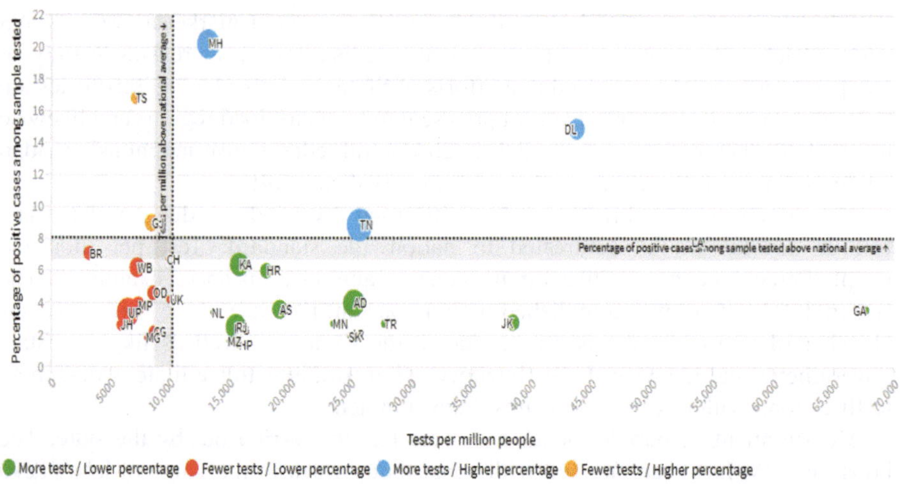

Fig. 8.9 Tests per million

8.3 shows the number of cases based on the tests conducted up to 790,000 above tests. The top pie charts represent the number of confirmed cases, while the bottom pie charts show the number of active cases, cured cases, and deaths (Fig. 8.10).

Table 8.2 COVID-19 tests

S. no.	Feature	Remarks
1	S. no.	Unique number for the country/province
2	Name of state/UT	Name of state or union territory in India
3	Total tested	Total COVID-19 tests conducted by each state
4	Positive	No. of positive cases based on tests
5	Negative	No. of positive cases based on tests
6	Active	No. of active cases present doing the treatment

Table 8.3 COVID-19 cases

S. no.	Feature	Remarks
1	S. no.	Unique number for the country/province
2	Name of state/UT	Name of state or union territory in India
3	Confirmed	No. of confirmed cases
4	Recovered	No. of recovered patients after treatment
5	Deaths	No. of deaths
6	Active	No. of active cases present under the treatment

8.5.3 Age Group and Gender Analysis

The natural perk of greater safety coming from COVID-19 fatalities that women in most different other countries possess seems to be completely losing out on for ladies in India.

The first-ever evaluation of gender differentials in COVID-19 fatalities in the country has uncovered that while the general assortment of infected men is higher, relative mortality resulting from the sickness is greater amongst ladies than guys—in conflict to the international pattern.

The evaluation by the researchers connected to the Institute of Economic Growth in Delhi, Institute of Health Management Research in Jaipur as well as additionally Harvard University in the United States has exposed that 3.3% of all gals contracting the condition in the country are perishing while this fee is actually 2.9% for males.

The difference is the starkest in the age of 40–49 years where 3.2% of the contaminated girls, as contrasted to 2.1% males, have succumbed to the transmittable illness and in addition in the grow older 5–19 years that has actually just found ladies casualties. The searching's for of the research equal threat, asymmetrical problem? Sex differential in COVID-19 mortality in India has been re-leased in the Journal of Global Health Science and is based upon COVID-19 deaths in India till 20 May when the full validated situations were 112,027 3433 fatalities at an occasion fatality percentage of 3.1%. Seventy-three thousand six hundred and fifty-four males and 38,373 girls were contaminated afterwards, while 2165 males and 1268 females had dropped their lives to the pandemic.

Notably, no infected male in the generation of 5–19 had really died in India whereas the death rate in generation one of the females was 0.6%. Globally com-

Table 8.4 Statewise COVID-19 case details

COVID-19 pandemic in India by state and union territory				
State/union territory	Cases	Deaths	Recoveries	Active
35/36	1,531,669	34,193	988,029	509,447
Andaman and Nicobar Islands	363.0	1.0	196.0	166.0
Andhra Pradesh	110,297.0	1148.0	52,622.0	56,527.0
Arunachal Pradesh	1330.0	3.0	617.0	710.0
Assam	34,947.0	88.0	26,618.0	8241.0
Bihar	43,843.0	269.0	28,856.0	14,718.0
Chandigarh	934.0	14.0	599.0	321.0
Chhattisgarh	8257.0	46.0	5439.0	2772.0
Dadra and Nagar Haveli and Daman Diu	982.0	2.0	596.0	384.0
Delhi	132,275.0	3881.0	117,507.0	10,887.0
Goa	5287.0	36.0	3595.0	1656.0
Gujarat	57,982.0	2372.0	42,412.0	13,198.0
Haryana	32,876.0	406.0	25,758.0	6712.0
Himachal Pradesh	2330.0	14.0	1234.0	1082.0
Jammu and Kashmir	18,879.0	333.0	10,885.0	7661.0
Jharkhand	9078.0	89.0	3868.0	5121.0
Karnataka	107,001.0	2055.0	40,504.0	64,442.0
Kerala	20,894.0	67.0	10,724.0	10,103.0
Ladakh	1327.0	6.0	1067.0	254.0
Lakshadweep	0.0	0.0	0.0	0.0
Madhya Pradesh	29,217.0	830.0	20,343.0	8044.0
Maharashtra	391,440.0	14,165.0	232,277.0	144,998.0
Manipur	2317.0	0.0	1612.0	705.0
Meghalaya	779.0	5.0	194.0	580.0
Mizoram	384.0	0.0	198.0	186.0
Nagaland	1460.0	5.0	577.0	878.0
Odisha	28,107.0	154.0	18,061.0	9892.0
Puducherry	3011.0	47.0	1782.0	1182.0
Punjab	14,378.0	336.0	9752.0	4290.0
Rajasthan	38,514.0	644.0	27,202.0	10,668.0
Sikkim	579.0	1.0	186.0	392.0
Tamil Nadu	227,688.0	3659.0	166,956.0	57,073.0
Telangana	57,142.0	480.0	42,909.0	13,753.0
Tripura	4269.0	21.0	2621.0	1627.0
Uttarakhand	6587.0	70.0	3720.0	2797.0
Uttar Pradesh	73,951.0	1497.0	44,520.0	27,934.0
West Bengal	62,964.0	1449.0	42,022.0	19,493.0
As of 30 July 2020				

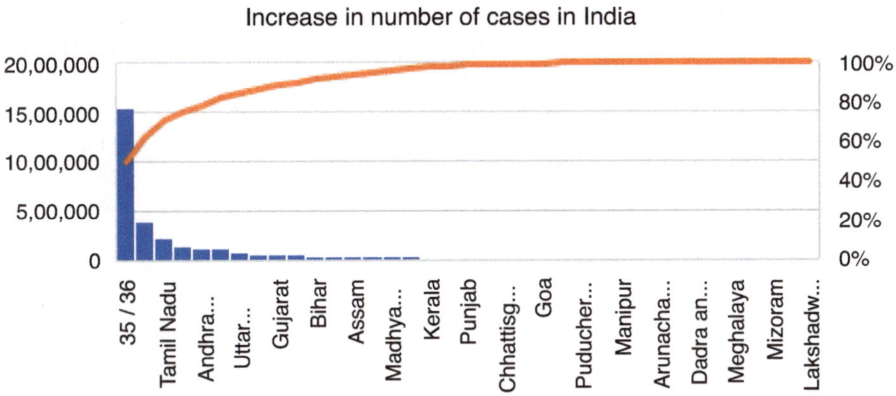

Fig. 8.10 Exponential increase of cases in India

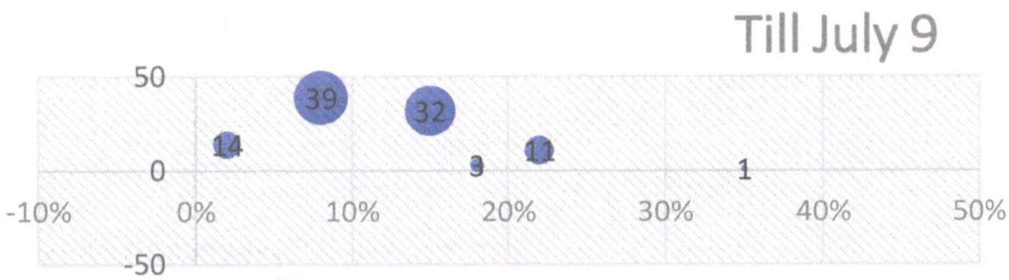

Fig. 8.11 Fatalities of young vs. old in India

parable analyses in countries like United States, China, and Italy have uncovered that the loved one fatality rate is higher amongst guys. The distinctions have been accepted to sex-based immunological differences due to girls hormones, a reduced frequency of smoking in women, and guys establishing co-morbid ailments such as hypertension at a much younger grow older than ladies. The researchers took note that 'although males share a greater trouble of fatality yet together it is actually essential to take note that women possess a pretty serious danger of COVID-19 death'. As numerous as 43% deaths have in fact occurred in the reasonably younger age bands of 30–44 and 45–59. Individuals in the age above 45 continue to become more at risk from Covid-19 in terms of victims. The section of deaths about age has not altered dramatically considered that 21 May. In regards to downright amounts, the fatalities have improved along with increase typically death (Fig. 8.11 and Table 8.5).

8.5.4 COVID-19 Impact on Indian Economy

The shopping market viewed a sag in development and stress on the source chain shipping's and likewise the assumptions of the consumers on the firms ahead of

Table 8.5 Fatalities amongst young and old in India

% Share in all COVID-19 deaths			
Age	Share in population (%)	Till 9 July	Till 21 May
≤14	35	1	0.5
15–29	18	3	2.5
30–44	22	11	11.4
45–59	15	32	35.1
60–74	8	39	40.2
≥75	2	14	10.3

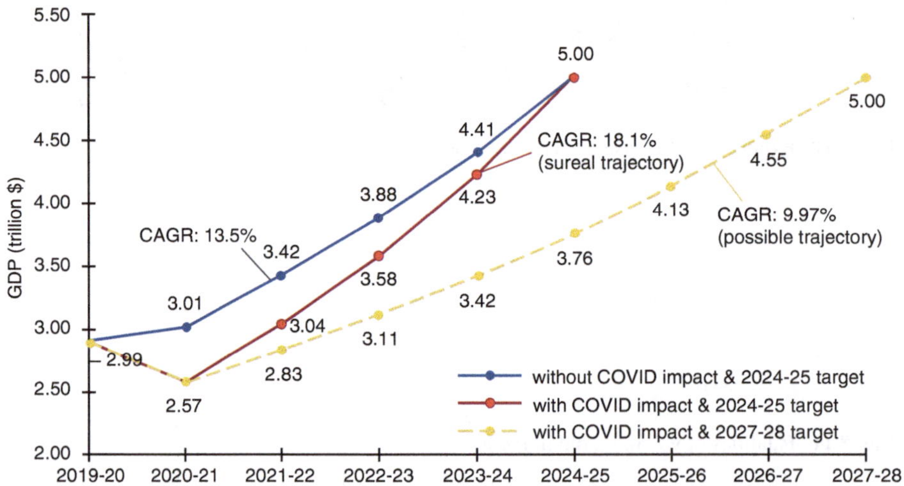

Fig. 8.12 GDP growth trajectory for $5 trillion objective

time up along with more recent circulation channels focusing on straight to client training courses. Within this escalating atmosphere, the regulating and preparing for of need will certainly play an important functionality in the buyer partnership area. Grouping the items into part i.e. non-essential assets and important commodities disclosed various feedbacks on the market (Fig. 8.12).

8.6 Prediction of COVID-19 Using Apache Spark

8.6.1 Apache Spark Architecture

Apache Spark, in easy phrases, circulated processing is only a dispersed unit, where various equipment's are performing particular work at the very same opportunity. While carrying out the job, equipment will connect through passing notifications between them. Distributed computer works, when there is criteria of rapid processing (calculation) on significant information.

Permit our team to take an easy analogy to reveal the idea. Let our team claim; you must count the number of publications in several segments of a sizable public library. And also you have to finish it in a lot less than an hour. This amount possesses to be particular as well as can easily not be estimated. What would certainly you carry out? If I resided in this position, I will phone as numerous good friends as I can easily and separate places/spaces amongst them. I'll partition the operate in non-overlapping ways and ask them to disclose back to be in 55 moments. I'll merely incorporate up the numbers to happen up along with a service once they happen back. This is exactly just how distributed computing works.

Apache Hadoop and also Apache Spark are widely known examples of Big records handling bodies. Hadoop and Spark are made for distributed processing of large information sets throughout bunches of computer systems. Although Hadoop is commonly used for rapid distributed processing, it has numerous disadvantages. As an example, it certainly does not utilise 'In-memory calculation', which is nothing but always keeping the information in RAM as an alternative of Hard Disk for rapid handling. The in-memory calculation makes it possible for a lot faster handling of Big records. When Apache Spark was created, it overcame this problem by using In-memory calculation for swift computer. MapReduce is likewise used commonly, when the task is actually to process massive quantities of records, in analogue (greater than one machines are doing a specific task simultaneously), on huge sets. In straightforward phrases, dispersed processing is only a circulated device, where numerous machines carry out certain work at the same time. Dispersed computing is beneficial when there is a requirement of fast processing (calculation) on huge records. Hadoop and Spark are made for dispersed processing of huge data collections all over sets of pcs.

8.6.2 Spark MLlib

Apache Spark also packages collections for applying artificial intelligence and chart evaluation approaches to information at a variety. Trigger MLlib includes a framework for generating machine learning pipe-lines, allowing for really effortless execution of feature extraction, options, in addition to changes on any sort of structured dataset. MLlib attributes distributed executions of clustering, and additionally, classification algorithms like k-means concentration and random rainforests can be exchanged basics of tailored pipe-lines very easily. Styles may be trained by info researchers in Apache Spark using R or even Python, spared utilising MLlib, and afterwards imported into a Scala-based or java-based pipe-line to create consumption.

Keep in mind that while Spark MLlib deals with fundamental equipment finding out including type, regression, concentration, as well as filtering, it does indeed not include centres for modelling as well as instruction deep neural networks.

8.7 Compartmental Models in Epidemiology

8.7.1 SEIR Model

For many significant contagions, here is a notable gestation retro throughout which individuals consume remained diseased but remain not contagious themselves. Throughout this duration, the person resides in section E (for subjected) (Fig. 8.13).

Presumptuous that the development retro is a chance mutable with exponential delivery with limit *a* (i.e. the average incubation period is *a*^{−1}*a*^{−1}), and also assuming the presence of vital dynamics with birth rate Lambda equal to death rate mu, we have the model:

$$\frac{dS}{dt} = \mu N - vS - \frac{\beta SI}{N} \tag{8.1}$$

$$\frac{dE}{dt} = \frac{\beta SI}{N} - vE - \sigma E \tag{8.2}$$

$$\frac{dI}{dt} = \sigma E - \gamma I - vI \tag{8.3}$$

$$\frac{dR}{dt} = \gamma I - vR \tag{8.4}$$

We followed the equation $X + Y + P + Q = S$, but this is first continuous because of the (degenerate) supposition that birth and death rates are equal; in general, S is a variable (Fig. 8.14).

8.7.2 ARIMA Model

ARIMA stands for Autoregressive Integrated Moving Average models. Univariate (solitary vector) ARIMA is an estimating procedure that expands the future evaluations of a setup dependent by itself inactivity. Its concept application remains

Fig. 8.13 Flow of SEIR model

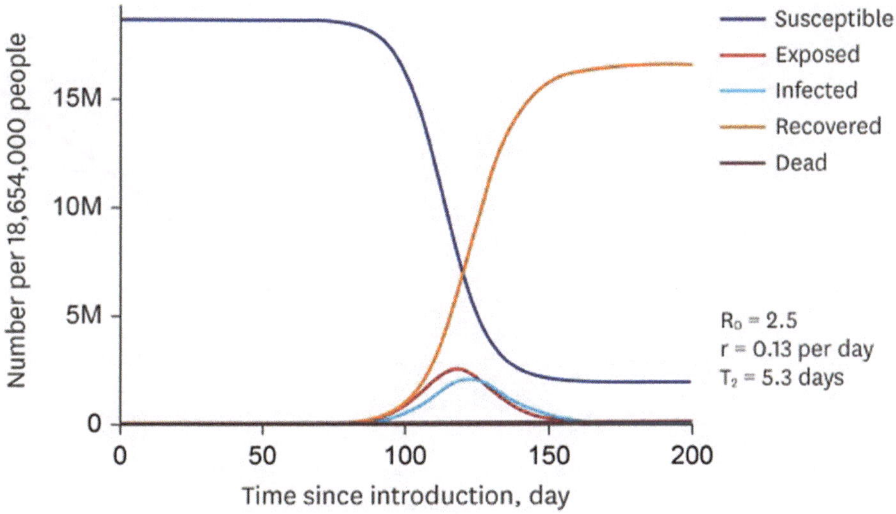

Fig. 8.14 SEIR model prediction of COVID-19

in the zone of short-lived gauging requiring at any rate 40 tape-recorded details concentrates. When your info shows a foreseeable or constant example after some time with a base procedure of exceptions, it functions best. ARIMA strategy undertakings to illustrate the advancements in a set time plan as a part of what is designated 'autoregressive as well as relocating regular' borders. These are alluded to as AR borders (autoregressive) and MA boundaries (relocating axes). An AR model with simply a single border might be composed as ... (Fig. 8.15)

$$X(t) = A(1) \times X(t-1) + E(t)$$

where

$X(t)$ = time series under investigation
$A(1)$ = the autoregressive parameter of order 1
$X(t-1)$ = the time series lagged 1 period
$E(t)$ = the error term of the model

Based on applied the ARIMA version to fit the historical data of the spread of COVID-19 in India. We got results reveals that we are experiencing the peak in these days. For the next 30 days, an increment is to be anticipated in the variety of infected, deceased and recouped individuals. Evidence of the design is provided by the price quotes of both the reproductive and implied incubation period acquired, which are similar to the values existing in literary works. An even more strong study must be applied.

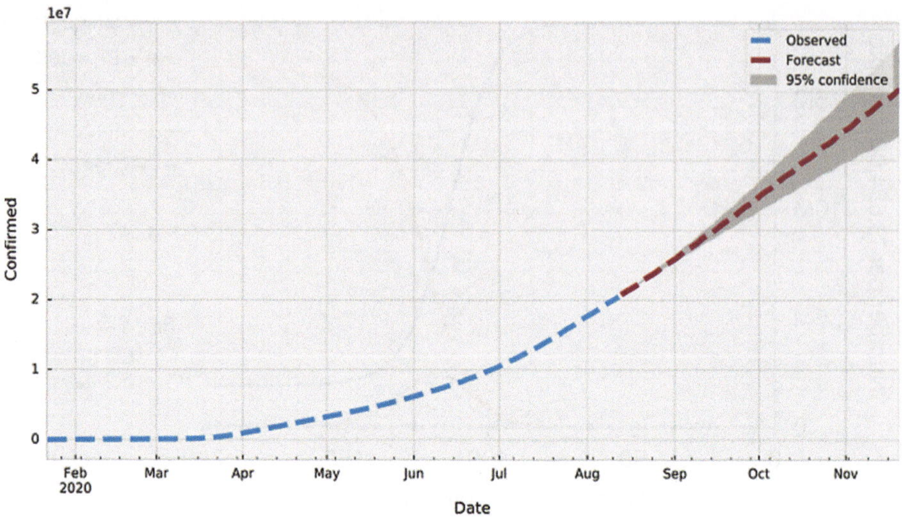

Fig. 8.15 ARIMA forecast

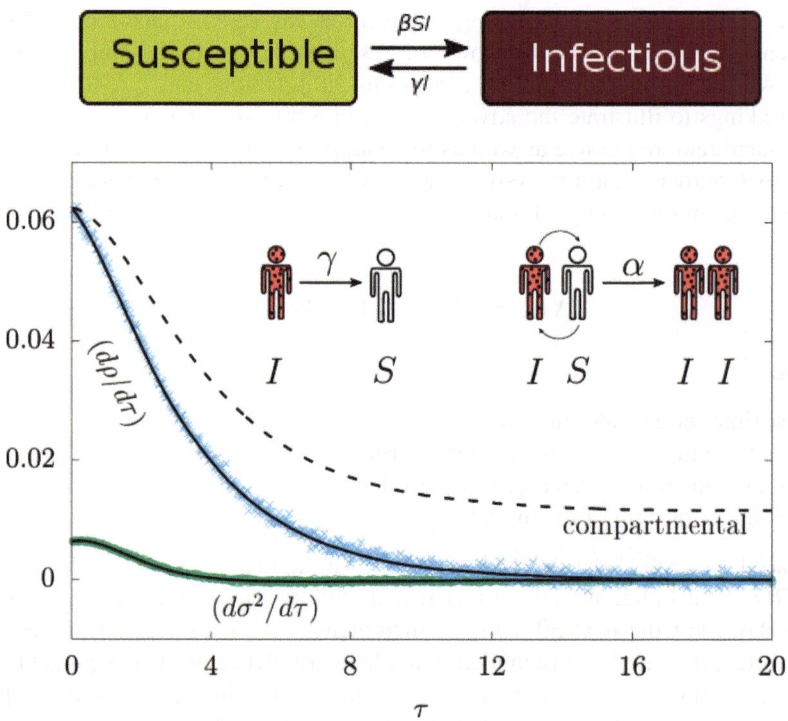

Fig. 8.16 SAS forecast

8.7.3 SIS Model

As an instance, some diseases, persons after the taciturn in addition to cold, prepare not to offer any permanent protection. Such contaminations carry out certainly not offer immunity upon healing coming from disease, and likewise, individuals find yourself being at danger once more. It is feasible to discover a logical answer toward this style (by creating an improvement of variables: $I = y\hat{}\{-1\}I = y\hat{}\{\{-1\}\}$ and relieving this into the mean-field reckonings), such that the rudimentary imitation rate is better than agreement (Fig. 8.16). The answer is assumed by way of

$$I(t) = \frac{I\infty}{1 + Ve} \tag{8.5}$$

8.8 Conclusion

In the present scenario, not having any immediate behaving foe of the popular supervisor and inoculations, the design exposed several vital ideas. Many essentially, the enormity of the prevalent is commonly under-reported. They predict that scenarios and deaths with 19 June 2020 are 13.8 and 2.48 times greater than the main records throughout the 85 states measured. Despite these raised statistics, the critics note that no republic stands from another location near developing herd immunity.

This chapter gives detailed knowledge of coronavirus's background, the outbreak of corona with in India and outside the world. It provides a statistical analysis of corona concerning age group and state wise. With this prediction, it will be expected that this Coronavirus COVID-19 outbreak may end in India by December 2020 based on the statistical data, prevention techniques and analysis done by using SEIR, ARIMA and SIS model.

References

1. V.C.C. Cheng, S.K.P. Lau, P.C.Y. Woo, Y.Y. Kwok, Severe acute respiratory syndrome coronavirus as an agent of emerging and re-emerging infection. Clin. Microbiol. Rev. **20**(4), 660–694 (2007). https://doi.org/10.1128/CMR.00023-07
2. J.-F. Dhainaut, Y.-E. Claessens, J. Janes, D.R. Nelson, Underlying disorders and their impact on the host response to infection. Clin. Infect. Dis. **41**(Suppl_7), S481–S489 (2005). https://doi.org/10.1086/432001
3. W. Li et al., Broad receptor engagement of an emerging global coronavirus may potentiate its diverse cross-species transmissibility. Proc. Natl. Acad. Sci. U. S. A. **115**(22), E5135–E5143 (2018). https://doi.org/10.1073/pnas.1802879115
4. A. Flahault, Has China faced only a herald wave of SARS-CoV-2? Lancet **395**(10228), 947 (2020). https://doi.org/10.1016/S0140-6736(20)30521-3

5. H.A. Mohd, J.A. Al-Tawfiq, Z.A. Memish, The Middle East Respiratory Syndrome Coronavirus (MERS-CoV) origin and animal reservoir Susanna Lau. Virol. J. **13**(1), 1–7 (2016). https://doi.org/10.1186/s12985-016-0544-0
6. World Health Organization (WHO) Eastern Mediterranean Regional Office, Laboratory confirmed cases of MERS reported in Eastern Mediterranean Region, July 2012–November 2019, https://www.who.int/emergencies/mers-cov/en/. Accessed 22 Feb 2020
7. V.C.C. Cheng, J.F.W. Chan, K.K.W. To, K.Y. Yuen, Clinical management and infection control of SARS: Lessons learned. Antivir. Res. **100**(2), 407–419 (2013). https://doi.org/10.1016/j.antiviral.2013.08.016
8. P. Wu et al., Real-time tentative assessment of the epidemiological characteristics of novel coronavirus infections in Wuhan, China, as on January 22, 2020. Eur. Secur. **25**(3), 1–6 (2020). https://doi.org/10.2807/1560-7917.ES.2020.25.3.2000044
9. C. Yeo, S. Kaushal, D. Yeo, Enteric involvement of coronaviruses: Is a fecal-oral transmission of SARS-CoV-2 possible? Lancet Gastroenterol. Hepatol. **5**(4), 335–337 (2020). https://doi.org/10.1016/S2468-1253(20)30048-0
10. US Centers for Disease Control and Prevention COVID-19 Response Team, Severe outcomes among patients with coronavirus disease 2019 (COVID-19): United States, February 12–March 16, 2020. MMWR Morb. Mortal Wkly Rep. (2020). https://doi.org/10.15585/mmwr
11. V.F. Corrales-Medina, M. Madjid, D.M. Musher, Role of acute infection in triggering acute coronary syndromes. Lancet Infect. Dis. **10**(2), 83–92 (2010). https://doi.org/10.1016/S1473-3099(09)70331-7
12. Centers for Disease Control and Prevention, SARS (10 Years After), https://www.cdc.gov/dotw/sars/index.html. Accessed 22 Feb 2020

Chapter 9
Visual Exploratory Data Analysis Technique for Epidemiological Outbreak of COVID-19 Pandemic

Joseph Bamidele Awotunde, Roseline Oluwaseun Ogundokun, Emmanuel Abidemi Adeniyi, and Sanjay Misra

9.1 Introduction

An occurrence of infectious disease is a disease that is not normally supposed to occur in a single population, geographic area or time [1]. An infectious disease usually entails accelerated dissemination, jeopardizing individuals' vast statistics' wellbeing, and therefore demands urgent intervention to prevent the spread of the illness at the population stage [2]. COVID-19 is triggered by a novel form of coronavirus earlier identified by the World Health Organization (WHO) as 2019-nCoV. MERS-nCoV and SARS-nCoV are among the seven documented human coronaviruses which are usually transmitted from human to human [3–5]. The infection signs include fever, coughing, shortness of breath and diarrhoea. COVID-19 also causes pneumonia and even death in more serious cases [5]. COVID-19's incubation cycle will last up to 2 weeks or longer [4]. The disease may also be contagious during the time of latent infection. The virus can spread by respiratory droplets and close contact from person to person [6–8].

COVID-19 is an infectious disease first detected in December 2019 in Wuhan, China, with the town's earliest recorded outbreak. The new strain was unclear until the epidemic started in December 2019, and about 80% of infections are at

J. B. Awotunde
Department of Computer Science, University of Ilorin, Ilorin, Nigeria
e-mail: awotunde.jb@unilorin.edu.ng

R. O. Ogundokun · E. A. Adeniyi
Department of Computer Science, Landmark University, Omu-Aran, Nigeria
e-mail: ogundokun.roseline@lmu.edu.ng; adeniyi.emmanuel@lmu.edu.ng

S. Misra (✉)
Department of Electrical and Information Engineering, Covenant University, Ota, Nigeria
e-mail: sanjay.misra@covenantuniversity.edu.ng

L. Garg et al. (eds.), *Healthcare Informatics for Fighting COVID-19 and Future Epidemics*, EAI/Springer Innovations in Communication and Computing,
https://doi.org/10.1007/978-3-030-72752-9_9

comparatively mild levels. The most prominent COVID-19 symptoms are fatigue, dry cough and fever. Certain patients also show other symptoms such as nasal congestion, runny nose, aches and pains, sore throat or diarrhoea. As many patients recorded in November having to see a resident fish and wildlife market in Wuhan, the transmission of animals to humans has surprisingly retained the root of epidemics. The disease has continued to be transmitted outside of China since 15 January 2020 after one outbreak in Japan and two incidents in Korea. After H1N1 (2009), polio (2014), Ebola in West Africa (2014), Zika (2016) and Ebola in the Democratic Republic of Congo (2019), the World Health Organization (WHO) publicized on 30 January 2020 that COVID-19 pandemic is the sixth public health emergency of a global proportion. As of 28 August 2020, there were 24,926,312 confirmed cases and 840,662 deaths.

The new hysteria created by COVID-19 has put nations in quarantine, and the epidemic has risen exponentially and has been transmitted to numerous areas of the biosphere. The astonishing prevention actions engaged by the worldwide administration to stop the transmission of the disease have been flushed down the trench [9]. As victims of fear and neglect of environmental problems, nations worldwide have gone to a complete shutdown. With an increase in infectious disease warnings because the spread of the virus progresses quickly, endangering the health of the wider community, the poor are the most affected. Immediate action is necessary at the root level to combat the virus [10, 11].

The coronavirus pandemic is a global health issue that threatens the entire world's peace since the start of the new year 2020 [12]. As the number of confirmed cases infected with the disease increases daily, the death rate cases recorded is low compared to the recovery cases, making the disease less deadly but more infectious. The daily increase of cases of this infectious disease has become a huge challenge to each country's socio-economic development across the globe.

The Secretary-General of the United Nations has advised that governments of various countries should take urgent measures to contain the outspread of the infectious disease [13, 14]. One of the United Nations Sustainable Development Goals is to discuss economic, social and environmental concerns between 2015 and 2030 and change towards sustainable growth [15, 16]. The UN SDGs include 17 aims and 169 objectives. The COVID-19 pandemic unswervingly challenges the accomplishment of the above wellbeing objectives as well as influenced the achievement of financial and societal advancement goals.

The transmission features of the COVID-19 pandemic have still not been properly familiar in the sense of worldwide environmental changes [15, 16]. Furthermore, the pace of global development, increased population size, more common and nuanced encounters and lack of medical security in emerging republics all contribute to the complexities of COVID-19 deterrence and regulation. COVID-19 seems to have a greater impact on the global economy than severe acute respiratory syndrome (SARS) in 2013.

The bone of contention is how to fight the spread of this infectious disease and how it is different from the 2003 contagion. Several nations depended on the observation of definitive phases to monitor illnesses and civic wellbeing to curtail the COVID-19 contagion, similar to the ones utilized with SARS in 2003 [17]. They cover from extreme seclusion actions in China (for instance, enclosing greater than 60 million of individuals in Hubei jurisdiction) to wide interaction management with hundreds of connection tracers (for instance, Singapore, Hong Kong and South Korea). Nevertheless, these interventions may not be successful in tackling the COVID-19 scale by 2020. Therefore, this chapter discusses the possible application of big data and analytics to improve conventional public health approaches to control, manage, identify and avoid COVID-19 and reduce its health effects implicitly.

To date, most reported cases globally have a travel history to Wuhan. Thus, the illness has spread widely globally since the early 2020. The WHO named the contagion COVID-19 which is triggered by 2019-nCoV on 11 February 2020. Day by day, the COVID-19 disease situation is getting serious and to further prevent and control this infectious disease, it is imperative to better understand the nature of this pandemic. For situational awareness and intervention, a rapid, quick and accessible epidemiological data are needed. The recent outbreak of COVID-19 underlines the significance of investigating the disease's epidemiological data and forecasting the dangers of contaminating individuals all over the world with this disease. Therefore, the investigation gathers and analyses epidemiological data of COVID-19 based on the Worldometer dataset for exploratory data analysis with imaging of the dataset to understand the number of cases recorded (confirmed, death, recovered, active and critical cases) globally. This was done to comprehend the risk and commence control actions to control this deadly novel virus; thus, it is extremely significant to willingly offer proper treatment, management and evaluation. The contribution of this study is as follows:

- The study on coronavirus could be useful as epidemiological data that is required if there are emergent contagions to forestall and best manage the transmission of ailments.
- The study on coronavirus infectious disease could be useful for governments and physicians to make decisions, thus lessening the danger of COVID-19 among the populace around the world.
- The study could be used as a reference for evaluation in future work.
- The study can be useful in COVID-19 treatment, awareness and management.
- The study be imperative for menace conveyance, supervision and assessment all through occurrences.
- The work provides deeper knowledge of the diagnosis and occurrence of coronavirus infection.

The paper is structured in five sections. Section 9.2 provides the background and literature review. The methodology is summarized in Sect. 9.3. Result and discussion and a conclusion drawn are given in Sects. 9.4 and 9.5, respectively.

9.2 Related Work

COVID-19 has quickly spread worldwide since this initial news. The WHO has declared a Public Health Emergency of International Concern (PHEIC) under the updated International Health Regulations on 30 January 2020 [18]. COVID-19 has been transmitted to all continents excluding Antarctica since the PHEIC announcement and has been a highly contagious pandemic with continuous population dissemination [19, 20]. The magnitude of the COVID-19 epidemic, with about 24,926,312 cases worldwide as of 28 August 2020, has much exceeded the previous coronavirus outbreaks, with the Middle East respiratory syndrome (MERS) having 2494 cases as of November 2019 and the 2003 SARS coronavirus having greater than 8000 cases which affected 26 nations [21, 22].

Whether virus mutations can cause outlines of yearly recurrence as perceived by infection strains is unclear. Efforts to forecast epidemiological characteristics (e.g. frequency, attack risk, rate of occurrence or regeneration, morbidity and mortality) of an epidemic are essential to notify infectious prevention and countermeasures for public health. This can be daunting in the initial periods of an epidemic with slight knowledge about the disease's aetiology, limited diagnosis and monitoring resources and inadequate epidemiological evidence on confirmed cases [22–24]. In the deficiency of data as mentioned earlier, the utilization of information in an automated setting, for instance, data procedural analysis and incidence visualization, will allow syndromic surveillance approaches to classify the spread of diseases and provide more rapid counts of accurate cases [9, 25, 26]. Dey et al. [25] assemble and scrutinize COVID-19 epidemiological epidemic statistics based on various free COVID-19 databases given by Johns Hopkins University, the World Health Organization, the Chinese Center for Disease Control and Prevention, the National Health Commission and DXY. Investigative data scrutiny with visualizations was used to gather and calculate the sum of confirmed, death and recuperated cases in various areas of China and globally. Identifying an epidemic like this is extremely critical to provide knowledge readily to begin the assessment which is necessary in recognizing the dangers and commencing restraint actions.

Authors [9] performed an exploratory COVID-19 analysis using the Kerala model. Data were obtained from various sources, and the study was split into three stages. The first stage starts from 30 January to 9 March 2020; the second stage begins from 10 March to 8 May 2020; and the third stage from 9 May to 31 May 2020. The data processing was carried out using MATLAB tools. The findings show that the government's actions have ensured that the virus is contained in the population affected. Communication tracking and home quarantine also limited group gatherings. During lockdown, health steps taken helped residents respond to the changes. Community-spreading abstinence still holds high. Aside from fighting the COVID-19 disease, Kerala has made the lives of Kerala residents happier with a set of welfare initiatives. Kerala's model for tackling COVID-19 could be viewed as a yardstick for how public health department should be adequately used.

Authors [25] proposed an investigative data scrutiny method to gather as well as interpret COVID-19 epidemiological outbreak data based on Bangladesh's initial openly accessible COVID-19 day-to-day dataset. For this report, numerous publicly available data antecedents on the outbreak of COVID-19 supported by the IEDCR, the World Health Organization (WHO), the Directorate General of Health Services (DGHS) and the Bangladesh Ministry of Health and Family Welfare (MOHFW) were used. The visual exploratory data analysis (V-EDA) was used between 8 March 2020 and 13 August 2020 to explain the epidemiological characteristics of COVID-19 outbreaks in various parts of Bangladesh, and these results were compared with those of other nations. Moreover, it is highly necessary to disseminate information promptly to identify the threats of this contagion and launch public restraint actions. Therefore, the availability of epidemiological data and its critical interpretation are essential in raising awareness of guiding policies and actions during the COVID-19 outbreak.

9.3 Methodology and Data Analysis

Secondary data collected from the Worldometer website was used as a dataset in this article, containing information on COVID-19 disease infections, i.e. confirmed, death, recovered and active cases. The data used were from January to April 2020 (4 months). The dataset consists of the furthermost accepted warning signs of COVID-19: fever, tiredness and dry cough. Aches and pains, sore throat, nasal congestion, runny nose or diarrhoea may also occur in some patients as discovered.

Computational scrutiny of the data was completed to visualize the incidence of the COVID-19 total confirmed, death, recovered and active cases to provide deeper knowledge of the occurrence and possible use by governments, private organizations and physicians to make decisions for future occurrence of any infectious disease. For the basic analysis of the dataset, linear regression was used. Data analysis is used to find the trends and future directives and applied in various application areas [27–29].

9.4 Results and Discussion

The COVID-19 epidemic was followed by an 'infodemic' which is simply an overabundance of information about it. Because some of the publicly accessible information might not be correct, it has been difficult for individuals to locate credible antecedent and trustworthy advice when they require it [30]. Owing to the strong request for accurate and dependable information on COVID-19, WHO's strategic risk coordination and social networking crews worked carefully to control and answer the mythologies and rumours about the disease through its head office in Geneva and its six district workplaces together with its associates. The organization is actively at work to recognize the utmost predominant myths that can affect the populace's wellbeing, such as misleading preventive programmes or cure reports. Then these theories are rebutted with the facts founded on evidence. The WHO provides information and recommendations on public health about COVID-19, like imaginary busters, accessible on its social networking platforms (like Weibo, Twitter, Facebook, Instagram, LinkedIn, Pinterest) and its Internet site [18]. The reaction of people to the broadcast of a transmitting communicable ailment is probable direct to the raised fear and increased expectations of the danger [31]. Social networking platforms have been operating as outlets for immediate statistics in which the community can access into if there are outbreaks of communicable illnesses. These networks also allow for easy and fast real-time exchange of information with families, colleagues and neighbours Oh, Lee, and Han [34].

COVID-19 daily event data were obtained from Worldometer's official website (https://www.worldometers.info/coronavirus/) from 15 January 2020 to 28 August 2020. Microsoft Excel package and Statistical Student Social Package (SSSP) were used to create a statistical table. A linear regression study was used to test the data collection, and detailed analyses were also carried out on the dataset. The data are listed under separate labels as overall cases, total deaths, total recovered, active cases and serious/critical cases per continent. To comprehend the sum of the various crises mentioned, data analysis with imaginations was given. Generally, it is very important to have details as soon as an epidemic like this starts, commence the assessment required to identify the threats and commence restraint actions.

The distribution of confirmed COVID-19 cases among the continents as of 28 August 2020 is shown in Tables 9.1, 9.2 and Fig. 9.1. The Oceania has the least case of COVID-19 follow by African with a higher different from what is obtainable in Oceania countries and Europe came third with a very higher case compared with Oceanic and African but very lower than the remaining (3) analysed continents. The sum of demises is very trivial compared to the number of confirmed cases in all the continents. The sum of recovered cases is very significantly higher than the sum of the established cases. The active cases are also very trivial when compared with severe/critical cases. Therefore, attributed to the low number of death cases recorded across all the continents compared with confirmed cases.

It means that the lockdown, international border closure instituted in some nations and sit at home reduce the rate of spread of COVID-19 globally when

Table 9.1 COVID-19 cases by continent

Continent	Overall cases	Total deaths	Total recovered	Active cases	Serious, critical
Europe	3,509,878	206,931	2,045,742	1,257,205	5639
North America	7,210,608	267,457	4,134,346	2,808,805	20,528
Asia	6,785,167	138,143	5,413,183	1,233,841	18,637
South America	6,131,708	198,378	4,709,004	1,224,326	15,117
Africa	1,233,365	29,141	964,846	239,318	1289
Oceania	28,148	612	22,674	4862	49

Table 9.2 Percentages of coronavirus cases by continent

Continent	% of total cases	% of total deaths	% of total recovered	% of total active cases	% of total serious, critical
Europe	14.08	24.62	11.83	18.57	9.21
North America	28.93	31.82	23.91	41.50	33.51
Asia	24.60	16.43	31.31	18.23	30.42
South America	27.33	23.60	27.20	18.09	24.68
Africa	4.95	3.47	5.58	3.54	2.10
Oceania	0.11	0.07	0.13	0.07	0.08

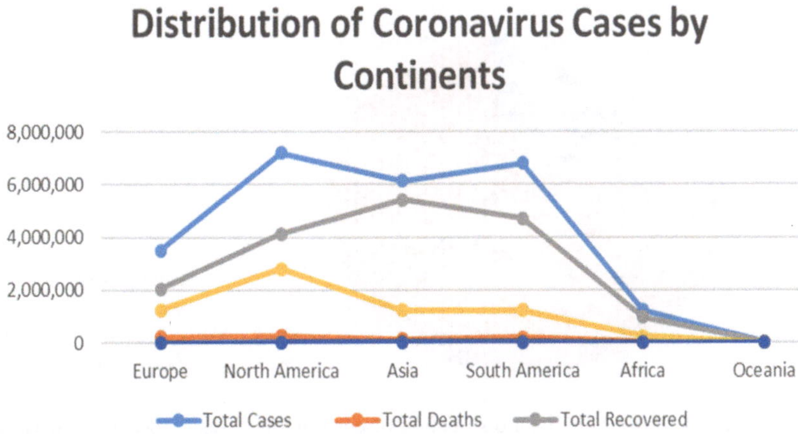

Fig. 9.1 Line graph showing the distribution of coronavirus cases by continent

comparing the index of the confirmed case in August to earlier months. Amazingly, the total recovered cases reported in August 2020 were significantly higher than the previous case globally, and it was around 17,289,795. It was around 69.36%, which more than 50% of the total confirmed cases. This shows significant improvement compared with the earlier case of the outbreak because the recovered case is very low and less than 50% of the total confirmed cases globally.

Table 9.3 describes the coefficient of total cases against the total deaths. The percentage of total death cases (total deaths, $b = 25.009$, $p = 0.025$) seems to be unrelated to the total cases confirmed. This shows that there are low death cases compared to the total cases confirmed daily. This is also related to Fig. 9.2, which shows a lower death rate of 3% of the total confirmed cases. Table 9.3 and Fig. 9.2 signify that there is hope of recovery from this deadly infectious disease when basic hygiene is maintained and rules are strictly followed.

Table 9.4 shows that the total recovered cases ($b = 1.325$) are not significant ($p = 0.003$). Its coefficient is positive, indicating that exertions have been set in place to reduce the number of active cases of COVID-19 globally. The measures put in place are yielding positively compared to the earlier outbreak of the pandemic. However, there is still room for improvement for the government, health workers,

Table 9.3 The coefficients of total cases and total deaths

Coefficients[a]						
Model		Unstandardized coefficients		Standardized coefficients	*t*	Sig.
		b	Std. error	Beta		
1	(Constant)	650,373.107	1,212,809.467		0.536	0.620
	Total deaths	25.009	7.129	0.869	3.508	0.025

[a]Dependent variable: total cases

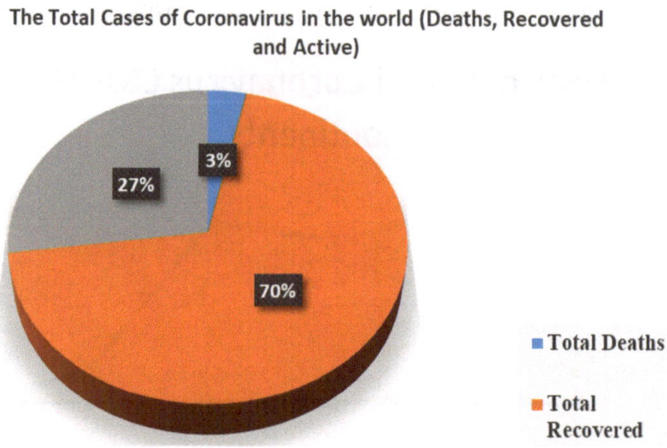

Fig. 9.2 Pie chart showing the total distribution of coronavirus cases by deaths, recovered and active

Table 9.4 The coefficients of total cases and total recovered

Coefficients[a]						
Model		Unstandardized coefficients		Standardized coefficients	*t*	Sig.
		B	Std. error	Beta		
1	(Constant)	335,401.483	750,356.974		0.447	0.678
	Total recovered	1.325	0.214	0.952	6.190	0.003

[a]Dependent variable: total cases

and individuals to get a higher recovery rate. According to Fig. 9.2, the rate of recovered cases is very high compared to the active cases in a mild or critical state.

According to Table 9.5, the active case is very low as compared to the total case. The effect of active cases ($b = 2.595$, $p = 0.034$) is significant that the greater active case proportion low when compared with the total case and the total recovered cases recorded. The active case is associated with the positive result of the measures put in place to fight the outbreak globally. The high number of transmissions proportionally reduced when compared with the active cases and the number of recovered cases is very high in recently; but this can still be reduced dramatically by the enforcement of total lockdown, isolation and the use of face mask imposed in most nations.

Table 9.5 The coefficients of total cases and total active cases

Coefficients[a]						
Model		Unstandardized coefficients		Standardized coefficients	*t*	Sig.
		B	Std. error	Beta		
1	(Constant)	1,227,368.781	1,185,596.904		1.035	0.359
	Active cases	2.595	0.820	0.845	3.165	0.034

[a]Dependent variable: total cases

Table 9.6 The coefficients of total cases and total serious/critical cases

Coefficients[a]						
Model		Unstandardized coefficients		Standardized coefficients	*t*	Sig.
		B	Std. error	Beta		
1	(Constant)	824,686.728	580,973.533		1.419	0.229
	Serious/critical	326.127	44.326	0.965	7.357	0.002

[a]Dependent variable: total cases

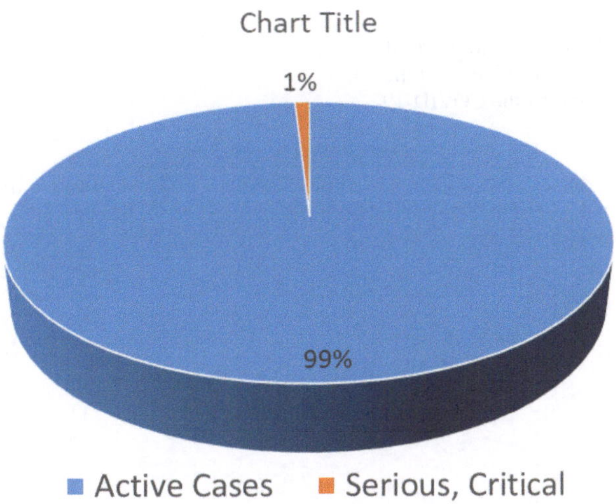

Fig. 9.3 Pie chart showing the total distribution of coronavirus cases by mild and critical cases

Table 9.6 shows the critical/serious case ($b = 326.127$); this variable is not significant ($p = 0.002$). However, more efforts are still needed to be put in place to maintain the lower critical cases than the mild cases, as displayed in Fig. 9.3. This can be achieved when people are tested for COVID-19 at an early stage. At all levels, the government makes the test available and affordable especially for the poor in the streets. By doing so, the COVID-19 disease with a higher recovery rate than the death rate (Fig. 9.4) will be, if not eliminated, controlled and contained to the nearest minimum in our streets (Table 9.7).

COVID-19 contagion situation may be unsolidified, and the 12 most countries worst hit by the virus are by now well-known. As of 28 August 2020, the United States has the highest confirmed cases with 5,811,519 (23.31%) followed by Brazil

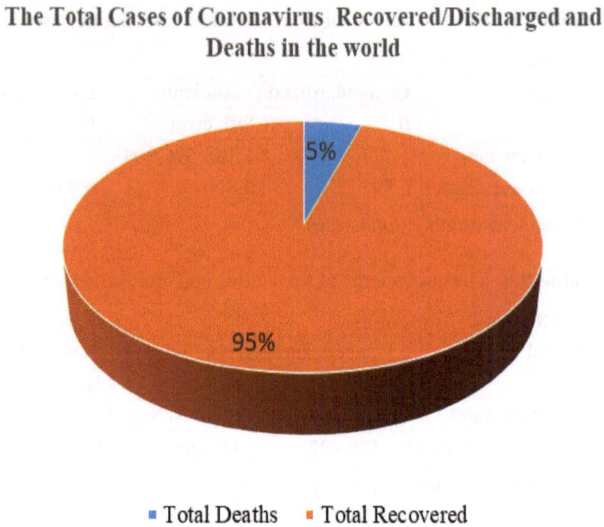

Fig. 9.4 The total distribution of coronavirus cases by recovered/discharged and death cases

Table 9.7 The 12 most affected countries of the world by the COVID-19

S. no	Country	Total cases
1	United States	5,811,519
2	Brazil	3,761,391
3	India	3,463,973
4	Russian Federation	985,346
5	Peru	621,997
6	South Africa	620,132
7	Colombia	582,022
8	Mexico	579,914
9	Spain	439,286
10	Chile	405,972
11	Argentina	380,292
12	Iran	369,911

with 3,761,391 (15.09%) and India with 3,463,973 (13.90%), making them the centres of the outbreak (Fig. 9.5).

The spread of COVID-19 virus appears to be slightly decreasing compared with earlier outbreaks in China. The most important tool any country has to track the impact of COVID-19 infection remains the number of deaths in test-positive cases [32, 33]. According to the results explained above, the virus appears to be highly contagious. Still, it seems less deadly than Ebola, Lassa fever and yellow fever, among others [22, 34] in parts of Africa and even worldwide. And there is no certainty that the behaviour of the disease will be the same or manifest to the same extent in Africa as described globally.

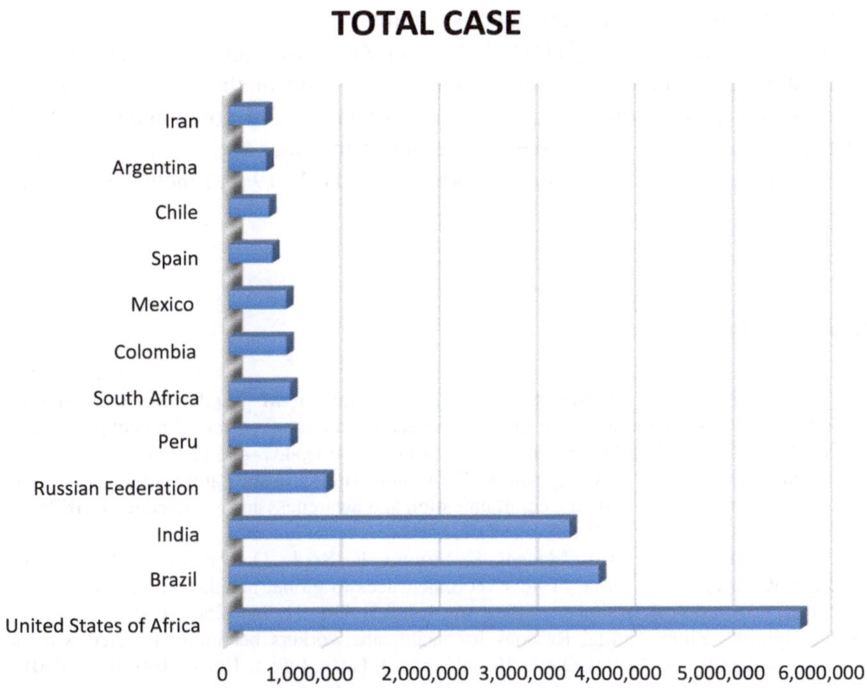

Fig. 9.5 The highest confirmed cases of COVID-19 by country

9.5 Conclusion

COVID-19 disease has been acknowledged as an international threat and, currently, has been recorded in 213 countries and regions around the world. The datasets were analysed using linear regression tools to picture those data to offer a satisfactory perception concerning the outbreak of COVID-19 globally. In this study, the data is visualized and analysed between 15 January and 28 August 2020. The United States has the highest confirmed cases with 5,811,519, while Brazil, India, Russian Federation, Peru and South Africa have 3,761,391, 3,463,973, 985,346, 621,997 and 620,132 confirmed cases, respectively. Other countries that were badly affected now comprise of Colombia with 582,022 confirmed cases, Mexico with 579,914 confirmed cases, Spain with 439,286 confirmed cases, Chile with 405,972 confirmed cases, Argentina with 380,292 confirmed cases and lastly Iran with 369,911 confirmed cases. Interestingly, six of these countries are from Europe, and Asia with three countries while the rest have high instances of COVID-19. From the scrutiny of the COVID-19 dataset, it could be concluded that the confirmed cases are increasing daily, with Europe topping the list of the region with the highest total confirmed and death cases. As of 28 August 2020, the total number of confirmed cases is 24,926,312, and the total number of death cases is 840,662. This showed that the

COVID-19 outbreak is very contagious but not too deadly compared to the previous pandemics such as Ebola, H1N1, Polio and Zika virus outbreaks. Therefore, the exploratory and data analysis using linear regression methods is a powerful tool for assisting government and public health planning and policymaking. The data visualization model also provides an interactive interface and will provide effective ways to understand the epidemic outbreak of COVID-19 and inclusively visualize every fact.

References

1. D. Toppenberg-Pejcic, J. Noyes, T. Allen, N. Alexander, M. Vanderford, G. Gamhewage, Emergency risk communication: Lessons learned from a rapid review of recent gray literature on Ebola, Zika, and Yellow Fever. Health Commun. **34**(4), 437–455 (2019)
2. L. Lin, R.F. McCloud, C.A. Bigman, K. Viswanath, Tuning in and catching on? Examining the relationship between pandemic communication and awareness and knowledge of MERS in the USA. J. Public Health **39**(2), 282–289 (2017)
3. D.S. Hui, E.I. Azhar, T.A. Madani, F. Ntoumi, R. Kock, O. Dar, et al., The continuing 2019-nCoV epidemic threat of novel coronaviruses to global health—The latest 2019 novel coronavirus outbreak in Wuhan, China. Int. J. Infect. Dis. **91**, 264–266 (2020)
4. J. Wang, M. Zhou, F. Liu, Reasons for healthcare workers becoming infected with novel coronavirus disease 2019 (COVID-19) in China. J. Hosp. Infect. **105**(1), 100–101 (2020)
5. World Health Organization, *Advice on the Use of Masks for Children in the Community in the Context of COVID-19: Annex to the Advice on the Use of Masks in the Context of COVID-19*, 21 August 2020 (No. WHO/2019-nCoV/IPC_Masks/Children/2020.1) (World Health Organization, 2020)
6. S. Bialek et al., Severe outcomes among patients with coronavirus disease 2019 (COVID-19)—United States, February 12–March 16, 2020. MMWR Morb. Mortal. Wkly Rep. **69**(12), 343–346 (2020) https://www.cdc.gov/mmwr/volumes/69/wr/mm6912e2.htm#contribAff
7. S. Bialek, R. Gierke, M. Hughes, T. Skoff, Coronavirus disease 2019 in children—United States, February 12–April 2, 2020. Morb. Mortal. Wkly Rep. **69**(14), 422 (2020) https://www.cdc.gov/mmwr/volumes/69/wr/mm6914e4.htm#contribAff
8. L. Garg, E. Chukwu, N. Nasser, C. Chakraborty, G. Garg, Anonymity preserving IoT-based COVID-19 and other infectious disease contact tracing model. IEEE Access **8**, 159402–159414 (2020)
9. S. Jayesh, S. Sreedharan, Analyzing the Covid-19 cases in Kerala: A visual exploratory data analysis approach. SN Compr. Clin. Med. **2020**, 1–12 (2020)
10. F.B. Hamzah, C. Lau, H. Nazri, D.V. Ligot, G. Lee, C.L. Tan, CoronaTracker: Worldwide COVID-19 outbreak data analysis and prediction. Bull. World Health Organ. **1**, 32 (2020)
11. S.K. Dey, M.M. Rahman, U.R. Siddiqi, A. Howlader, Analyzing the epidemiological outbreak of COVID-19: A visual exploratory data analysis approach. J. Med. Virol. **92**(6), 632–638 (2020)
12. M. Ienca, E. Vayena, On the responsible use of digital data to tackle the COVID-19 pandemic. Nat. Med. **26**(4), 463–464 (2020)
13. S. Chen, J. Yang, W. Yang, C. Wang, T. Bärnighausen, COVID-19 control in China during mass population movements at New Year. Lancet **395**(10226), 764–766 (2020)
14. L. Peng, W. Yang, D. Zhang, C. Zhuge, L. Hong, Epidemic analysis of COVID-19 in China by dynamical modeling, arXiv preprint arXiv:2002.06563 (2020)
15. A.E. Ling, Y.S. Leo, Potential presymptomatic transmission of SARS-CoV-2, Zhejiang Province, China, 2020. Emerg. Infect. Dis. **26**(5), 1052–1054 (2020)

16. C. Zhou, F. Su, T. Pei, A. Zhang, Y. Du, B. Luo, et al., COVID-19: Challenges to GIS with big data. Geogr. Sustain. **1**, 77–87 (2020)
17. D.S.W. Ting, L. Carin, V. Dzau, T.Y. Wong, Digital technology and COVID-19. Nat. Med. **26**, 459–461 (2020)
18. World Health Organization, *Novel Coronavirus (2019-nCoV): Situation Report, 13* (World Health Organization, Geneva, 2020)
19. V. Surveillances, The epidemiological characteristics of an outbreak of 2019 novel coronavirus diseases (COVID-19)—China, 2020. China CDC Week. **2**(8), 113–122 (2020)
20. Epidemiology Working Group for NCIP Epidemic Response, Chinese Center for Disease Control and Prevention, The epidemiological characteristics of an outbreak of 2019 novel coronavirus diseases (COVID-19) in China. Zhonghua Liu Xing Bing Xue Za Zhi **41**(2), 145 (2020)
21. C. Wang, P.W. Horby, F.G. Hayden, G.F. Gao, A novel coronavirus outbreak of global health concern. Lancet **395**(10223), 470–473 (2020)
22. R.O. Ogundokun, A.F. Lukman, G.B. Kibria, J.B. Awotunde, B.B. Aladeitan, Predictive modeling of COVID-19 confirmed cases in Nigeria. Infect. Dis. Model. **5**, 543–548 (2020)
23. R.O. Ogundokun, J.B. Awotunde, Machine learning prediction for COVID 19 pandemic in India, medRxiv (2020)
24. C.D. Kelly-Cirino, J. Nkengasong, H. Kettler, I. Tongio, F. Gay-Andrieu, C. Escadafal, et al., Importance of diagnostics in epidemic and pandemic preparedness. BMJ Glob. Health **4**(Suppl 2), e001179 (2019)
25. S.K. Dey, M.M. Rahman, U.R. Siddiqi, A. Howlader, Exploring epidemiological behavior of novel coronavirus (COVID-19) outbreak in Bangladesh. SN Compr. Clin. Med. **2020**, 1–9 (2020)
26. J. Li, Q. Xu, R. Cuomo, V. Purushothaman, T. Mackey, Data mining and content analysis of the Chinese social media platform Weibo during the early COVID-19 outbreak: Retrospective observational infoveillance study. JMIR Public Health Surveill. **6**(2), e18700 (2020)
27. S.I. Popoola, A.A. Atayero, O.F. Steve-Essi, S. Misra, Data analytics: Global contributions of world continents to computer science research, in *International Conference on Computational Science and Its Applications*, (Springer, Cham, 2019), pp. 512–524
28. O. Jonathan, S. Misra, E. Ibanga, R. Maskeliunas, R. Damasevicius, R. Ahuja, Design and implementation of a mobile webcast application with google analytics and cloud messaging functionality. J. Phys. Conf. Ser. **1235**(1), 012023 (2019)
29. M.Y. Patil, C.A. Dhawale, S. Misra, Analytical study of combined approaches to content based image retrieval systems. Int. J. Pharm. Technol. **8**(4), 22982–22995 (2016)
30. World Health Organization, *2019 Novel Coronavirus (2019-nCoV): Strategic Preparedness and Response Plan* (World Health Organization, Geneva, 2020)
31. C. Chew, G. Eysenbach, Pandemics in the age of Twitter: A content analysis of Tweets during the 2009 H1N1 outbreak. PLoS One **5**(11), e14118 (2010)
32. M.C. Read, Rapid risk assessment: outbreak of Ebola virus disease in West Africa, 8 April 2014 (ECDC, edited) (2016)
33. K.M. Edwards, S. Kochhar, Ethics of conducting clinical research in an outbreak setting. Annu. Rev. Virol. **7**(1), 475–494 (2020)
34. D. Benvenuto, M. Giovanetti, L. Vassallo, S. Angeletti, M. Ciccozzi, Application of the ARIMA model on the COVID-2019 epidemic dataset. Data Brief **29**, 105340 (2020)
35. S.H. Oh, S.Y. Lee, C. Han, The effects of social media use on preventive behaviors during infectious disease outbreaks: The mediating role of self-relevant emotions and public risk perception. Health Commun., 1–10 (2020)

Chapter 10
Machine Learning Approach Using KPCA-SVMs for Predicting COVID-19

Micheal Olaolu Arowolo, Roseline Oluwaseun Ogundokun, Sanjay Misra, Akeem Femi Kadri, and Tahir Olanrewaju Aduragba

10.1 Introduction

The world has met numerous epidemics in the past decades. Lately, a deadly sickness identified as COVID-19 has surfaced from China [1, 2]. Inimitable public health adversity is triggered by severe acute respiratory syndrome coronavirus 2 (SARS-CoV-2) [2–4]. The World Health Organization (WHO) termed the new epidemic as COVID-19. It is acknowledged as a Public Health Emergency of International Concern since the beginning of 2020. It was considered an epidemic around the first quarter of 2020 [5–7], as Americans joined forces with investigative institutions and scientific concerns for global artificial intelligence (AI) investigators' activities in evolving groundbreaking machine learning measures that will help tackle COVID-19 linked surveys [3]. COVID-19 is a novel solitary intelligent ribonucleic acid (RNA) germ comprising of a huge pathological genomic sequence. It alters advances fast with no specific limitation for evaluating or investigating techniques or suitable medications. Secluding infected individuals by quarantining is the utmost way of safeguarding the universe from more escalation of the deadly COVID-19 [8].

Currently, the utmost reliable analytical examination takes time as far as a week, hence, vulnerable to unevenly accurate, raising the risk of unproductive

M. O. Arowolo · R. O. Ogundokun
Department of Computer Science, Landmark University, Omu-Aran, Nigeria
e-mail: ogundokun.roseline@lmu.edu.ng

S. Misra (✉)
Department of Electrical and Information Engineering, Covenant University, Ota, Nigeria
e-mail: sanjay.misra@covenantuniversity.edu.ng

A. F. Kadri · T. O. Aduragba
Department of Computer Science, Kwara State University, Malete, Nigeria

L. Garg et al. (eds.), *Healthcare Informatics for Fighting COVID-19 and Future Epidemics*, EAI/Springer Innovations in Communication and Computing,
https://doi.org/10.1007/978-3-030-72752-9_10

dissemination of medical kits and resources. There is a necessity for instantaneous findings for medical and precautionary actions [9].

Machine learning has proven to be an advanced method for discovering relevant information for the society of forthcoming immoderations and inconsistent discovery of outliers through developing data-driven health conditions, calculating risk scores, utilizing machine learning models for testing and training purposes, utilizing classification approaches, and developing application platforms, among others [10]. In a rapid period of COVID-19 occurrence, innovative machine learning procedures have been proposed in classifying COVID-19 genomes [11], subsistence prognosis of acute COVID-19 patients [12], and CRISPR-based COVID-19 discovery evaluation [13] and realizing probable medication candidates counter to COVID-19 [14]. Continuous efforts are ongoing to progress innovative investigative methods using machine learning procedures such as machine learning-built transmission of SARS-CoV-2 analytical strategies with a CRISPR-built infectious discovery structure [10]. Neural network classifiers approach important information about COVID-19-infected persons built on their diverse breathing design [15]. A deep learning analytical approach for thoracic CT images was carried out to perceive and control COVID-19 patients automatedly [16]. The readiness of COVID-19-associated medical data for processing detailed reachable records has been a crucial existing barrier [3].

This study proposes a machine learning method and exploits for prediction approach for COVID-19 occurrence in humans as artificial intelligence and machine learning are healthily incisive for prediction and diagnostics methods to fight COVID-19 pandemic. An enhanced kernel principal component analysis (KPCA) is used to fetch relevant kernel latent component features of genes that clinicians can efficiently use by clinicians to discover prescriptions, predictions, and diagnosis of patients suspected to be infected. Extracted features are classified by passing them into SVM-RBF classifier to classify the COVID-19 for prediction and the system performance is evaluated using the confusion matrix.

The remaining part of the paper is structured as thus: Sect. 10.2 addressed the overview of the investigation and of related investigations. Section 10.3 provides research materials and methods. Section 10.4 provides experimental research outcomes. Section 10.5 provides the conclusion of the investigation.

10.2 Background and Related Works

Machine learning is a statistical and mathematical method for predictions [17]. Prediction is a significant aspect of interest in healthcare, such as the kind of virus, which is probably predominant in the coming influenza period. What ampoules of virus vaccination to prepare ahead? Relatively, prediction is not the same as treatment properties. Numerous machine learning approaches can evaluate treatment properties, although there are discrepancies between treatment-effect and prediction assessment, which concern machine learning works.

Significant machine learning includes preprocessing, segmenting datasets into validation, and learning procedures to develop high developed classification accuracy algorithms on the proposed full dataset for prediction purposes. Machine learning approaches contain different systems, such as classification trees [17, 18].

Machine learning has increased and extracts general concepts from massive datasets in algorithms to predict outcomes, especially in healthcare. It is an emerging field promising for data preparation, preprocessing, normalization, evaluation, and parameter erudition. The purpose is to acquire an evaluation that corresponds participations to a result. Predicting impending hospitalization and pandemic cases as we witness them is crucial, and analysts gather evidences for successful measurements and forecasts. Machine learning uses a predictor and learner to perform its task by measuring how often the learned predictor appropriately labels patients' readmissions [19]. Machine learning methods are efficient to health facility investigators looking forward to improving the prediction of a healthcare result to train and improve the machine learning prediction algorithm. This approach can support comprehensive data driven by offering significant encounters for medical results that are of value. Computational enhancements in hardware and cloud computing knowledge have made machine learning approaches progressively available to medical investigators and medical industries. In a period of an epidemic as we presently observe, evolving machine learning procedures are possibly valuable for the healthcare practitioners if a forecast is a momentous and eloquent attempt. The prognosis could be joint with a fundamental investigation to advance consideration as machine learning approaches advance. Several machine learning algorithms have evolved and can be adopted for the novel COVID-19, such as the deep learning approach, SVM, and decision trees [18–23].

As shown in Fig. 10.1, the proposed workflow consists of a proposed machine learning model, which can be used to train a test several implementation processes that can enhance the prediction and detection of COVID-19 to help for proper medications and future occurrence.

Several research abstracts evolve from COVID-19 with several dataset repositories like Kaggle updating their outlets daily on the novel COVID-19. These documents help in extracting richer content for the application of machine learning [24]. Dimensionality reduction is a vital aspect of machine learning. It allows summary data from the curse of dimensionality and reduces computational complexity without halting the information's performance. Examples of efficient dimensionality reduction models include kernel principal component analysis (KPCA), ISOMAP, partial least square, and independent component analysis, among others [25].

KPCA is a kernel principal component analysis. It has played an essential role in dimensionality reduction by removing irrelevant information from a given unique dataset as a preprocessing phase in machine learning. It is executable and operative when working with mutual instances commonly encountered. Complex cases are unproductive using PCA. Recently KPCA is a modified PCA that has been proposed to confront the nonlinearity difficulties. As a nonlinear PCA method, KPCA could resourcefully calculate principal constituent in extreme dimensional prominence space using essential operators and nonlinear kernel purposes [26].

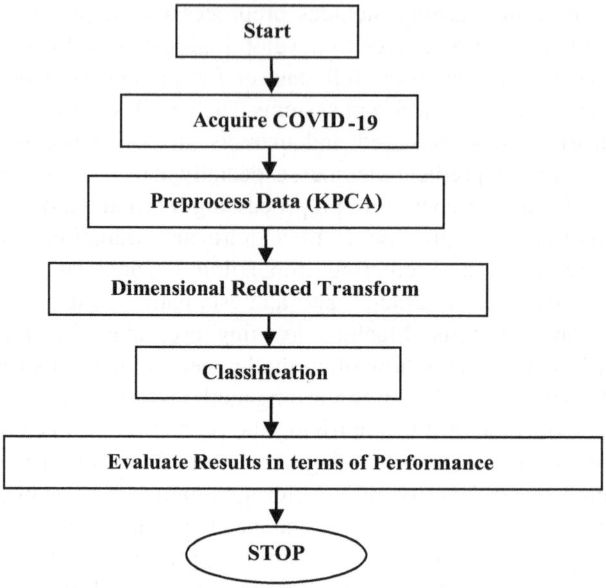

Fig. 10.1 Workflow approach for proposed methodology

PCA suffers from a probabilistic understanding, with no fundamental probability density model. PCA suffers from the predictable covariance matrix and turn out to be rank lacking. Case like this in the previous study is identified as small illustration delinquent in extreme dimensions. Due to the curse of dimensionality, classical multivariate approaches degenerate and break down. The data covariance matrix cannot be calculated and obtained ones classify poorly, due to high noise formed by irrelevance and redundancy of genetic factor (i.e., features) existing in the data.

This study addresses this limitation of PCA to develop and introduce a novel dimension reduction technique for gene expression analysis classification. This study introduces and uses probabilistic kernel principal component analysis (KPCA) as an alternative to the classic PCA.

KPCA methods enable the construction of different nonlinear versions of the algorithm and reduce dimensionality, thereby improving linear PCA.

Before applying the same optimization as PCA, kernel PCA (KPCA) maps the data into a higher dimensional feature space [46–48]. The mapping can be done implicitly by using a kernel function. The Gaussian kernel $K(xi, xj) = \exp(-\|xi - xj\|2\sigma 2)$ was applied in our study.

Clustering techniques are unsupervised learning methods for creating groups of similar samples from a population. Several clustering methods exist, such as the k-means and hierarchical agglomerative clustering, among others [23], intending to find the best clustering representation for a whole data sample space. Deep learning is a feature representation used to learn rich, informative illustrations of information and extract highly representative features for overcoming overfitting, training, and augmentation of data and detecting inferences on clinical applications [27, 37].

The classification approach in machine learning helps discover class separations of samples for meaningful interpretations in substantive theory context. Several efficient classifiers exist, such as the support vector machine (SVM) [45], KNN, decision trees, and ensemble, among others, which can be proposed to help in the diagnosis and prediction of COVID-19 [28]. Machine learning techniques help the computer learn the use of training information processes to predict and make intelligent decisions. Several studies of its approaches and algorithms for modelling and performing tasks are of the essence.

An SVM is a robust classification algorithm with superior performance in several applications such as medical and educational, among other machine learning approaches. Due to its better understanding, it has been used for classification and analysis. Several machine learning methods have been proposed in predicting the diagnosis and threats of COVID-19, such as random forest and neural networks [9].

SVM move features to developed dimensions that can be distinguishable by a hyperplane by maximizing this hyperplane for more accurate classification. Consider a series of data points $D = [xi, di]\ i\ n$ where n is the size of data, di represents the target value, and xi represents the input space vector of the sample.

The SVM evaluates the function as given in the following two equations:

$$(x) = \omega\varphi(x) + b \tag{10.1}$$

where $\varphi(x)$ is the high-dimensional space feature, b is a scalar, and ω is a normal vector.

10.2.1 Related Work

Adegboye et al. [29] proposed a main advance detail of new COVID-19 in Nigeria by providing a preliminary epidemiological study of COVID-19 eruption in Nigeria by approximating the original contagious over time, varying imitation total constructed on the Bayesian method with uncertainty in the dispersion of serial discontinuity of indications in individuals and used for virus access. They test the transcription volume every day for the prevalence, and assessments suggested that Nigeria's COVID-19 occurrence is reduced than probable. The limitation of this study is the robustness of the study and analyzing the records.

Ohia et al. [30] suggested a COVID-19 and Nigeria certainties in the situation for critical need in positioning into perceptions, certainties strange globally by discovering joint procedures and conciliations for conveying the epidemic. The gaps in this study are coming up with relevant decision-making approach. Introducing statistical and computational learning is of the essence.

Ozili [31] suggested a COVID-19 epidemic, financial predicament knowledge and operational reasons. The globe is in an economic predicament by examining overabundance to countries like Nigeria and operational faintness in organizations with the present disaster and predictions for transformation. The limitation of this study calls for the survey and statistical approaches for boosting the economy in post-COVID era.

Dutta and Bandyopadhyay [5] suggested a machine learning method for checking COVID-19 occurrence, with neural network deep learning procedure, efficient prediction, and faster achievable detailed virus recognition. Further insight is of the essence by consulting more efficient machine learning techniques.

Alimadadi et al. [3] discoursed on the necessity for artificial intelligence and machine learning to fight COVID-19, imperative developments of cyberinfrastructure in powering international associations and creations of links with creativities, and linking COVID-19-associated health information with predominant biorepositories that can utilize endeavors in the direction to a nearer and attainable technique for meaningful data mining by bioinformaticians and computational scientists, to progress predictive, diagnostic, and valuable methods against COVID-19 and similar future outbreaks.

Alom et al. [32] suggested an advanced determinate study method to control the amount of infested zones in x-ray and CT pictures on COVID-19 case discovery, with deep learning multi-task methods by using CNN with a transfer learning (TL) technique for COVID-19 detection; NABLA-N network was demonstrated to section areas COVID-19 has infested. Their template achieved an accuracy of 85% and 99%. This study requires further improvement by employing other data forms to the knowledge apart from the CT and x-ray images.

Pinter et al. [33] proposed a COVID-19 overall evaluation for Hungary with a combination machine learning technique for the prognosis of COVID-19 and signifying its concealed features using Hungarian data on an ANFIS-MLP-ICA integrated procedure to predict the period classification of ailing individuals and demise ratio. For future works, gaps in this study need to tackle computational time and accuracy enhancement.

Batista et al. [9] proposed a COVID-19 investigation evaluation in emergency convalescent care. Using the machine learning technique, by predicting COVID-19-positive investigation risks, they collected patient's information and established a helpful verdict of COVID-19 from RT-PCR tests. Random forests, neural networks, logistic regression, gradient boosting trees, and SVM algorithms were used to train patients' samples, and the presentation was verified on novel unobserved data. SVM outperforms other classification algorithms with an 85% AUC and found out that targeted choices for getting COVID-19 tests with data habitually composed are a capable, innovative part using machine learning procedures. Future works require the optimization of the classifier, as it should be further improved.

Rhadhawa et al. [11] proposed a machine learning method with intrinsic genomic signatures by merging supervised machine learning with digital signal processing (MLDSP) for gene calculations, enhanced by a decision tree and a Spearman's rank correlation persistent study for result evaluation with enormous limited epidemiologic gene classification dataset. Their method achieves 100% classification accuracy and understands relevant genetic genes' relations with raw chromosome system data with no precise genetic data, training, protein sequence, or gene annotations. The alignment-based method limitations consist of a comparison of approaches to complement classification taxonomic is of the essence.

Onoja [10] worked on the machine learning process for treating persons medical extent on COVID-19 crisis, by using an imposing end-to-end data determined signifying technique for exploiting review privileges for information gatherings feeding Supervised Machine learning plans for determining person's medical status, by evolving an effective way determining, categorizing, and predicting their medical rank. They were supporting medical care personnel to identify cases and acknowledge suitable medical attention in their localities. There is a further necessity required for current state and need for minimizing COVID-19 spread.

Zhang et al. [1] used an in-depth learning approach for COVID-19 suppository profiling by gathering RNA-Seq disease with GISAID data by screening RNA-Seq records into protein sequences and then building a 3D protein model with homology modelling. COVID-19 primary protease is a critical, valuable goal and is occupied on medication screening grounded on the exhibited COVID-19 protease structure. DFCNN procedure was used to rank and recognize protein-ligand communications with high accuracy. The mechanism between the molecular dockings is a limitation and requires an important biological understanding of COVID-19.

Beck et al. [34] proposed a predicting antiviral drug that may be made for current or present COVID-19 pandemic with a deep-learning method with a proficient medication-target Fragment Transformer-Drug Target Interaction to discover saleable prevailing drugs that can accomplish pathological proteins of COVID-19. Antiretroviral medication for giving and averting HIV was suggested as the superlative biological composite, although there is no applied suggestion to back up the proposal. This study's limitation requires the development of useful control of spreading COVID infections by proposing prediction approached that will help experimental therapy identify the infection.

Ardabili et al. [35] worked on a machine learning comparative study for predicting COVID-19 prevalence as an auxiliary for SIR and SEIR illustrations. Two models obtained proficient results between the proposed machine learning designs identified as the MLP and ANFIS methods. Due to the complicated way of the COVID-19 existence and its interactive inconsistency worldwide, their study suggested machine learning as an effective method for demonstrating the prevalent by providing standards for indicating the likelihood of machine learning for impending investigations and originalities in general predictions can be realized with machine learning and SEIR methods. Modelling for the mortality rate is essential to plan for facilities, by integrating machine learning with the proposed model, to enhance existing study in terms of accuracy.

Xu et al. [36] operated on a deep learning method for COVID-19 and attained 87% accuracy for vigorous cases. This study presented a novel method for screening CT images of COVI-19 using deep learning. The model mechanism requires enhancement in terms of its accuracy, and it will be a promising, supplementary diagnostic approach by using robust data (Table 10.1).

Table 10.1 Comparison of existing works on COVID-19

S/No	Authors and work done	Findings	Deduction
1.	Adegboye et al. [29]	Assessed the replica amount of daily outbreak using a three weekly space through fine-tuning the cases	Requires relevant analysis
2.	Dutta and Bandyopadhyay [5]	Uses deep learning neural network with long short-term memory (LSTM) and gated recurrent unit (GRU) for training the data and the prediction results for COVID-19 cases	Call for accuracy enhancement
3.	Alom et al. [32]	An efficient COVID-19 patient identification approach using multi-task deep learning was proposed. CT scan and x-ray image dataset were evaluated. An inception recurrent residual convolutional neural network with transfer learning (TL) method for COVID-19 discovery and NABLA-N network model to segment infected regions were used	Call for further classification approaches with dimensionality reduction techniques
4.	Pinter et al. [33]	Proposed hybrid machine learning method for predicting COVID-19 using Hungary data. An adaptive network-based fuzzy inference system (ANFIS) and multi-layered perceptron-imperialist competitive algorithm (MLP-ICA) were utilized	Enhancement of the machine learning approach
5.	Beck et al. [34]	Proposed deep learning approach for drug-target interaction model for COVID-19	Prediction result enhancement
6	Raveendran et al. [38]	Random forest and support vector regression methods are used for the COVID-19 contagion dataset and compared the prediction accuracy. PCA fetched the relevant features classified	Call for enhanced dimensionality approaches for better classification
7.	Ardabili et al. [35]	Compared machine learning approaches using the susceptible, infected recover and susceptible exposed infectious removed model, with ANFIS using COVID-19 dataset	Enhancement of the accuracy
8.	Xu et al. [36]	Proposed a deep learning approach for screening COVID-19 from IAVP and pulmonary images	Accuracy enhancement

10.3 Materials and Methods

Recent helpful methods are essential for treating COVID-19 carriers globally. There is no definite, recognized medication. It is risky to establish inventive methods to repurpose tolerable health drugs or propose innovative drugs for SARS-CoV-2. Machine learning-built inversion and persistence context is proposed to rank present drugs for SARS-CoV-2 investigational examinations. Machine learning-built drug unearthing vessel has been projected for designing and producing advanced drug-like compounds for SARS-CoV-2. Probable protein structures associated with COVID-19 methods have been proposed to help as an indication for the COVID-19 vaccine plan. Countless COVID-19 management data in hospitals all-inclusive desires innovative machine learning methods to examine improved beneficial properties for evaluating patient's prediction and improved care for patients and communications and suitable provisions. Diverse machine learning methods exist for various responsibilities such as detection and prediction [46–48] and segmentation models.

10.3.1 Database

Since the arrival of COVID-19, scholars have been gathering associated data for the prevalence. Several datasets for engaging machine learning methods have been proposed, such as the pneumonia detection models from openly accessible datasets [3, 9, 20, 21, 34, 39], to support the fast and extensive distribution of study for the COVID-19 epidemic. Numerous bodies like the World Health Organization have been fetching investigators and health consultants together to speed exploring procedures and growths to advance values that can hold the spread of this deadly epidemic and support care for the affected people. The dataset from the COVID-19 medical record worldwide sample of the available data online given by WHO is concerned about patients diagnosed positively with COVID-19 [40].

The upper airway gene expression differentiates COVID-19 from other acute respiratory diseases in this analysis. It shows the suppression of innate immune responses by the SARS-CoV-2 dataset from the University of California San Francisco after August 2020.

The data involves high-throughput sequencing expression profiling with GPL24676 234 samples of *Homo sapiens* species. Out of 234 patients with COVID-19 ($n = 93$), other acute respiratory diseases (ARIs) are infectious ($n = 100$) or non-viral ($n = 41$). Compared to other viral ARIs, COVID-19 patients displayed substantially decreased amounts of neutrophils, macrophages, and increased amounts of goblet, dendritic, and B cells [41].

S/No	COVID-19 data archives
1.	https://github.com/ieee8023/covid-chestXray-dataset
2.	www.worldometers.info/coronavirus/country/hungary/
3.	www.kaggle.com/sudalairajkumar/novel-corona-virus-2019-dataset
4.	data.humdata.org/dataset/novel-coronavirus-2019-ncov-cases
5.	dataverse.harvard.edu/
6.	www.who.int/tb/country/data/download/en/
7.	github.com/datasets/covid-19
8.	ourworldindata.org/coronavirus-testing
9.	springernature.com/gp/researchers/campaigns/coronavirus/research-data
10.	https://www.ncbi.nlm.nih.gov/geo/download/?acc=GSE156063
11.	https://github.com/owid/covid-19-data/tree/master/public/data

10.3.2 Economy

Since the global economic tragedy, the world has been brought into the middle of the nastiest recession. The economic downturn of countries like Nigeria has been impelled by the incorporation of worsening oil value and spillovers from the COVID-19 widespread and engaged to a radical lineage in the cry for oil products and still economic events from taking place when communal hostility strategies were required.

Anxiety thrives concerning the new epidemic and its consequences as cumulative records losses surge with costs owing to loss of production, and comorbidities are of concern [42]. The financial results are unfavorable to employment, health, travel, sport, trading, agriculture, market world, and merchandise, among others [43]. Some of the recommended strategic solutions are positive administration methods, health strategy basis to address societal causes of health, education, administration, knowledge, nationwide and global modifications in investments, private and public corporations, and World Technical Council establishments on COVID-19. Operative application of policy keys will necessitate the total backing of all investors, such as governments, the mass media, NGOs, health specialists, public, and persons. An extensive socioeconomic progress strategy in sector diplomacies and an environment encouraging enterprise are required to enhance commercial productions. It is wise for administrations and economic institutes to always evaluate the situation and ensure a better living [17, 44].

10.4 Experimental Results

In this study, KPCA was used to fetch out relevant information from the high-dimensional data comprising of 234 attributes and 15,979 instances of COVID-19 sample genes. SVM classification algorithms were used as a model to test the experiment's prediction; Fig. 10.2 shows the dataset information.

KPCA fetched relevant information from the data with 33 latent component attributes of the relevant genes. Figure 10.3 shows the extracted features. The extracted features projects relevancy with the irrelevant information been eliminated. The KPCA aids nonlinearity. It helps classify improvements by representing and integrating the input variables to reveal interpretability.

Figure 10.4 shows the computational time it takes for KPCA to execute and 15.0318 s was recorded as the time taken. The extracted features are then passed to the classifier for evaluation.

The findings discovered from this study can help clinicians in decision-making. Figure 10.5 shows the classification scattered plot; it represents the individual values of the data point with their variable relationships. KPCA output result is also shown in Fig. 10.5.

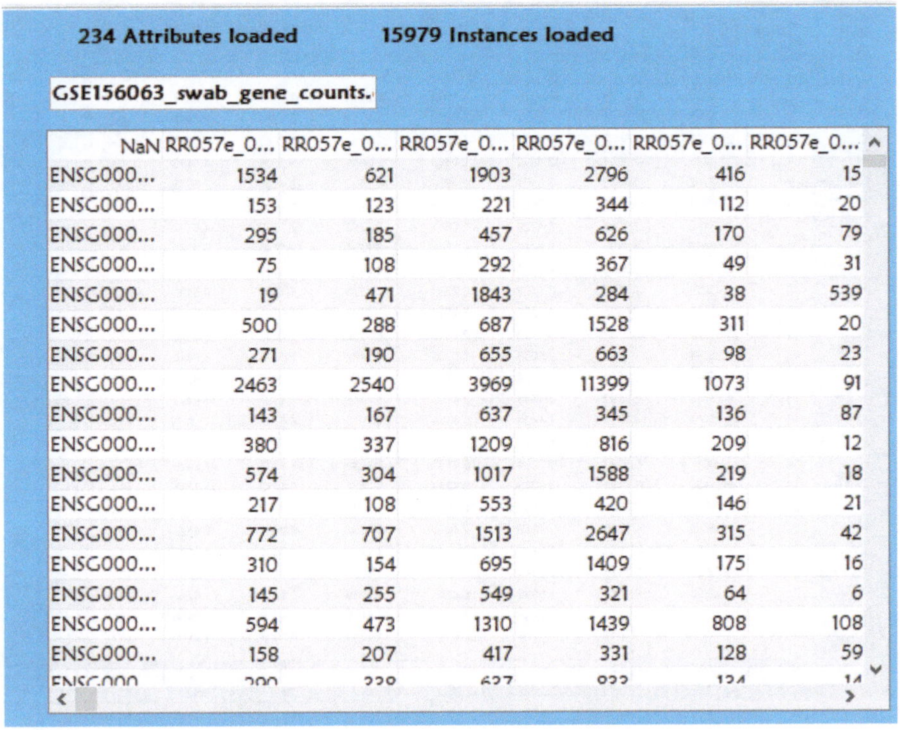

234 Attributes loaded 15979 Instances loaded

GSE156063_swab_gene_counts.

NaN	RR057e_0...	RR057e_0...	RR057e_0...	RR057e_0...	RR057e_0...	RR057e_0...
ENSG000...	1534	621	1903	2796	416	15
ENSG000...	153	123	221	344	112	20
ENSG000...	295	185	457	626	170	79
ENSG000...	75	108	292	367	49	31
ENSG000...	19	471	1843	284	38	539
ENSG000...	500	288	687	1528	311	20
ENSG000...	271	190	655	663	98	23
ENSG000...	2463	2540	3969	11399	1073	91
ENSG000...	143	167	637	345	136	87
ENSG000...	380	337	1209	816	209	12
ENSG000...	574	304	1017	1588	219	18
ENSG000...	217	108	553	420	146	21
ENSG000...	772	707	1513	2647	315	42
ENSG000...	310	154	695	1409	175	16
ENSG000...	145	255	549	321	64	6
ENSG000...	594	473	1310	1439	808	108
ENSG000...	158	207	417	331	128	59

Fig. 10.2 The COVID-19 dataset

SVM-kernels using radial basis function and linear SVM were employed for classification with tenfold cross-validation using MATLAB. The confusion matrix is further used for the evaluation procedure, and their results were compared. Figure 10.6 shows the KPCA-L-SVM classification confusion matrix, used for evaluating the performance metrics for the experiment.

Figure 10.7 depicts the KPCA-SVM-RBF classification confusion matrix; it is used for evaluating the performance metrics for the experiment.

In this study, the reduction and classification of high-dimensional COVID-19 data were developed. The experiment used the KPCA to reduce the data and classify the experiment using the L-SVM and SVM-RBF classifiers. The experimental results are tabulated in Table 10.2.

In this study, KPCA and SVM were used for COVID-19 clinical data provided online to predict the pandemic. The result achieved 93% and 87% accuracy, respectively. With this prediction, this study can help clinicians' decision-making process by translating the data analysis using the machine learning perspectives. Presently with the data available, there are cumulated challenging issues and needs

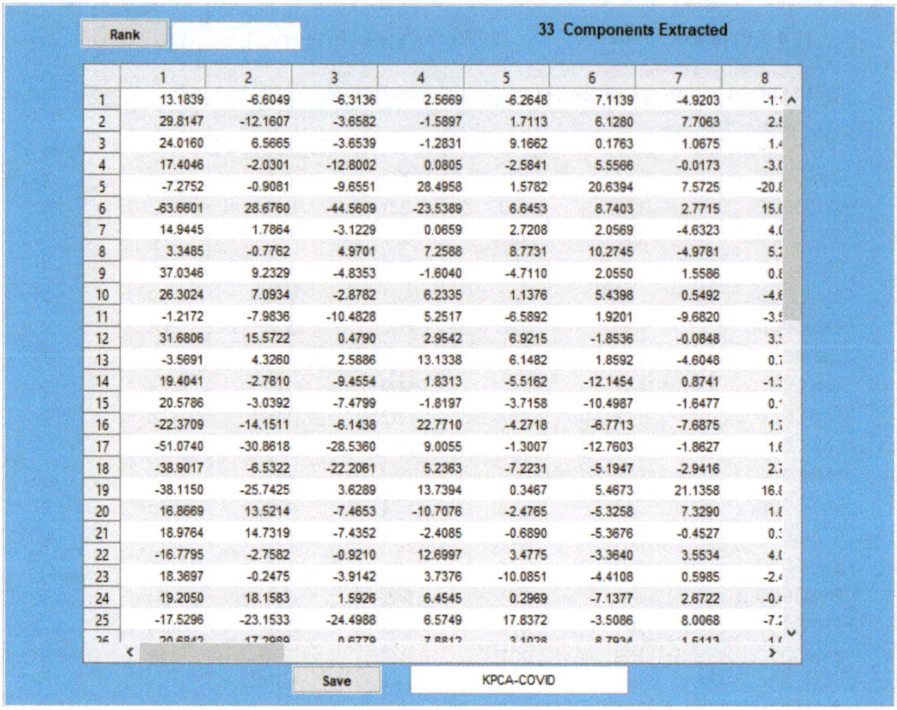

	1	2	3	4	5	6	7
1	13.1839	-6.6049	-6.3136	2.5669	-6.2648	7.1139	-4.9203
2	29.8147	-12.1607	-3.6582	-1.5897	1.7113	6.1280	7.7063
3	24.0160	6.5665	-3.6539	-1.2831	9.1662	0.1763	1.0675
4	17.4046	-2.0301	-12.8002	0.0805	-2.5841	5.5566	-0.0173
5	-7.2752	-0.9081	-9.6551	28.4958	1.5782	20.6394	7.5725
6	-63.6601	28.6760	-44.5609	-23.5389	6.6453	8.7403	2.7715
7	14.9445	1.7864	-3.1229	0.0659	2.7208	2.0569	-4.6323
8	3.3485	-0.7762	4.9701	7.2588	8.7731	10.2745	-4.9781
9	37.0346	9.2329	-4.8353	-1.6040	-4.7110	2.0550	1.5586
10	26.3024	7.0934	-2.8782	6.2335	1.1376	5.4398	0.5492
11	-1.2172	-7.9836	-10.4828	5.2517	-6.5892	1.9201	-9.6820
12	31.6806	15.5722	0.4790	2.9542	6.9215	-1.8536	-0.0848
13	-3.5691	4.3260	2.5886	13.1338	6.1482	1.8592	-4.6048
14	19.4041	-2.7810	-9.4554	1.8313	-5.5162	-12.1454	0.8741
15	20.5786	-3.0392	-7.4799	-1.8197	-3.7158	-10.4987	-1.6477
16	-22.3709	-14.1511	-6.1438	22.7710	-4.2718	-6.7713	-7.6875
17	-51.0740	-30.8618	-28.5360	9.0055	-1.3007	-12.7603	-1.8627
18	-38.9017	-6.5322	-22.2061	5.2363	-7.2231	-5.1947	-2.9416
19	-38.1150	-25.7425	3.6289	13.7394	0.3467	5.4673	21.1358
20	16.8669	13.5214	-7.4653	-10.7076	-2.4765	-5.3258	7.3290
21	18.9764	14.7319	-7.4352	-2.4085	-0.6890	-5.3676	-0.4527
22	-16.7795	-2.7582	-0.9210	12.6997	3.4775	-3.3640	3.5534
23	18.3697	-0.2475	-3.9142	3.7376	-10.0851	-4.4108	0.5985
24	19.2050	18.1583	1.5926	6.4545	0.2969	-7.1377	2.6722
25	-17.5296	-23.1533	-24.4988	6.5749	17.8372	-3.5086	8.0068

Fig. 10.3 The extracted features using KPCA

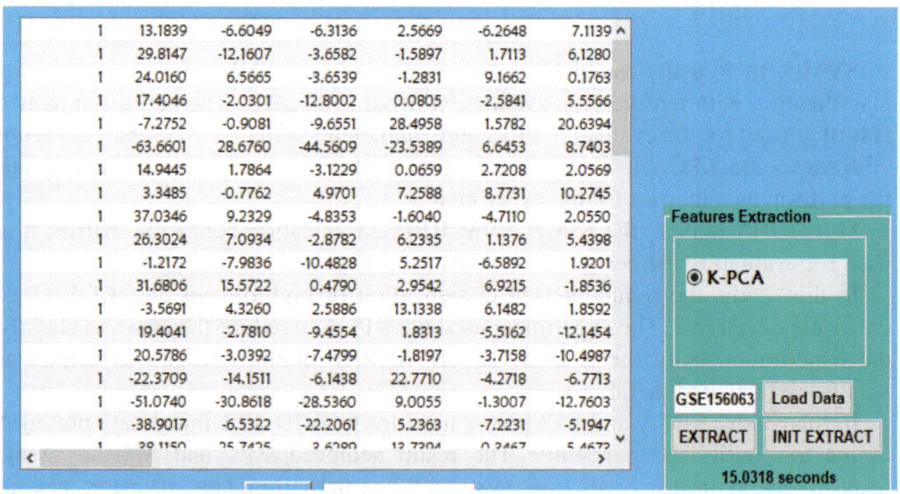

1	13.1839	-6.6049	-6.3136	2.5669	-6.2648	7.1139
1	29.8147	-12.1607	-3.6582	-1.5897	1.7113	6.1280
1	24.0160	6.5665	-3.6539	-1.2831	9.1662	0.1763
1	17.4046	-2.0301	-12.8002	0.0805	-2.5841	5.5566
1	-7.2752	-0.9081	-9.6551	28.4958	1.5782	20.6394
1	-63.6601	28.6760	-44.5609	-23.5389	6.6453	8.7403
1	14.9445	1.7864	-3.1229	0.0659	2.7208	2.0569
1	3.3485	-0.7762	4.9701	7.2588	8.7731	10.2745
1	37.0346	9.2329	-4.8353	-1.6040	-4.7110	2.0550
1	26.3024	7.0934	-2.8782	6.2335	1.1376	5.4398
1	-1.2172	-7.9836	-10.4828	5.2517	-6.5892	1.9201
1	31.6806	15.5722	0.4790	2.9542	6.9215	-1.8536
1	-3.5691	4.3260	2.5886	13.1338	6.1482	1.8592
1	19.4041	-2.7810	-9.4554	1.8313	-5.5162	-12.1454
1	20.5786	-3.0392	-7.4799	-1.8197	-3.7158	-10.4987
1	-22.3709	-14.1511	-6.1438	22.7710	-4.2718	-6.7713
1	-51.0740	-30.8618	-28.5360	9.0055	-1.3007	-12.7603
1	-38.9017	-6.5322	-22.2061	5.2363	-7.2231	-5.1947

Fig. 10.4 KPCA computational time

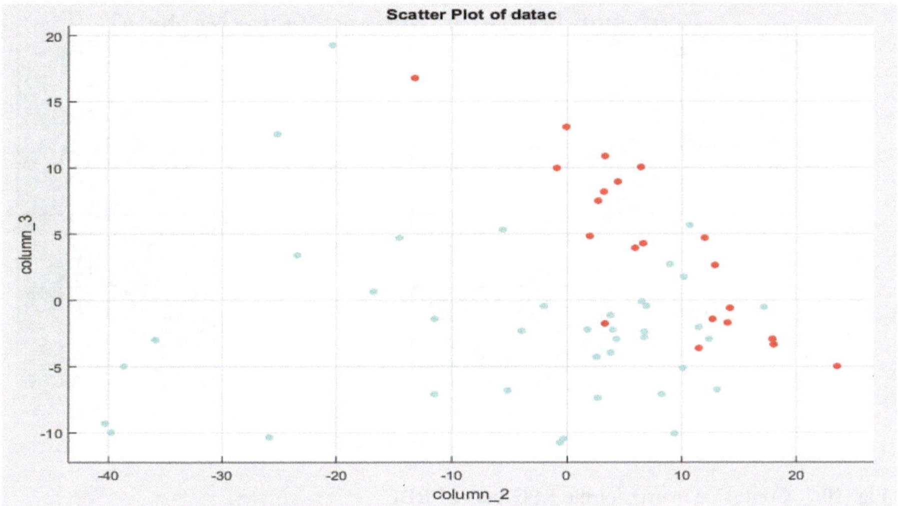

Fig. 10.5 Classification scattered plot

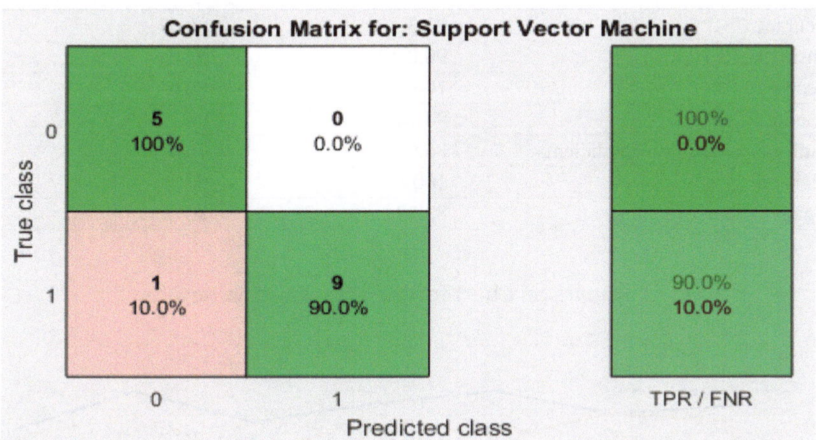

Fig. 10.6 Confusion matrix for the KPCA-L-SVM

relevant to genetic information to help predict and detect the epidemic. Prediction correctness of models is essential for hospitals and immune systems of infected persons. KPCA-L-SVM has proven to be an efficient approach for predicting the COVID-19 outbreak; the comparative chart for the experiment is depicted in Fig. 10.8.

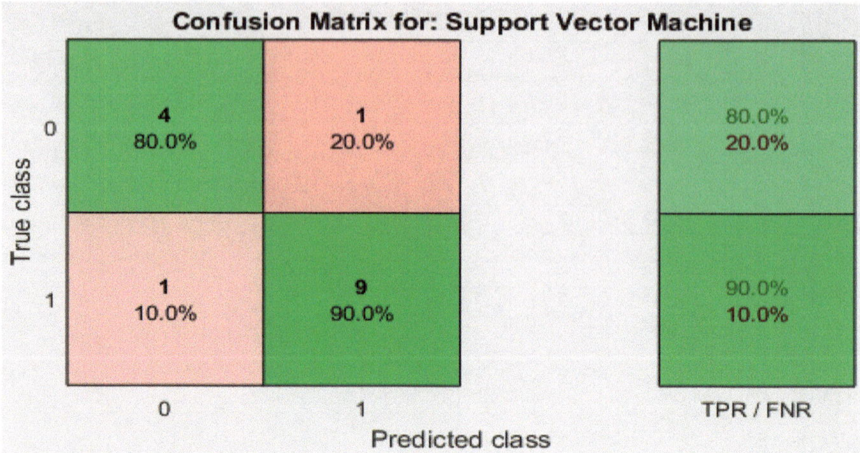

Fig. 10.7 Confusion matrix for the KPCA-SVM-RBF

Table 10.2 Experimental results

Performance metrics	KPCA-L-SVM	KPCA-RBF-SVM
Accuracy (%)	93.3	86.67
Sensitivity (%)	90.0	90.0
Specificity (%)	100	80.0
F-Score (%)	94.74	90
Matthews correlation coefficient	86.6	70
Precision	100	90
Negative predictive value	83.33	80

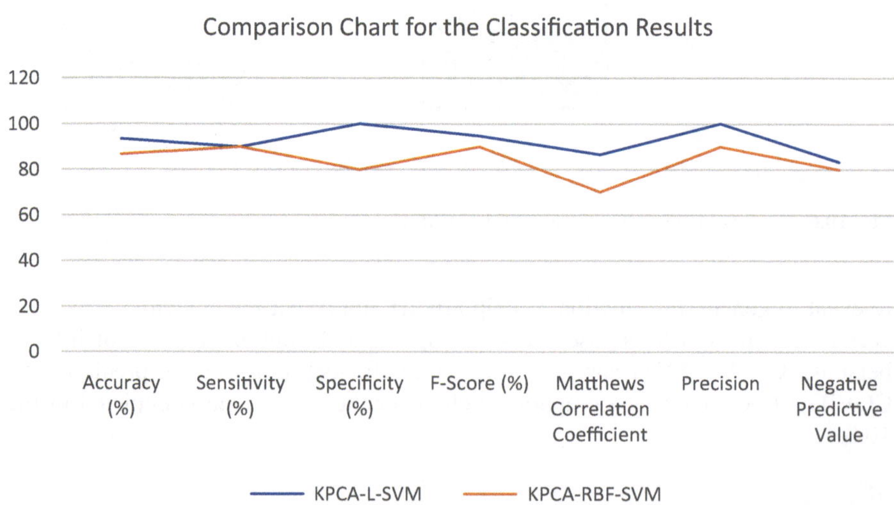

Fig. 10.8 Result comparison chart

10.5 Conclusion

Machine learning is a popular approach for predictive modelling, yet it does not significantly combat COVID-19. Machine learning can help define treatment effects, pharmaceutical views, and diagnostic prediction and improve several facets such as the economy the recent worldwide pandemic can bring. Improving proposed approaches with its risk factors should concern and present efficient algorithms for rapid prediction, and improvement should be considered. In this study, KPCA-SVM was used for predicting the novel COVID-19, and an accuracy of about 93% and 87% was attained. Frameworks have assisted healthcare to evaluate the strength of suggestions over the years. Several algorithms for assessing and understanding machine learning have been proposed, and significant public categories of learners can help predict and analyze COVID-19. In the future, several Machine learning algorithms can be used to enhance the performance and compared with the state-of-art. Using other approaches such as probabilistic PCA, Probabilistic Partial Least Square with classifiers such as SVM an KNN could also be employed.

References

1. H. Zhang, K.M. Saravanan, Y. Yang, M.T. Hossain, J. Li, X. Ren, Y. Wei, Deep learning based drug screening for novel coronavirus 2019-nCov. Preprints **2020**, 2020020061 (2020). https://doi.org/10.20944/preprints202002.0061.v1
2. R.O. Ogundokun, A.F. Lukman, G.B. Kibria, J.B. Awotunde, B.B. Aladeitan, Predictive modelling of COVID-19 confirmed cases in Nigeria. Infect. Dis. Model. **5**, 543–548 (2020)
3. L. Garg, E. Chukwu, N. Nasser, C. Chakraborty, G. Garg, Anonymity preserving IoT-based COVID-19 and other infectious disease contact tracing model. IEEE Access **8**, 159402–159414 (2020)
4. E.A. Adeniyi, J.B. Awotunde, R.O. Ogundokun, P.O. Kolawole, M.K. Abiodun, A.A. Adeniyi, Mobile health application and covid-19: Opportunities and challenges. J. Crit. Rev. **7**(15), 3481–3488 (2020)
5. S. Dutta, S.L. Bandyopadhyay, Machine learning approach for confirmation of COVID-19 cases: Positive, negative, death and release. medRxiv Preprint (2020). https://doi.org/10.1101/2020.03.25.20043505
6. R.O. Ogundokun, J.B. Awotunde, Machine learning prediction for COVID 19 pandemic in India. medRxiv (2020)
7. A.F. Lukman, R.I. Rauf, O. Abiodun, O. Oludoun, K. Ayinde, R.O. Ogundokun, COVID-19 prevalence estimation: Four most affected African countries. Infect. Dis. Model. **5**, 827–838 (2020)
8. W. Guan, Z. Ni, Y. Hu, W. Liang, C. Ou, J. He, L. Liu, H. Shan, C. Lei, D.S.C. Hui, Clinical characteristics of 2019 novel coronavirus infection in China. MedRxiv (2020)
9. A.F.M. Batista, J.L. Miraglia, T.H.R. Donato, C.A.D.P. Filho, COVID-19 diagnosis prediction in emergency care patients: A machine learning approach. medRxiv. https://doi.org/10.1101/2020.04.04.20052092
10. A.A. Onoja, A Proposed Machine Learning Approach for Monitoring Individual's Health Status on Corona Virus, researchgate.net/publication/339827100

11. G.S. Randhawa, M.P.M. Soltysiak, H.E. Roz, C.P.E.D. Souza, K.A. Hill, L. Kari, Machine learning using intrinsic genomic signatures for rapid classification of novel pathogens: COVID-19 case study. PLoS One **15**(4) (2020). https://doi.org/10.1371/journal.pone.0232391
12. L. Yan, H.T. Zhang, Y. Xiao, M. Wang, C. Sun, J. Liang, S. Li, M. Zhang, Y. Guo, Y. Xiao, Prediction of survival for severe Covid-19 patients with three clinical features: Development of a machine learning-based prognostic model with clinical data in Wuhan. medRxiv (2020). https://doi.org/10.1101/2020.02.27.20028027
13. H.C. Metsky, C.A. Freije, T.-S.F. Kosoko-Thoroddsen, P.C. Sabeti, C. Myhrvold, CRISPR-based COVID-19 surveillance using a genomically comprehensive machine learning approach. bioRxiv (2020). https://doi.org/10.1101/2020.02.26.967026
14. Y. Ge, T. Tian, S. Huang, F. Wan, J. Li, S. Li, H. Yang, L. Hong, N. Wu, E. Yuan, L. Cheng, Y. Lei, H. Shu, X. Feng, Z. Jiang, Y. Chi, X. Guo, L. Cui, L. Xiao, Z. Li, C. Yang, Z. Miao, H. Tang, L. Chen, H. Zeng, D. Zhao, F. Zhu, X. Shen, J. Zeng, A data-driven drug repositioning framework discovered a potential therapeutic agent targeting COVID-19. bioRxiv (2020). https://doi.org/10.1101/2020.03.11.986836
15. Y. Wang, M. Hu, Q. Li, X.-P. Zhang, G. Zhai, N. Yao, Abnormal respiratory patterns classifier may contribute to large-scale screening of people infected with COVID-19 in an accurate and unobtrusive manner. Arxiv2002.05534 (2020)
16. O. Gozes, M. Frid-Adar, H. Greenspan, P.D. Browning, H. Zhang, W. Ji, A. Bernheim, E. Siegel, Rapid AI development cycle for the coronavirus (COVID-19) pandemic: Initial results for automated detection & patient monitoring using deep learning CT image analysis. arXiv2003.05037 (2020)
17. W.H. Crown, Potential application of machine learning in health outcomes research and some statistical cautions. Value Health **18**(2), 137–140 (2015)
18. T. Zheng, W. Xie, L. Xu, X. He, Y. Zhang, M. You, G. Yang, Y. Chen, A machine learning-based framework to identify type 2 diabetes through electronic health records. Int. J. Med. Inform. **97**, 120–127 (2017)
19. P. Doupe, J. Faghmous, S. Basu, Machine learning for health services researchers. Value Health **22**(7), 808–815 (2019). https://doi.org/10.1016/j.jval.2019.02.012
20. S. Basu, J.H. Faghmous, P. Doupe, Machine learning methods for precision medicine research designed to reduce health disparities: A structured tutorial. Ethn. Dis. **30**(1), 217–228 (2020). https://doi.org/10.18865/ed.30.s1.217
21. Y. Chen, V.V. Chirikov, X.L. Marston, J. Yang, H. Qiu, J. Xie, N. Sung, C. Gu, P. Dong, X. Gao, Machine learning for precision of health economics and outcomes research. Methodol. Health Care Policy **7**(1), 1–10 (2020)
22. H. Storm, K. Baylis, T. Heckelei, Machine learning in agricultural and applied economics. Eur. Rev. Agric. Econ.. https://doi.org/10.1093/erae/jbz033
23. S. Vollmer, B.A. Mateen, G. Bohner, Machine learning and artificial intelligence research for patient benefit. BMJ Res. Methods Report. **368** (2020). https://doi.org/10.1136/bmj.l6927
24. A. Doanvo, X. Qian, D. Ramjee, H. Piontkivska, A. Desai, M. Majumder, Machine learning maps research need in Covid-19 literature. bioRxiv preprint (2020) https://doi.org/10.1101/2020.06.11.145425
25. S.K. Sonbhadra, S. Agarwal, P. Nagabhushan, Target specific mining of COVID-19 scholarly articles using one-class approach. arXiv:2004.11706v1
26. Y. Zhou, B. Sun, F. Li, W. Song, NC machine tools fault diagnosis based on kernel PCA and K-nearest neighbor using vibration signals. Shock Vibrat. **2015**, 139217 (2015)
27. J.B. Awotunde, R.O. Ogundokun, F.E. Ayo, O.E. Matiluko, Speech segregation in background noise based on deep learning. IEEE Access **8**, 169568–169575 (2020)
28. S. Anto, S. Chandramathi, Supervised machine learning approaches for medical dataset classification. A review. IJCST **2**(4), 234–240 (2011)
29. O.A. Adegboye, A.I. Adekunle, E. Gayawan, Early transmission dynamics of novel coronavirus (COVID-19) in Nigeria. Int. J. Environ. Res. Public Health **17**(9) (2020). https://doi.org/10.3390/ijerph17093054

30. C. Ohia, A.S. Bakarey, T. Ahmad, COVID-19 and Nigeria: Putting the realities in context. Int. J. Infect. Dis. **95**, 279–281 (2020)
31. P.K. Ozili, COVID-19 pandemic and economic crisis: The Nigerian experience and structural causes (2020). https://doi.org/10.2139/ssrn.3567419
32. M.Z. Alom, M.M.S. Rahman, M.S. Nasrin, T.M. Taha, V.K. Asari, COVID_MTNet: Covid-19 detection with multi-task deep learning approaches. Electr. Eng. Syst. Sci.. arXiv:2004.03747
33. G. Pinter, I. Felde, A. Mosavi, P. Ghamisi, R. Gloaguen, COVID-19 pandemic prediction for Hungary; a hybrid machine learning approach. https://doi.org/10.20944/preprints202005.0031.v1
34. B.R. Beck, B. Shin, Y. Choi, S. Park, K. Kang, Predicting commercially available antiviral drugs that may act on the novel coronavirus (2019-nCoV), Wuhan, China through a drug-target interaction deep learning model. bioRxiv preprint (2020). https://doi.org/10.1101/2020.01.31.929547
35. S.F. Ardabili, A. Mosavi, P. Ghamisi, F. Ferdinand, A.R. V-Koczy, U. Reuter, T. Rabczuk, P.M. Atkinsion, COVID-19 outbreak prediction with machine learning, Health Economics and Outcomes Research Artificial Intelligence and Machine Learning (2020) https://doi.org/10.21203/rs.3.rs-27130/v1
36. X. Xu, X. Jiang, C. Ma, P. Du, X. Li, S. Lv, L. Yu, Y. Chen, J. Su, G. Lang, Y. Li, H. Zhao, K. Xu, L. Ruan, W. Wu, Deep learning system to screen coronavirus disease 2019 Pneumonia. Appl. Intelligence **22**, 1–7 (2020)
37. A.A. Adeyinka, M.O. Adebiyi, N.O. Akande, R.O. Ogundokun, A.A. Kayode, T.O. Oladele, A deep convolutional encoder-decoder architecture for retinal blood vessels segmentation, in *International Conference on Computational Science and Its Applications*, (Springer, Cham, 2019), pp. 180–189
38. S. Raveendran, P. N. Indi, S. Agrahari, S. Menon, D. A. Sathia Seelan, Machine Learning Based Prognostic Model and Mobile Application Software Platform for Predicting Infection Susceptibility of COVID-19 Using Health Care Data (2020)
39. Coronavirus-Dataset, Version 1, https://www.kaggle.com/kimjihoo/coronavirusdataset-old. Accessed 17 Mar 2020
40. E.H. Aboul, S. Aya, D. Ashraf, Artificial intelligence approach to predict the COVID-19 patient's recovery
41. https://www.ncbi.nlm.nih.gov/geo/download/?acc=GSE156063
42. O. Evans, Socio-economic impacts of novel coronavirus: The policy solutions. BizEcons Q. **7**, 3–12 (2020)
43. M. Nicola, Z. Alsafi, C. Sohrabi, A. Kerwan, A.A. Jabir, C. Iosifidis, M. Agha, R. Aghaf, The socio-economic implications of the coronavirus pandemic (COVID-19): A review. Int. J. Surg. **78**, 185–193 (2020)
44. https://github.com/owid/covid-19-data/tree/master/public/data
45. R.O. Abolade, S.O. Famakinde, S.I. Popoola, O.F. Oseni, A.A. Atayero, S. Misra, Support vector machine for path loss predictions in urban environment, in *International Conference on Computational Science and Its Applications*, (Springer, Cham, 2020), pp. 995–1006
46. S.I. Popoola, S. Misra, A.A. Atayero, Outdoor path loss predictions based on extreme learning machine. Wirel. Pers. Commun. **99**(1), 441–460 (2018)
47. R.K. Behera, S.K. Rath, S. Misra, M. Leon, A. Adewumi, Machine learning approach for reliability assessment of open source software, in *International Conference on Computational Science and Its Applications*, (Springer, Cham, 2019), pp. 472–482
48. G. Blessing, A. Azeta, S. Misra, F. Chigozie, R. Ahuja, A machine learning prediction of automatic text based assessment for open and distance learning: A review, in *International Conference on Innovations in Bio-Inspired Computing and Applications*, (Springer, Cham, 2019), pp. 369–380

Chapter 11
COVID-19 Epidemic Impact on Various Society Sectors

Mohandas V. Pawar, J. Anuradha, Asha M. Pawar, Sudarshan Sanap, Rajneesh Kaur Sachdeo, Kishore Ravande, Jyoti Malhotra, H. R. Bhapkar, and Pranav Pawar

11.1 Introduction

The novel coronavirus (COVID-19) travels rapidly worldwide, emerging in Wuhan, China, at the end of December 2019, and has a significant effect on all facets of culture across all industries. The COVID-19 epidemic has brought our planet to a standstill. It has a disruptive, unexpected impact on our lives, markets, communities, and livelihoods, and chances of global recession and significant employment losses are on the rise. When policymakers adapt dramatically to the COVID-19 epidemic, companies readily react to their employees, consumers, and suppliers' evolving demands and resolve financial and organisational challenges. The possible change to be addressed may be overwhelming if any sector, feature, and geography are affected. A global novel virus in our homes could redirect our interaction with the nation, the outside environment, and even each other for months to come [1, 2].

These experts sound uncertain or disturbing in the coming months or years regarding any changes: Are nations remain closed? Is contact going to be taboo? How are restaurants going to happen? Yet times of turmoil often bring opportunities: new and more versatile applications of technologies, fewer fragmentations, a renewed love of the world, and other pleasures of existence [3]. Nobody knows just what is happening, so here is our only roadmap to how culture, education, economy,

M. V. Pawar (✉) · A. M. Pawar · S. Sanap · R. K. Sachdeo · K. Ravande · J. Malhotra
H. R. Bhapkar
MIT School of Engineering, MIT ADT University, Pune, India
e-mail: mohandas.pawar@mituniversity.edu.in

J. Anuradha
School of Computer Science and Engineering, VIT University, Vellore, India

P. Pawar
Bar-Ilan University, Tel Aviv, Israel

L. Garg et al. (eds.), *Healthcare Informatics for Fighting COVID-19 and Future Epidemics*, EAI/Springer Innovations in Communication and Computing,
https://doi.org/10.1007/978-3-030-72752-9_11

habits, and more will shift [4, 5]. This chapter offers you professional perspectives combined with concrete steps through which the enterprise can turn enormous uncertainty into positive progress. The pandemic COVID-19 remains a health and humanitarian issue, but it also has significant market impacts. If policymakers react dramatically to the COVID-19 virus, corporations adapt quickly to their staff, consumers, and vendors' evolving demands and tackle the financial and operating challenges. The number of possible adjustments may be overwhelming if any sector, feature, and geography are affected [6].

This chapter is designed in the following manner: Sect. 11.2 describes the motivation for writing this chapter. Section 11.3 specifies the related work and discusses the challenges of COVID-19 in various sectors and some solutions. Proposed solutions are mentioned in Sect. 11.4. Moreover, Sect. 11.5 describes the limitations of technological solutions in a short time of this epidemic. Finally, the conclusion is shown in Sect. 11.6.

11.2 Motivation

We are surrounded by the unpredictable, uncertain, and decisions of all sorts, which ultimately leave a mark in short to long-term manner in which we push things. During any situation, technological solution providers have two equally essential responsibilities: address and avoid the immediate problem. The pandemic of COVID-19 is an obvious example. The world will now save lives and change how we respond to outbreaks generally. The first is more immediate, but the second has significant long-term consequences. We began to develop and revive this concept primarily because of the interactions we have encountered in the last couple of weeks.

11.3 Related Work and Discussion

Pandemic and consequent lockdown have hit various sectors throughout the world.

Areas affected due to COVID-19 are as follows:

- Auto
- Pharma
- Oil, gas, and chemical executive
- Supply chain
- Tourism
- Global economy and GDP
- Human mental health
- Information technology
- Food and agriculture
- Textiles (Fig. 11.1)

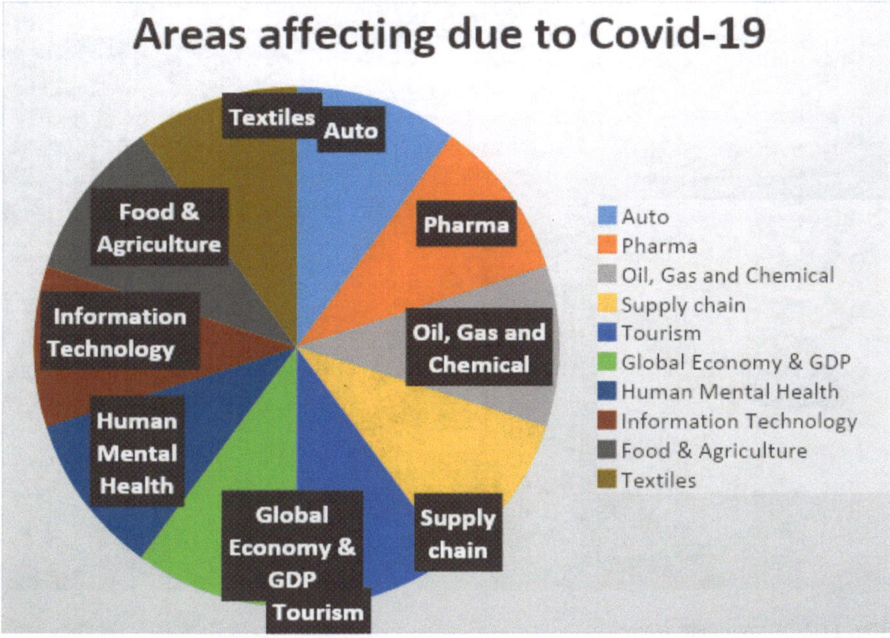

Fig. 11.1 Areas affected due to COVID-19

11.3.1 Auto

COVID-19 has either stopped activities or worked on a limited staff to avoid the global automobile sector. Development cycles are static and designed for performance in fast-moving mass-producing industries such as automobiles. Similarly, based on production forecasts, supply chains have been operating on the timetable weekly. Car manufactures are still seeking to upgrade these devices to suit uncertain market conditions. Automakers continue to monitor flexible manufacturing processes and supply chains quickly as they brace themselves in reaction to the global pandemic of COVID-19 for a dynamic world of demand. Informatics firms supporting car producers have obtained proposals from businesses pursuing quick transformation to agile manufacturing methods and supply chains, along with efforts to reduce costs. Two measures are obviously of concern to carmakers, and the first is to maintain the fragmented supply chain and render manufacturing more agile. Emphasis switches from mere output efficiency to living in unexpected changes to rapidly respond to rising market conditions. Smaller lot sizes, faster selling cycles, and reduced development prices would enable carmakers to embrace flexible and lean manufacturing.

The COVID-19 pandemic rapidly and severely impacted the internationally industrialised automotive industry. Symptoms include failure of Chinese shipments of parts, large-scale interruptions of the product throughout Europe, and suspensions

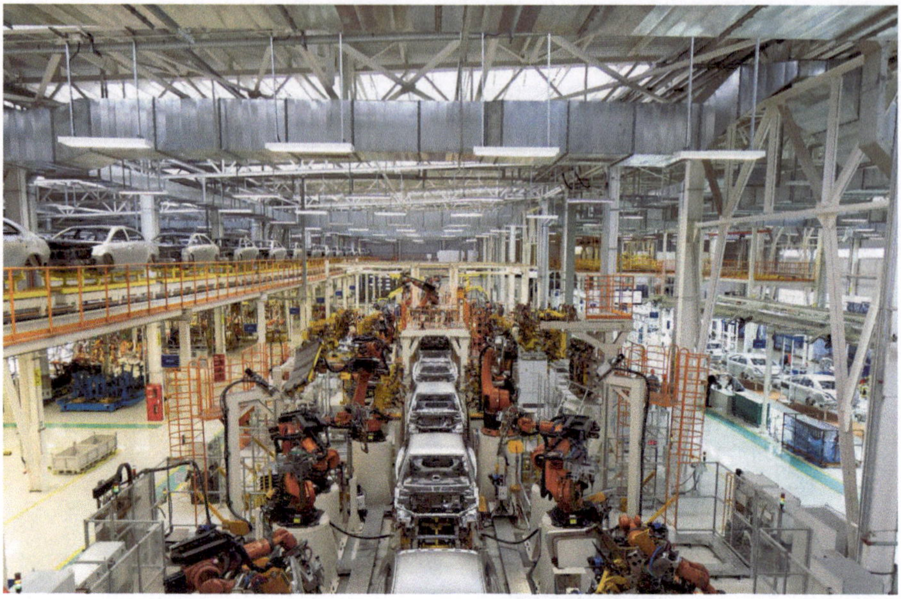

Fig. 11.2 Automobile sector

of manufacturing plants in the United States. This places tremendous strain on a sector that already faces a change in global demand and undoubtedly contributes to further merger and acquisition (Fig. 11.2).

11.3.1.1 Potential Long-Term Impact on the Automotive Sector

1. Prolonged truncation of market demand when creating multiple lock scenarios will contribute to an overall slowdown, culminating in a general lack of customer interest, which would directly affect automaker sales and productivity.
2. Car companies may be required to redirect money to support operations, famine R&D funds for new development programs, and other budgetary ventures.
3. Strategic decisions to leave unprofitable world markets and product models may be improved, substantially reduced by streamlining/consolidated production capability.
4. Liquidity manufacturers will quickly change market conditions, creating significant instability and possibly disastrous implications for the entire world automotive manufacturing climate.

A considerable volume of consolidation in the automobile retail industry can be anticipated because dealers cannot adapt fast enough to adjust market conditions.

11.3.1.2 Overcome in this the COVID-19 Epidemic

1. Determine, prioritise, and ramp up company-wide costing steps.
2. Optimise working capital to have fast and measurable benefits to cash flows.
3. Revision of prediction assumptions, with priority despite existing market uncertainties and downside scenarios.
4. Identify alternative funding outlets to gain access to alternative financing options if successful scenario preparation suggests that liquidity is a concern.
5. Engaged employees will concentrate on the well-being and care of workers as possible rehabilitation.

For example, supply disruption from China has been severely affected. China accounts for 27% of the manufactured automotive parts of India and global automobile producers worldwide. Due to the closure, vehicles' production and distribution, including Bharat Stage 4 (BS-IV) compatible models, have reportedly been postponed.

11.3.2 Pharma

Pharmaceutical companies react to the swift challenges of changes to supply chains and adjust the processes of operation during this extraordinary era. If the present COVID-19 pandemic is medium to long term, the availability of active ingredients to materials (mainly from China) and the import and export of pharmaceutical goods would be impacted. There is also a possible adverse effect on R&D and production operations, both short and long term and time expended on non-core supply chain/data processing initiatives/ventures. While it is still uncertain of the global pandemic's full impact, pharmaceutical companies will adapt, survive, and prosper.

11.3.2.1 Key Signs That During this Crisis Companies Should Take Note

- Crisis management team
- People management
- Compensation to casual labour due to temporary layoffs
- Remote work and cybersecurity concerns
- Plant and warehousing operations
- Supply chain management
- Research and development (R&D)
- Insurance
- Financial management (Fig. 11.3)

The effect of COVID-19 has raised the odds of shooting the cost of raw materials and medicines in China and of lockdowns in Asia, the United States, and

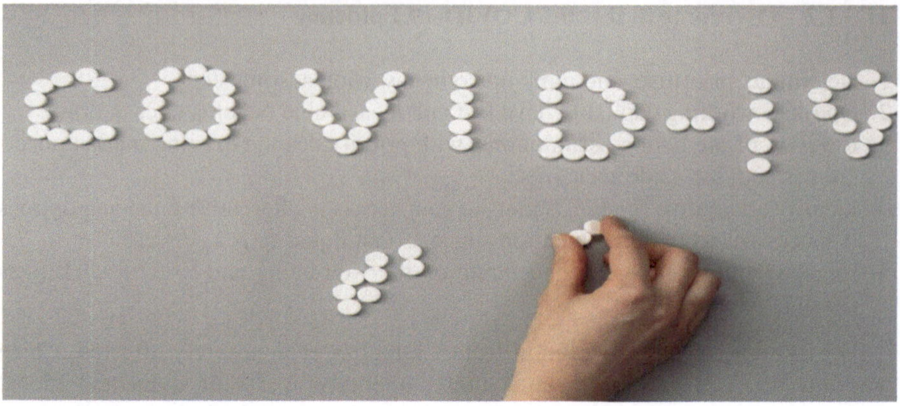

Fig. 11.3 Pharmaceutical sector

other nations. In 2018, 24% of medications and 31% of medicinal products have been manufactured from Asia. Thirteen percent of the pharmaceutical and genetic modification firms are headquartered outside of China, according to the FDA.

11.3.2.2 Example

1. Paracetamol prices have risen to between 400 and 450 Indian Rupees per kilogram from 250 to 300 Rupees per kilogram in India.
2. The prices of penicillin and vitamins rose in India by 40–50%.
3. The rising price of drugs.
4. Failure to have active pharmaceuticals or finished Chinese medicines.
5. Interstate transport challenges.

The prices of prescription medicines might also increase in the United States and other nations through prolonged prolongation.

11.3.2.3 Overcome in this COVID-19 Epidemic

1. The government is exploring ways to promote APIs' domestic development by building a country's correct ecosystem.
2. The FDA collaborates with the local manufacturer to alleviate the shortage. FDA aims to ensure that others can substitute. No lack of goods has been established.
3. The government has also limited the immediate export of diagnostic kits and ensured that medical tools are not permitted in any conditions to be exported by the firms.

4. Through lowering the expense of sanitising and surgical gloves, the government has taken a crucial measure. Nevertheless, connectivity is a huge hindrance to the public.
5. The government aims to expand in the future the API market.

11.3.3 Oil, Gas, and Chemical Executive

The effect of COVID-19 and fuel markets' battle has revealed that the crude, gas, and chemical industries have been experiencing a double crisis. Failure to agree on on-demand reductions implies a decline in oil prices, and industrial slowness and travel constraints resulting from the global pandemic are slowing down the need for chemical and finished goods.

Through the middle of a two-way situation, the crude, gas, and pharmaceutical industries face an energy price battle and the effects of COVID-19. A few weeks ago, OPEC and Russia struggled to decide on supply reductions, so petroleum prices fell sharply. In tandem with the need for chemicals and refinements arising from the production slowdowns and travel restrictions following COVID-19, such imbalances in oil supply/demand exist. Consequently, the short- to medium-term forecast continues to be more daunting than ever for high-cost firms, smaller players, and high-end debt businesses.

There is a range of problems confronting existing or new ventures through the petroleum and gas chain regarding project delivery, preparation, and pandemic risk management. Therefore, it is necessary to pay attention to the way the EPC industry cope with COVID-19 to remain afloat. This deterioration in the control of the workers and expenses of existing and future ventures will be quite tricky for the industry (Fig. 11.4).

11.3.3.1 Potential Long-Term Impact on Oil, Gas, and Chemical Companies

Big oil, gas, and chemical firms respond by reducing capital and operating costs to manufacturers and oilfield services. This suggests the following:

1. Inefficient companies that are heavily leveraged can face liquidity crises, with some being put out of business.
2. US shale producers would be particularly stressed if they continue to have supply surplus and rising rates.
3. Some of the bigger, more stable businesses may alter or speed up their efforts to diversify into other energy markets, triggering a business model transition.
4. After redundancies and disappearances, businesses can face a shortage of qualified staff until the economy recovers.

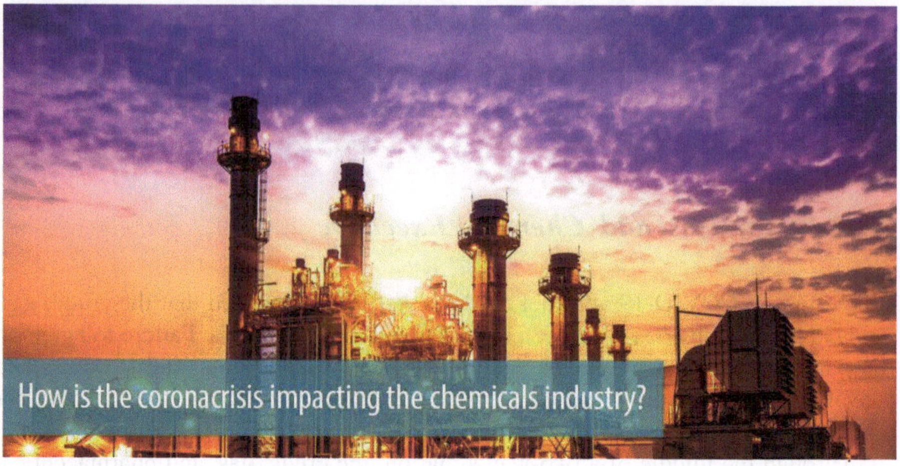

Fig. 11.4 Oil, gas, and chemical sector

11.3.3.2 Practical Next Steps

The leaders of oil, gas, and chemicals can be identified in crisis management three dimensions: reacting, healing, and flourishing. Several essential next moves are as follows:

1. Assess how the business should proceed with its financing, maintaining the gap between its current requirements and its expected returns, dividends, equity buybacks, etc. on the sector.
2. Consider how the recession is to be seen as a tool for rethinking how the job has been performed, such as speeding up digital capability adoption.
3. Assess the direction of jobs and complement emerging global expertise approaches.

We are strengthening this circumstance by mobilising and solving the public safety issue, stabilising and mitigating financial consequences, strategising and creating bold campaigns for catching the individual chances of this problem, and establishing viable value chains.

11.3.4 Supply Chain

This chapter discusses the potential short-term steps that businesses may take in reaction to the transformation of the market and supply chain issues arising from the global growth of COVID-19. Will COVID-19 be the Black Swan case compelled to reconsider and change its global supply chain paradigm for other businesses and the whole industry in the long run? In particular, it has exposed the weaknesses of many

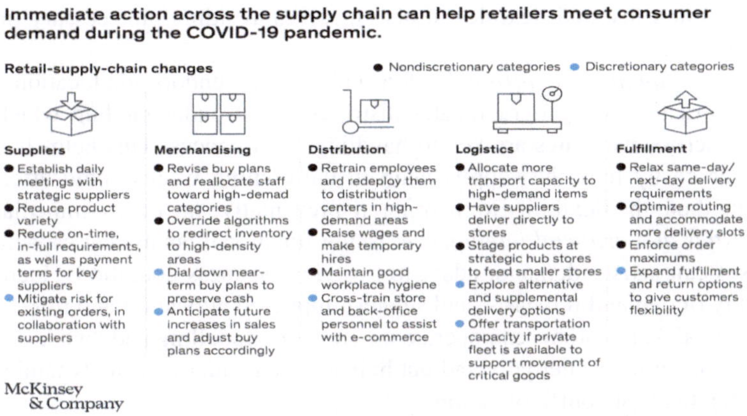

Fig. 11.5 Supply chain overcome during the COVID-19 pandemic

organisations for those who are highly reliant on China to meet their requirements for raw materials or finished goods. A decades-long emphasis on the management of supply chains to mitigate prices, cut inventories, and maximise stock usage has reduced reserves and absorption efficiency, and the COVID-19 demonstrates that many companies are not entirely conscious of the weakness of their supply chains in the face of global shocks.

Fortunately, new technologies have emerged in the supply chain, which significantly boosts the entire supply chain's exposure to these shocks and allows firms to cope with them. The linear supply chain's modern model has been turned into a digital supply network (DSN), disassembling physical silos and linking companies along the supply chain to ensure end-to-end connectivity, alignment, accessibility, and performance.

DSNs have been designed to avoid and solve new technical challenges such as IoT, AI, robotics, and 5G. Regardless of whether a "Black Swan" case such as COVID-19, trade war, war or extremism, regulatory changes, labour disputes, a rapid increase in competition, or collapse of manufacturers, organisations operating DSNs are willing to address the unpredictable [7].

The epidemic has prompted others to rapidly change their supply chains, while the supply chain business confronts various obstacles, including changing market demand, constraints, and possible commodity shortages (Fig. 11.5).

Organisations will focus on approaches promoting strategic preparation in the future and reducing the effects of related incidents.

Among the areas of improvement are as follows:

1. *End-to-end stock visibility*: Organisations will know what is on offer in their stores, and when, and they can respond rapidly to evolving circumstances and consumer demands. A centralised platform includes standardised inventory representation across platforms. This helps companies to replenish and product

movement's fast and flexible—it also involves avoiding unnecessary inventory expenses.
2. *Complex supplier monitoring*: Understanding how vendors and locations of their subcontractors are geographically distributed and understanding which goods move across such sites are key to handling disturbances. This helps businesses foresee easily how the supply chain in the coming weeks could affect them, giving them the flexibility to incorporate preventative measures immediately.
3. *Analytics and artificial intelligence*: Using functional, analytical capacity, businesses can satisfy demand, adapt to evolving business conditions, increase the quality of demand forecasts, and suggest improved allocation and refurbishment strategies. Applications can operate on scenario modelling and "what-if" scenarios by integrating internally and publicly assisted data to create dynamic models to track the best course of action.
4. *Process automation*: Automation of process ensures the replenishment becomes much faster and more agile. Systems that have low-stock warnings, for instance, will quickly and efficiently order items for a specific shop from the correct location.

11.3.5 Tourism

The COVID-19 pandemic could lose millions of jobs in the world's tourism industry, which, like no other case in history, has disrupted travel and rendered 96% of all destinations worldwide restrictions in reaction to the epidemic, says UNWTO. In recent years, UNWTO has been tracking travel facilitation and witnessing a continuous movement towards more transparency as a professional United Nations department for tourism. Since January 2020, almost all foreign destinations have implemented travel limits, including full travel bans, as they seek to combat the pandemic. Ninety-six percent of all global destinations imposed travel limitations as a consequence of the epidemic as of April 6. Roughly or in part 90 destinations have closed their borders to visitors, while some 44 additional targets remain closed to other visitors, depending on their home country. The government placed public safety first and imposed full or limited limits on transport. COVID-19 has a significant effect in the past of transportation and transport like any other case before.

Aeroplanes and hotels have been shut down, and the worldwide pandemic has impacted tourism in several respects. However, travel have already rendered the virus a global problem, so it is essential to focus on the role of travel in modern societies (Figs. 11.6 and 11.7).

The tourism sector accounts for 10% of GDP, generating over 50 million workers. Throughout the industry, there would be a 12–14% decline. All concerned would be impacted. Asia is the world's biggest continent. The tourism value chain spanning accommodation, travel agents, tour facilities, attractions, restaurants, family entertainment places, and transport from air, ground, and sea would decline.

Estimated impact of COVID-19 on air transport in 2020
(RPKs and air passenger revenue loss), IATA

Region of airline registration	% Change in RPKS (2020 vs. 2019)	Est. Impact on pass. revenue 2020 vs. 2019 (US$ billion)
Africa	-32%	-4
Asia Pacific	-37%	-88
Europe	-46%	-76
Latin America	-41%	-15
Middle East	-39%	-19
North America	-27%	-50
Industry	-38%	-252

Fig. 11.6 Air transport impact due to COVID-19. (Source: IATA)

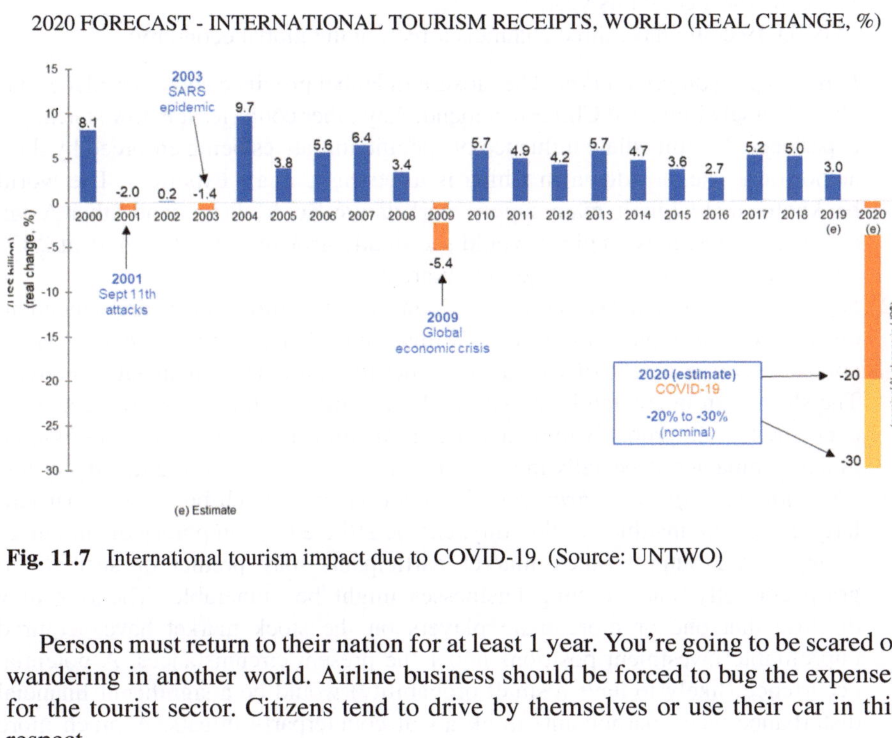

Fig. 11.7 International tourism impact due to COVID-19. (Source: UNTWO)

Persons must return to their nation for at least 1 year. You're going to be scared of wandering in another world. Airline business should be forced to bug the expenses for the tourist sector. Citizens tend to drive by themselves or use their car in this respect.

11.3.6 Global Economy and GDP

The COVID-19 can have three significant impacts on the global economy: directly impacting output, building a supply chain and upsetting markets, and having a financial influence on businesses and capital markets. Nonetheless, the public's reaction to the disease depends a lot.

This expanded through more than 190 nations in all US states after the original COVID-19 epidemic was detected. The pandemic has a pronounced influence on global economic development. Estimates to date suggest that if current circumstances continue, the virus could lower global economic growth up to 2.0% each month. Depending on the global financial crisis's magnitude and scale, world trade could also decline by 13–32%. Also, the consequences of the pandemic outbreak can be completely understood. This study analyses the rising global economic impacts and the answer to these consequences from policymakers and foreign bodies [2].

COVID-19 has a more extended and more extreme economic effect than predicted, with macro forecasts again being lowered. We have already seen a 2.4% decrease in world GDP this year.

COVID-19 could have three channels affecting the global economy:

1. *Direct impact on production*: The closure in Hubei province and other places has also adversely impacted Chinese demand. Any other countries are now starting to experience the immediate influence of specific initiatives being enforced by their authorities. The slowdown in China is affecting China's exporters. The world banknotes that China's main supply markets are Korea, Japan, and other Asian countries. Thus, these regions would see steady growth in the first half of 2020 without the advent of new epidemic outbreaks.
2. *Supply chain and market disruption*: Many manufacturing firms are dependent on intermediate input imports from China and other affected countries. Many companies often depend on China's revenues to achieve their financial objectives. The slowdown in economic activity and transport constraints—in the countries concerned—will probably influence the production and profitability of individual global companies, especially in manufacturing and manufacturing raw materials.
3. *The financial impact on firms and financial markets*: Such businesses, particularly those with insufficient liquidity, can be afflicted by temporary disturbances in input and output. Stock market participants may predict or struggle to grasp correctly, and growing businesses might be vulnerable. The risk may disclose that one or more main players on the stock market have acquired unprofitable investment positions under the present circumstances. A potential occurrence (likely to have a small probability) would be a significant financial disturbance when participants think about counterparty threats. A much more significant risk is that the financial markets and corporate bond markets would decrease considerably, with investors tend to keep state securities (particularly US Treasuries) due to the pandemic instability.

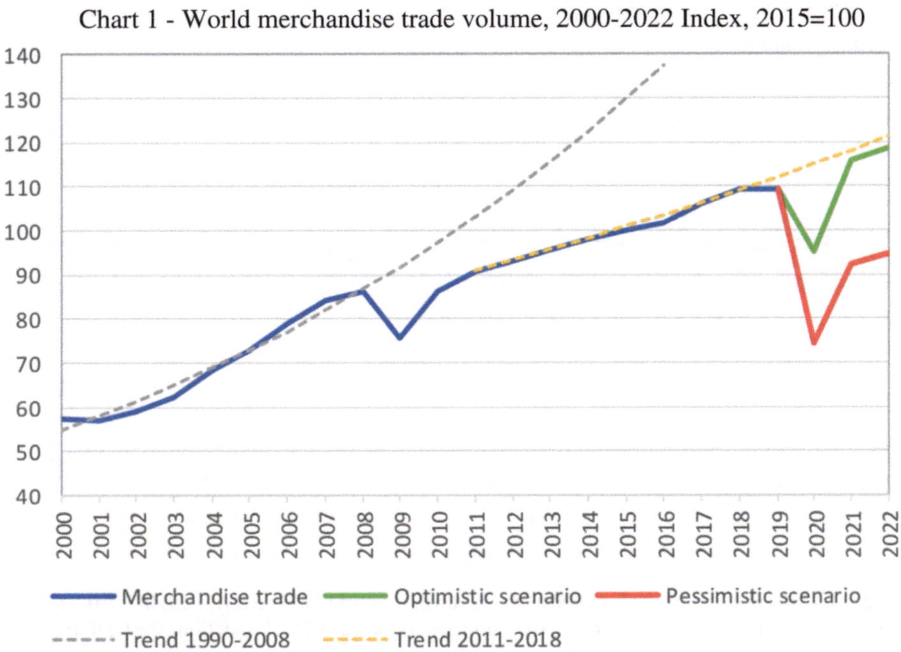

Fig. 11.8 World merchandise trade volume, 2000–2022. (Source: WTO Secretariat)

The wide variety of explanations for the downturn was attributed to the extraordinary complexity and ambiguity of the health problem's exact economic effects. Yet WTO analysts agree that the fall is likely to surpass the 2008–2009 trade slump (Figs. 11.8 and 11.9).

The continually evolving complexity of the COVID-19 crisis poses many challenges, which allows calculating the maximum expense of global economic operation challenging.

Such issues are not limited to but include:

- The situation will continue for how long?
- How many workers are temporarily and permanently affected?
- How many countries are infected, and how much will be reduced economic activity?
- When are the economic impacts going to peak?
- What is the amount of economic activity lost following the viral inflammation?
- What are the most successful national and global monetary and fiscal strategies to address the crisis?
- How does the crisis briefly and permanently affect how businesses manage their staff?
- Numerous public health initiatives, such as Italy, Taiwan, South Korea, Hong Kong, and China, have significantly impacted these countries' economies

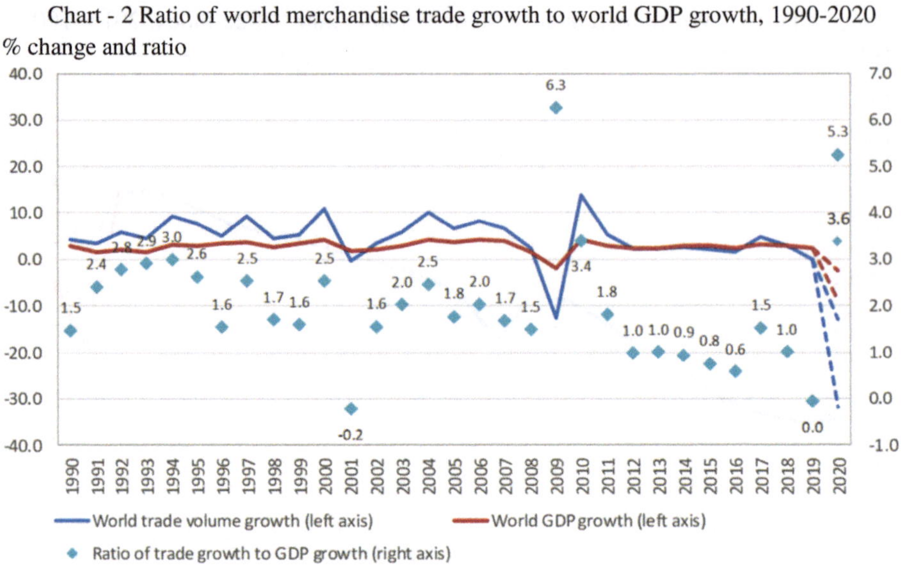

Fig. 11.9 Ratio of world merchandise trade growth to world GDP growth, 1990–2020. (Source: WTO Secretariat for trade and consensus estimates for actual GDP. Projections for GDP based on scenarios simulated with WTO Global Trade Model)

(including plant closures and travel restrictions). What are the trade-offs between public health and the economic implications of strategy to reduce the virus's spread?

11.3.7 Human Mental Health

The pandemic level of COVID-19 has now been reached. In biomedical and psychological terms, the WHO has guided the management of the question. Although preemptive and surgical steps are the most critical in this process, psychological emergency management strategies are often essential for people experiencing COVID-19. This encompasses patient primary, families, healthcare professionals, and skilled services indirect [8, 9, 10].

Firstly, there are five details regarding pain, the brain, and mental well-being that can support. There is almost no behavioural health-friendly disorder, disorder, or accident.

1. This is a useful link between our minds and our digestive system. Environmental factors such as bacteria, chemicals, and notorious COVID-19 are mainly regulated in the immune system. It is closely connected to our mood and several brain diseases ranging from Alzheimer's disease to stroke and depression.

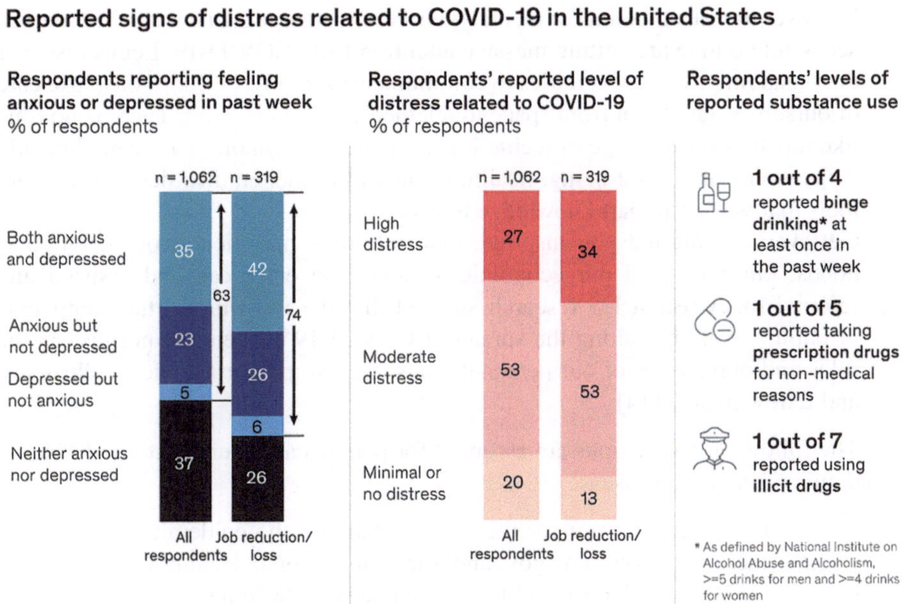

Fig. 11.10 Distress in the United States due to COVID-19

2. Stress is natural and can be useful (and encourage positive behaviour; think of a zebra that wants to flee the lion fast), just not too much tension. High and unchecked pressures have multiple adverse impacts on the brain and immune and vascular system that contribute to blood sugar imbalances, blood pressure, and compromised immune and inflammatory responses—the almost exact opposite of the possible influence of COVID-19 [11].
3. Physical activity has been associated with improvements in neural connectivity and rises in brain development factors in both physical and mental well-being and daily exercise.
4. Carefulness and calming strategies may enhance morale and sleep quality by growing awareness and concentration on the body's anticipation and worries.
5. Investing in countries with long-term benefits in behavioural well-being. Studies have shown that the potential for physical and behavioural well-being is related to past mental and physical health investments. The more reliable, the faster—though never too late [12, 13] (Fig. 11.10).

Three habits for good mental hygiene to beat COVID-19, a healthier new normal, are as follows:

1. Take what you should do every day and take action—how low that can be. There is a lot of industry for small technology and also no-tech options. Go out of nature and enjoy the slowest physical exercise speed, relaxation, and vitamin D every day.

2. Discover the latest toolkit for mental well-being—including its form. Those tools accessible online are getting massive attention from COVID-19. Let us discover the broad range of opportunities to communicate socially, be conscious, take care of ourselves, and learn from space to telemedicine and beyond. There is no time like this to test our usage of technology, especially technology in mental health. Apps won't offer well-being, health, or an end to mental disorder, but they are tools that we can impart knowledge to use.
3. Get everyone around you inspired. Our cultures—our friends, our neighbourhoods, our jobs, and our economies—should be embraced and assisted and referred to. A recent US research showed that the most influential campaigns of public health in halting the spread of COVID-19 concentrate not just on the roles and obligations of our personal goals but also on our families, colleagues, and fellow people [14].

The following instructions are essential for patients and their relatives during an epidemic of infectious disease:

1. *Stay updated*: Keep aware for the latest details on the epidemic from reliable outlets, including www.cdc.gov and the International Health Organization's Centers for Disease Control and Prevention, at www.who.int.
2. *Teach-educate*: To prevent diseases such as hand washing and coughing, monitor and exchange essential knowledge on hygiene.
3. *Correct disinformation*: Correct facts. Medical professionals' sharing of credible and established public health resources helps correct inaccurate information and misperception.
4. *Limit media access*: Use media sufficiently to make rational choices and shut it off.
5. *Anticipate and address stress reactions*: Be mindful that it is normal for you or family members to experience anxiety as a response to the spread of infectious illness and recognise the signs of stress. Take efforts to alleviate and minimise tension such as following daily habits, taking part in enjoyable events, concentrating on the best qualities of your life and issues you can manage, searching for help from family and friends, and engaging in physical and tension-reduction strategies [15].

11.3.8 Information Technology

COVID-19 impacted the technology market negatively, such as the impact on raw material stocks, interruptions in the electronics supply chain, and commodities' price inflation. From the constructive perspective, the intrusion has allowed the remote process to intensify, and the end-to-end value chain is quickly measured. Potential cuts in carbon emissions can also contribute to a renewed emphasis on sustainable practices.

Digital contact tracing is effective and efficient, but not widely used in the western world due to strict privacy regulations and patient rights. Current infection control and tracing measures do not include animals and moving objects like cars despite evidence that these moving objects can be infection carriers. This model solution will allow moving objects to receive or send notifications when they are close to a flagged, probable, or confirmed diseased case, or flagged place or object [16]. Artificial intelligence (AI) is a weapon in the battle against the infectious pandemic that has impacted the whole planet since early 2020. Data scientists use social media, web, and other knowledge machine learning techniques for subtle signs that the disease may spread. Advances on AI software such as natural language processing, expression understanding, and data mining are used [17]. Novel coronavirus (COVID-19) outbreak has raised a calamitous situation all over the world. Deep learning techniques proved themselves to be a powerful tool in the arsenal used by clinicians. This paper aims to overview the recently developed systems based on deep learning techniques using different imaging modalities [18]. In addition to these initiatives, integrating COVID-19-related clinical data with existing biobanks, such as the UK Biobank, could maximise efforts towards a faster and feasible approach for meaningful data mining [19]. Remote patient monitoring [20] and remote working [21] might also be beneficial.

11.3.8.1 Potential Long-Term Impact on Technology Subsectors

1. *Hardware/Software*
   (a) New mobile releases may be delayed due to constraints in the supply chain. Cell phone users will delay the replacement of their devices because of decreased customer trust in contracts.
   (b) After the reopening of factories in Asia, businesses face the task of entirely operating production. There may be significant short-term and future long-term consequences.
   (c) Unlike the shortage of parts and the unpredictability of supply chains, the software is a production driver.
   (d) Remote work solutions businesses are now seeing rising demand as organisations increase their ability for remote work.
   (e) Third-party monitoring tools have the benefits of rising remote staff. As companies continue to protect terminals, in particular cloud-based applications, log monitoring, and VPNs, IT expenditure on protection technologies may be increasing.
   (f) Computer vendors may see a strong demand from businesses placing large orders for laptops and connectivity products to benefit home-based workers.
2. *IT Services*
   (a) Outlook for IT usage shows continuing cloud computing services demand and a future rise in tech expenditure. Forecasts often foresee growing

competition for communications equipment as companies support workers' role and shift to online classes in schools.
   (b) The software infrastructure with a robust corporate continuity strategy is not effective for most companies. IT departments will play a more significant role in future PCOs because of improved remote operational scenarios. They would require IT service providers to support acquiring equipment and create a robust, scalable, and stable network, recovery systems, IT protection, etc.
   (c) The requirement for rapidly accelerated connectivity and integration of network hardware and communications will intensify the emphasis as well and speed up 5G network rollout and 5G technology acceptance.

3. *Semiconductors*
   (a) Road materials like titanium, copper, and chemicals are vulnerable to intrusion, with up to a quarter gap of supply, and are not easy to reinvent.
   (b) Within the short term, production and output fluctuations occur in the upward and downward technological value chain. This may cause a part scarcity (or lack) and trigger shock points in the development of boards and systems.
   (c) New launch plans can be delayed over the longer term, and product development approaches may need adjustments to match the supply chain pace (designs, decision-making, etc.). Delays may contribute to reduced consumer engagement, organisational meetings, and public events.
   (d) In the long run, the threats of regional fragmentation and durability will be expected to be tackled by businesses, to avoid the single failure points to restrict potential disruption.
4. *Network Equipment*
   (a) Increased telecommunication tools are more development firms embrace telecommuting would have possible advantages for businesses that already have applications in place.
   (b) The requirement for rapidly accelerated data connectivity and integration would intensify the emphasis of 5G network deployment and 5G system implementation on the network hardware and communications.

11.3.8.2 Practical Next Steps

Leaders of technology will be identified by addressing a crisis in three dimensions: reaction, recovery, and development.

Some vital next steps include the following:

- Evaluate the supply chain and disruptions in potential incidents.
- Accelerate progress and technical development in favour of the "new" scenarios.
- Find M&A prospects for technological development and production.
- Comprehend and improve inventory techniques for buffer uncertainty and risk, including supply-side shocks.

- Incorporate technologically activated potential technologies, like company and back-office software.

11.3.9 Food and Agriculture

Any 820 million people worldwide are reportedly struggling with extreme poverty—they do not consume enough adequate resources to lead everyday lives. Among these, 113 million faces acute severe poverty starvation so intense that it presents an urgent threat to their life or livelihoods and leaves them reliant on external aid. We could not risk any further delays or exposure to products brought on by COVID-19. The implications may be dramatic if COVID-19 situations, already present in most world regions, increase in the 44 countries that need international food assistance or 113 million acute food scarcity in 53 nations. Many of whose public safety and social welfare programs are faced by capacity restriction.

COVID-19 disrupts dozens of other farming and supply chain operations. Preliminary reports indicate that migration labour's unavailability, especially in north-western India where wheat and pulses are harvested, is interrupting some harvesting activities. Supply chains become broken owing to logistics issues and other challenges. Prices for maize, vegetables, and other commodities have fallen. However, customers spend more regularly.

Some steps are essential here to ensure the functionality of the agricultural and supply chains:

1. The challenges affecting labour shortages and dropping rates should be fixed.
2. To ensure food health, ensuring supply chains work well.
3. As far as possible, agricultural communities will be shielded from the coronavirus through monitoring and social isolation.
4. The government should promote commerce by removing export bans and limits on imports.

11.3.10 Textile

The COVID-19 pandemic is projected to have primarily adverse effects on exports and second-class effects in both exports and local sales in domestic markets. The epidemic has affected the export markets, with around 60% of all clothing exports from India in terms of revenue (the United States, the EU combined making up). It results in orders being cancelled, contributing to inventories and hopes that export receivables will be slower to sell due to higher demands for working capital.

According to the Clothing Manufacturers Association of India, there may be as many as one crore employment losses in the textile industries severely impacted by the ongoing lockout, if no assistance and recovery packages are required from the government. CMAI, which employs around 3700 people and 7 lakhs, reported that most of its leaders do not have the kind of assets they need to see approximately 80% of the cloak market, mainly micro-, small-, or medium-sized enterprises.

11.4 Proposed Solutions

- AI and big data analytics are the crossroads of public health planning, epidemiology, science development, and IT. Their goal is to give specialists in these fields an exciting opportunity to work together and meet standards for an efficient and timely response.
- Media reports indicate that a couple of days before the outbreak's official announcement, BlueDot, a Canadian artificial intelligence company, raised the first warning regarding an outbreak of an air condition [22].
- AI researchers may use machine learning techniques to collect data on fever polluting people from social media chats on the Internet, where doctors and other data track and detect cases on subtle signs of disease transmission. In reality, several viewing methods were developed to demonstrate the spread of the coronavirus [23].
- Smart AI testing kits.
- AI-based quarantine system.
- AI-based application for contact tracing.
- AI-based system improving diagnostic efficiency and classifying patient.
- AI-based mobile information-sharing software.

11.5 Technological Limitations in Short Time

COVID-19's rapid spread has prompted countries to use every trick in the book to contain the disease. During their battle against the pandemic, this wide variety of technology poses concerns about unnecessary surveillance and the infringement of people's privacy.

Location tracing, mobile apps, CCTVs, smart imaging, robots, and drones can be used, but every technology has its limitations. Telehealth software is at the forefront of treatment for coronavirus. And it does improve. It is difficult to provide the necessary technological resources in a short time.

11.6 Conclusion

The COVID-19 pandemic has impacted multiple industries. Businesses respond quickly, thus managing the financial and organisational problems, to rising demands of the employees, consumers, and suppliers. The number of possible improvements to the paradigm may be overwhelming for all markets, roles, and geographies impacted. This chapter has covered the COVID-19 epidemic impacts and suggestions to overcome it. It is not shocking that industries are influenced to various degrees. Several industries, such as transportation, leisure, and hotels, have reduced interest. This market cannot be restored in a significant proportion. Delays are likely to exist in other industries. This is a crisis without precedent and raises unparalleled threats to all industries' freedoms, stability, and growth worldwide. We need to work together to advance intelligence, unity, and action on these three fronts. We have a chance to solve this pandemic and change our way of fostering and engaging in the young generation. We have an opportunity to address this pandemic and change our way of promoting and participating in the young age by providing solutions using big data and AI. But now we must move and take swift and wide-ranging steps. This is not a gradual question but an invitation to clarify the world's future in all its sectors.

Declaration of Competing Interest None.

References

1. World Health Organization, *Countries Agree Next Steps to Combat Global Health Threat by MERS-CoV* (WHO, Geneva, 2019)
2. W. Qiu, C. Chu, A. Mao, J. Wu, The impacts on health, society, and economy of SARS and H7N9 outbreaks in China: A case comparison study. J. Environ. Public Health **2018**, 2710185 (2018)
3. J.C. Morganstein, R.J. Ursano, C.S. Fullerton, H.C. Holloway, Pandemics: Health care emergencies, in *Textbook of Disaster Psychiatry*, ed. by R. J. Ursano, C. S. Fullerton, L. Weisaeth, B. Raphael, 2nd edn., (Cambridge University Press, Cambridge, UK, 2017), pp. 270–283
4. G.W.K. Wong, T.F. Leung, Bird flu: Lessons from SARS. Paediatr. Respir. Rev. **8**(2), 171–176 (2007)
5. Smith, Responding to global infectious disease outbreaks: Lessons from SARS on the role of risk perception, communication, and management. Soc. Sci. Med. **63**(12), 3113–3123 (2006)
6. R.J. Scarfone, S. Alexander, S.E. Coffin, et al., Emergency preparedness for pandemic influenza. Pediatr. Emerg. Care **22**(9), 661–671 (2006)
7. S. Hahn, Coronavirus (COVID-19) Supply Chain Update [Internet]. US Food and Drug Administration (FDA), February 27, 2020, https://www.fda.gov/news-events/press-announcements/coronavirus-covid-19-supply-chain-update. Cited 24 Mar 2020
8. X. Huo, L.-L. Chen, L. Hong, et al., Economic burden and its associated factors of hospitalized patients infected with A (H7N9) virus: A retrospective study in Eastern China, 2013–2014. Infect. Dis. Poverty **5**(1), 79 (2016)
9. Z.A.Z. Hu, L. Zhao, A comparative study of public-health emergency management. Ind. Manag. Data Syst. **109**(7), 976–992 (2009)
10. M. Xu, S.-X. Li, Analysis of good practice of public health emergency operations centers. Asian Pac J Trop Med **8**(8), 677–682 (2015)
11. A.M. Zaki, S. Van Boheemen, T.M. Bestebroer, A.D.M.E. Osterhaus, R.A.M. Fouchier, Isolation of a novel coronavirus from a man with pneumonia in Saudi Arabia. N. Engl. J. Med. **367**(19), 1814–1820 (2012)

12. Y. Bai, C.-C. Lin, C.-Y. Lin, J.-Y. Chen, C.-M. Chue, P. Chou, Survey of stress reactions among health care workers involved with the SARS outbreak. Psychiatr. Serv. **55**(9), 1055–1057 (2004)
13. J.T.F. Lau, X. Yang, H.Y. Tsui, E. Pang, Y.K. Wing, Positive mental health-related impacts of the SARS epidemic on the general public in Hong Kong and their associations with other negative impacts. Infection **53**(2), 114–124 (2006)
14. L. Du, B. Luo, J. Wang, B. Pan, J. Chen, J. Liu, Study on social burden of ASRS in Guangzhou. Chin. J. Public Health Manage. **22**(4), 274–276 (2006)
15. M. Bults, D.J. Beaujean, O. de Zwart, G. Kok, P. van Empelen, J.E. van Steenbergen, et al., Perceived risk, anxiety, and behavioral responses of the general public during the early phase of the influenza A (H1N1) pandemic in the Netherlands: Results of three consecutive online surveys. BMC Public Health **11**, 2 (2011). https://doi.org/10.1186/1471-2458-11-2
16. L. Garg, E. Chukwu, N. Nasser, C. Chakraborty, G. Garg, Anonymity preserving IoT-based COVID-19 and other infectious disease contact tracing model. IEEE Access **8**, 159402–159414 (2020). https://doi.org/10.1109/ACCESS.2020.3020513
17. M.V. Pawar, J. Anuradha, A. Pawar, Machine learning solutions to COVID 19, in *Data Science for COVID 19*, (Elsevier, Amsterdam, 2020) ISBN: 9780128245361
18. Md. Milon Islam, F. Karray, R. Alhajj, J. Zeng, A review on deep learning techniques for the diagnosis of novel coronavirus (COVID-19)
19. A. Alimadadi, S. Aryal, I. Manandhar, P.B. Munroe, B. Joe, X. Cheng, Artificial intelligence and machine learning to fight COVID-19. Physiol. Genomics **52**, 200–202 (2020). https://doi.org/10.1152/physiolgenomics.00029.2020
20. M. Jayalakshmi, L. Garg, K. Maharajan, K. Srinivasan, K. Jayakumar, A.K. Bashir, K. Ramesh, Fuzzy logic-based health monitoring system for COVID'19 patients. Comput. Mater. Continua (2022)
21. A.K. Bhardwaj, L. Garg, A. Garg, Y. Gajpal, E-Learning during COVID-19 outbreak: Cloud computing adoption in Indian Public Universities. Comput. Mater. Continua **66**(3), 2471–2492 (2022). https://doi.org/10.32604/cmc.2021.014099
22. This Canadian Start-Up used A.I. to Track Coronavirus and Raised Alarm days Before the Outbreak, https://economictimes.indiatimes.com/magazines/panache/this-Canadian-startup-used-ai-to-track-coronavirus-and-raised-alarm-days-before-the-outbreak/articleshow/74203640.cms. Accessed 19 Feb 2020
23. How A.I. is tracking the Coronavirus Outbreak, https://www.wired.com/story/how-AI-tracking-coronavirus-outbreak/. Accessed 18 Feb 2020

Chapter 12
A New Collaborative Platform for Covid-19, Benchmark Datasets

Olivier Debauche, Saïd Mahmoudi, Sidi Ahmed Mahmoudi, and Pierre Manneback

12.1 Introduction

The need to share data between research teams is crucial and requires the implementation of specific security measures to guarantee the security of the exchanged data, the results, and applications produced. Security measures that should be implemented are the more important as the data processed is sensitive. In the medical field, in particular, due to the sensitivity of data, specific measures of protection of the private life are added. These measures use the anonymization of the data to prevent patients' identification. The establishment of an exchange and referencing platform for datasets and benchmarks is a tool that facilitates the establishment of new researches. However, to gain the support of users and gain the confidence necessary for its use, it must offer high-level data security mechanisms. In fact, IT developments in terms of security must therefore be important to guarantee security to the best of current possibilities and sufficiently solid to perpetuate it for years to come. Indeed, the results of any security threats resulting in sensitive data forgery, leakage, loss, or tampering must be prevented in a sharing data platform.

However, this issue can be overcome by the task of sharing data between secured networks through a common interface to data from multiples origins such as storage systems, and data backup. The system must be fault-tolerant to interrupted data transfer and reconcile large volumes of data and limited bandwidth between institutions [1].

O. Debauche (✉) · S. Mahmoudi · S. A. Mahmoudi · P. Manneback
University of Mons, Mons, Belgium
e-mail: olivier.debauche@umons.ac.be; said.mahmoudi@umons.ac.be; sidi.mahmoudi@umons.ac.be; pierre.manneback@umons.ac.be

L. Garg et al. (eds.), *Healthcare Informatics for Fighting COVID-19 and Future Epidemics*, EAI/Springer Innovations in Communication and Computing,
https://doi.org/10.1007/978-3-030-72752-9_12

Our platform was born from our own need in matter of data sharing during the Covid-19 crisis in order to develop and train specific artificial intelligence algorithms. In explanation, there were several teams of researchers to work in different aspects of the detection of Covid-19 patterns in X-ray and CT-scan images of lungs. The centralization of our research applications and results has made it possible to facilitate their dissemination and emulate collaborations with other research teams.

Following the subsequent paragraphs, this chapter will be structured as follows: In Sect. 12.2, we analyze the pros and cons of the existing works in matter of datasets sharing. Then, in Sect. 12.3, we present the conceptualization of our dataset benchmark sharing platform based on the analysis of various use cases, technological choices, and their implementation. Afterward, in Sect. 12.5, we test our platform in different use cases. Additionally, Sect. 12.6 will be dedicated to address constraints and limitations of the platform. Finally, we sum up and give an overview of our future developments in Sect. 12.7.

12.2 Related Works

This section is organized into following three parts: in the first part, important conceptualization aspects and issues must be clearly identified in order to be addressed. The second part focuses on the existing works dedicated to the security and the sharing of sensitive platform. Finally, the third part studies the best ways to ensure an optimal security to sensitive data.

12.2.1 General Principles of Platform Conceptualization

Dong et al. have proposed a framework based on the four aspects that must be considered to guarantee the safety: the first factor is the transmission from data owner to the platform; the second factor is computing at platform level and the security problem storage; the third factor concerns internal issues present in cloud platform; and finally, the fourth factor is the secure data destruction[2]. Niu et al. have proposed a framework based on cloud computing restful to secure a big data platform following the eight aspects of security: application, management, interface, network, platform software, server, storage, and virtualization platform[3]. We are inspired by this framework to develop our platform.

12.2.2 Existing Platforms to Manage Sensitive Data

Sharing sensitive data platforms can be categorized into cloud-centric and distributed platforms.

12.2.2.1 Cloud-Based Platforms

They use the cloud to process, encrypt and decrypt, and store sensitive data. This approach assumes that it is easier to manage data from a central point. However, cloud does not offer always all guarantees in terms of security and privacy.

Among the well-known and established research systems, we can mention the following major contributions:

The *COllaborative Informatics and Neuroimaging Suite (COINS)* is a toolkit dedicated to innovation and technology in order to handle a diverse set of data that offer to the scientific community an open-source application to deal with research, imagery, and medical data [4].

The *Alzheimer's Disease Neuroimaging Initiative (ADNI)* aims to investigate topics related to elderly's health, Mild Cognitive Impairment (MCI), and Alzheimer's disease to improve the technical capabilities for optimization, analysis, and acquisition [5].

The Mind Research Network (MRN) Clinical Imaging Consortium (CIC) is an institutional program that involves several partners to advance technology in terms of multisite with data coming from heterogeneous sources for outstanding capabilities to supply analyzing, archiving, exporting, querying, reporting, security, and summarizing [6].

The *Neuroimaging Informatics Tools and Resources Clearinghouse (NITRC)* is a website for organizing knowledge about the resource publicly available. It provides a common environment to download, discuss, educate, rate, and document a tremendous amount of resources [7].

The *Longitudinal Online Research and Imaging System (LORIS)* is a secure and user-friendly data automation based on a website that allows to manage all the chain from data acquisition, data storage, processing, and dissemination. LORIS facilitates the coordination and real-time management of input and output data, archiving, requesting, and exchanging with outer data [8].

The Cancer Imaging Archive (TCIA) is an open-source resource of knowledge providing help to diverse activities such as study, improvement, and assessment using cancer imaging [9].

The *Extensible Neuroimaging Archive Toolkit (XNAT)* is an open website that aims to receive, archive, manage, process, and share data of images that provide accessible services via REST API [10].

The *Quantitative Imaging Network (QIN)* encourages research, development, and clinical validation of better study cancer in clinical trial settings [11].

Among recent major contributions, we retained:

Dong et al. [2] have proposed to encrypt data store on the cloud storage in AES 256; the symmetric key is then encrypted with a Heterogeneous Proxy Re-Encryption (H-PRE) that transforms Identity-Based Encryption (IBE) into Public-Key Encryption (PKE). Moreover, they secure the sharing of sensitive data throughout the private procedure based on the XEN Virtual Machine Monitor (VMM).

GIFT-Cloud is a medical imagery data-sharing platform proposed by Doel et al. [1] composed of a server and an uploader. The role of this server is to secure the storage of anonymized data, hosts a web-based interface which allows a direct data access, and a REST API to provides integration to external software. The uploader achieves an automated anonymization and encryption on-site and data upload.

12.2.2.2 Distributed Platforms

These platforms are based on the repartition of sensitive data on multiple sites locally responsible for the encryption and decryption of data. The storage and the processing can be achieved locally or be distributed among many nodes. But, this approach is dependent on the security policy carried out at the level of each node.

Among major contributions in matter of distributed platforms, we retain the following ones:

The *Biomedical Informatics Research Network (BIRN)* is a collaborative effort to develop a federated and distributed new software-based platform to store, retrieve, analyze, and document biomedical imaging data in order to offer a service of data sharing to researchers specialized in biomedicine [12, 13].

Ozyurt et al. [14] defined the *Human Clinical Imaging Database* (HCID) as a collaborative effort of a combination of imaging and clinical data stored in a federated and distributed environment in which the database is able to provide help for storing new data types without changing the system. HCID addresses the needs to collaborate and create multisite projects taking into account high performance, usability, robustness, and extensibility.

Castiglione et al. [15] proposed an architecture composed of four modules: (1) a 3D adaptive lossless compression algorithm and digital embedded watermark module using a 3D adaptive lossless algorithm to healthcare data; (2) a Virtual infrastructure-less Cloud (VC) that is a cloud-based software as a service (SaaS) contains a set of node stacks running on a peer-to-peer overlay network; (3) a retention module based on the combination of MySQL and CryptDB; and (4) a front-end interface module that receives the inputs, shows patients' information kept in Virtual Cloud, and triggers the discovery and data transfer operation.

12.2.3 *Large Sharing Databases*

During the platform development in various domains, different large shareable databases have been built to understand diverse thematic among them: The Human Genome Project (HGP) for the genetic material [16]. The *Human Connectome Project (HCP)* aims to understand brain function [17, 18]. The *Cancer Genome Atlas (TCGA)* collects tissue samples and generates maps of the genetic changes in 20 cancers [19]. The collection and provision of very large amounts of data open up new possibilities in knowledge extraction and new fields of research.

12.2.4 *Best Ways of Secularization for Sensitive and Private Data*

Generally, a firewall is placed between the source and the cluster but has no control over inside activity. It is also necessary to detect internal attacks inside the cluster [20].

Apache Metron is a cybersecurity framework for big data that provides a centered and monitored tool to analyze quickly and answer to potential abnormalities. The framework contains four components: (1) a security Data Lake storing enriched telemetry data used to do feature engineering; (2) a pluggable framework providing a resourceful set of parsing for standard security data for common sources (fireye, netflow, pcap, snort,[1] sourcefire, Zeek[2] (formerly bro)) extensible to custom parsers; (3) a security application providing standard SIEM (agents to ingest data sources, alerting, threat intelligence framework); and (4) a Threat Intelligence Platform is a real-time machine learning algorithm to detect anomalies.

Paul et al.[20] have proposed a testbed in order to generate threats at same time internal and external, as well as to create large amounts of data for big data cluster. Moreover, they used hing3 tools to generate network protocol attacks such as DOS, ICMP Flooding, etc. While TestDFSIO allows to generate a tremendous amount of I/O operation, YARN REST API produces an important network activity [20].

12.3 Milestones of a Collaborative Platform

According to Niu et al. sensitive data attracts more potential attackers; consequently, it is necessary to have a strong platform security strategy [3] (Fig. 12.1).

[1]https://www.snort.org/.

[2]https://zeek.org/.

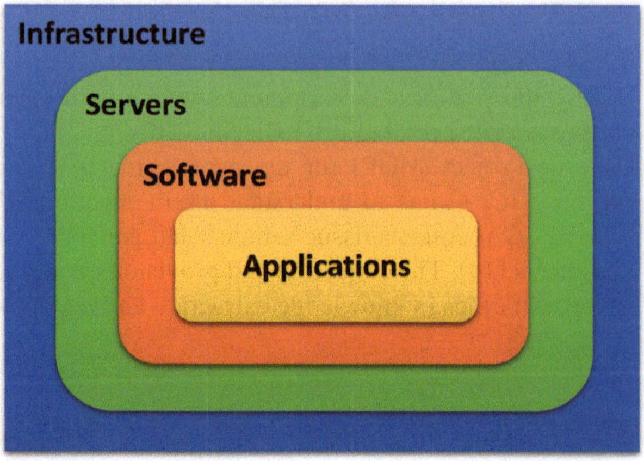

Fig. 12.1 Principle aspects of the platform

The main aspects that must be studied in detail are located at four levels: the infrastructure, the configuration of the servers with its software, and the developed applications. The infrastructure level contains two main aspects that are the network security and the data storage. This first level is generally controlled by a provider, and we rarely have a total control of this level. Servers rely on infrastructures in the data center. We have a greater or lesser degree of mastery over the servers depending on the type of services used: from the weakest with Virtual Private Server (VPS) to the largest with Dedicated Servers (DS) and their software configuration. The choice of Operating System and kernel and its configuration impact directly performances and the level of security. Generally, we have a complete mastery of software installed on servers and full responsibility for the quality of the applications developed.

12.4 Our Collaborative Platform

Our collaborative platform is called Covid Engineering (https://covid.engineering). This platform aims to allow the sharing of dataset and benchmark of medical images, epidemic data, and models and applications developed by research teams. It presents a cloud-centric platform replicated in three data centers to ensure high-availability services and a distributed replication of data. The main specificity of our platform is to integrate a same time high level of encryption to guarantee the data privacy, protection IDS/IPS/NIDS to guard against attacks from inside and outside. The following paragraphs describe the key aspects of our platform.

12.4.1 Network Security

The transfer of data is located between backbone routers, and each data center router analyzes DDoS attack signatures on netflow sent by routers measured in packets per second or in bytes on the following protocols: ACK, DNS, ICMP, IP fragmentation, Null and Private, RST, SYN, TCP Null, and UDP. The mitigation is based on a pre-firewall that filters coarsely the traffic and then on a firewall that filters more finely the flow. Afterward, attacks by amplifications such as DNS amp, NTP amp, SNMP amp, and Smurf are filtered. Finally, the most sophisticated attacks are treated. Figure 12.2 shows a global scheme of the implementation of network security.

12.4.2 Storage Security

The availability of data is essential; therefore, we have ensured the high availability of data with multiple replications of datasets in many geographical regions. In case of disaster, we implante a protocol of IP failure that changes the datastose in few secondes. Moreover, daily, 2 days, 3 days, and 1 week distant backup are automatically achieved to provide the recovery in case of a major disaster. For instance, in case of illegal access and/or theft, we use a double encryption to sense the non usability of data. A regular hash control of all files allows to verify that they have not been forged or tampered.

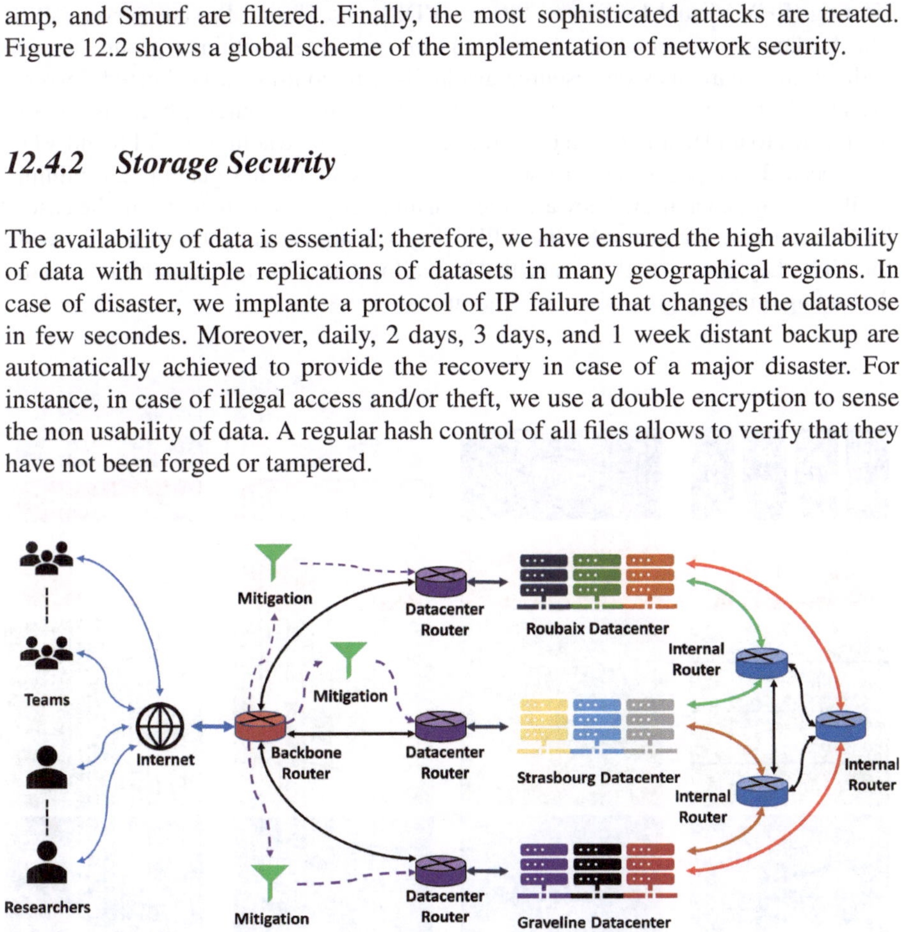

Fig. 12.2 Network security scheme

12.4.3 Server Security

On servers present in each of the three data centers, the operating system is installed with a grsecurity-patched kernel that contains a full suite of synergistic defenses. Furthermore, minimum configuration of the required components and applications are only installed. Moreover, anti-virus, anti-malicious code, and root kits are installed to ensure that servers are free of threats.

Figure 12.3 shows the differences between Dedicated Server (DS), Shared Hosting (SH), Virtual Dedicated Server (VDS), and Virtual Private Server (VPS). The Dedicated Server (DS) shares common resources within a group of users without any guarantees on resource availability. In contrast, a Dedicated Server is exclusively reserved for a single user who has all the resources, but this solution often leads to under-utilization of resources. Intermediate solutions (VPS and VDS) have been developed to better use of server's resources and guarantee a minimal availability for each user. They are often assimilated to each other, but in the case of VDS resources, for example, the CPU, they are allocated 100% to a user, while for VPS they are virtual servers that are allocated with an availability variable depending on the degree of use of other users.

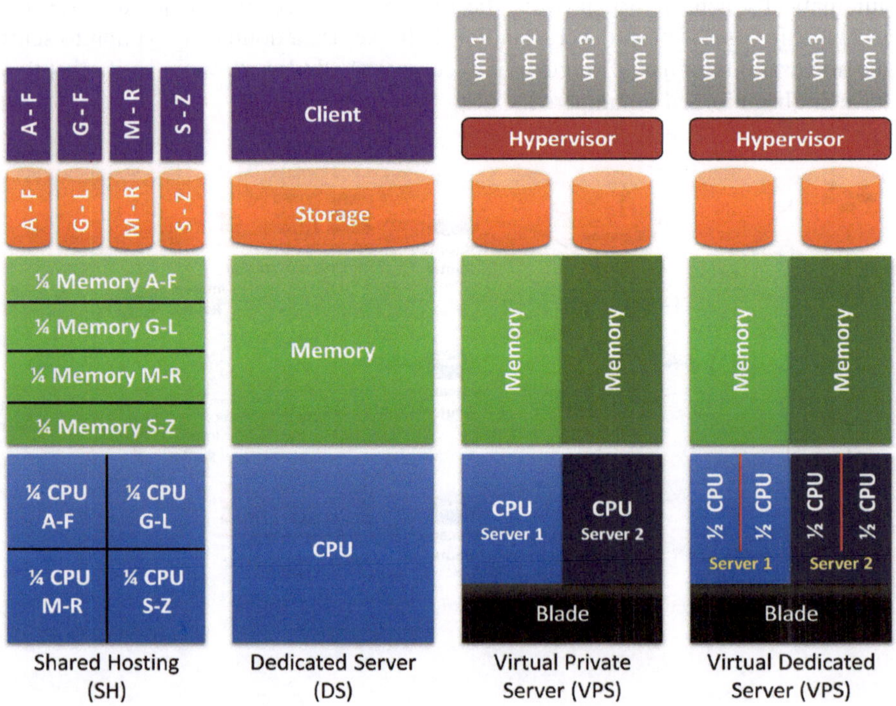

Fig. 12.3 Main ways of using servers

We use Virtual Dedicated Server (VDS) that brings advantages of Dedicated Server (DS) with computing power not shared and Virtual Private Server (VPS) offering the sharing of disk space hosting operating system (OS) and software, RAM, and network between multiple users in an isolated way. Software is installed in Docker containers to ensure a rapid deployment and adapt a number of instances in function of the load on the cluster.

12.4.4 Platform Security

We have implemented https protocol with TLS 1.3 and http 2 to secure and accelerate the loading between the platform and the users. Furthermore, fields of forms are obfuscated and regenerated at each call. Their lifetime is limited for 10 min. After this delay, the form is invalided. Each form also contains an authentication key saved in the database to avoid the theft of data by session fixation. Moreover, we have verifed by means of comparison of files hash to periodically detect code alterations by modification, new file addition, or code deletion. All actions achieved by users on the platform are recorded and include date-time, information source, event identifier, descriptions, parameters, and outcomes.

12.4.5 Users Management

Each user is identified by 2-factor authentication. The first authentication uses a couple user/password, and the second factor is a code sent by Short Message Service (SMS) on the user's cell phone. User password is hashed with Argon2id algorithm. The algorithm was designed by researchers from the University of Luxembourg that is a hybrid between Argon2i that maximizes resistance to GPU cracking attacks and Argon2d that maximizes resistance to side-channel attacks. We have implemented Argon2id by means of Sodium library. Users can be associated in groups to facilitate access to sharing data. A team can be authorized by IP restriction and common password for the team.

12.4.6 Dataset Management

When an individual user or a team of researchers deposits a new dataset on the platform, they must complete a form to describe the new dataset. Afterward, an individual FTP access is automatically created to upload the new dataset and the companion files such as metadata, annotation, and license file, etc. Each upload space is independent and only accessible by this Secure FTP (SFTP) access. In the next step, the user must identify each file and specify its nature, give a tiny description, and specify its privacy level (private, public, or shared). If images are also uploaded, they are used to create a carousel of images that show a sample of the proposed data. Dataset files are then individually encrypted with the Advanced Encryption Standard (AES) 256-GCM algorithm with the own key of the user that shares the dataset. We used the OpenSSL library to encrypt the dataset files. Symmetric key of each file encrypted with AES-256-GCM is then encrypted with XChaCha20Poly1305 algorithm, a hardened version of Chacha20Poly1305 against nonce misuse, thanks to Sodium library. The proposed datasets published in public mode are first validated by an administrator.

12.4.7 Developed Application Management

Platform users and research teams can publish their own models, applications, and pipelines. A proposed application must first be validated by an administrator before being available in public mode. When the application is offered in private or shared mode, it is accessible by people who have been designated by the owner for private mode (individual authentication) or by research teams for shared mode (IP restriction).

12.4.8 Integrity Verification

The integrity of the platform is checked regularly to ensure that no file in the application part has been modified. A checksum of each of the files is performed with SHA3-384 algorithm and compared with the one stored in the database. This verification is achieved every hour. It also allows to detect added code, altered or deleted parts on each file by comparison with the size of the original file one. If one or more corrupted files are detected, the platform manager is immediately notified. The system isolates, corrupts files, and restores the original ones.

12.4.9 Scalability

The cloud is potentially scalable at vertical extension of the infrastructure. However, physical limits constrain the possibilities of expansion such as the size of the data center, the network capacities in terms of backbone, and the possibilities of power supply.

12.5 Experimentation

Experimentation was conducted, based on the three use cases that allow us to evaluate the operation of our platform according to different configurations. The Covid-19 research uses mainly, on one hand, medical images to train various algorithms and establish models to detect the presence/absence of Covid-19 or localization of lesions due to the Covid-19. On the other hand, researchers work on the prediction. Researchers are also working on predicting the evolution of the Covid-19 at different local, national, continental, and global scales, but also on factors related to the virus. In addition, they also have needs in terms of sharing models, pipelines, and applications.

12.5.1 The Sharing of Covid-19 Image Benchmarks

The first case is the sharing among users the medical images (X-ray and CT scan) in order to train artificial intelligence algorithms to elaborate a rapid diagnostic of a possible Covid presence on X-ray and identify suspicious areas on slides of CT-scan to help the radiologist to quickly confirm Covid-19 cases.

New medical data (images and metadata) are continuously added to rise the dataset to diversify the data to improve the robustness of the algorithms developed and enhance their accuracy and/or validate prediction on new datasets by calculating the confusion matrix.

Each authorized user can load a complete dataset or differentiate them by adding and updating the last downloaded ones. These latter limit the amount of data needed to generate user-specific sub-dataset, which are resource-consuming. Sub-datasets are deleted after 7 305 days tosave the disk space required for data storage.

12.5.2 Covid Epidemic Dataset Sharing

The second use case focuses on sharing daily epidemic data used to ensure the following of Covid-19 pandemic and develops predictive models on the evolution of the numerous new cases, deaths, hospitalizations, and more particularly patients in intensive care. All data are stored in a database, plain text file, or CSV files according to the origin of the data. Data must be queryable on a selected time range when it is possible.

Several teams of researchers elaborate models on the basis of this data to predict the evolution of the Covid-19 with and without containment measures. These models are particularly important to inform policy makers during deconfinement phases by estimating the impact of these measures on the spread of the virus within the population.

This data is a matter of privacy and must therefore be encrypted using strong algorithms and signed using a hash algorithm in order to be protected against attempted theft, misappropriation, modification, and/or voluntary or unintentional alterations.

12.5.3 Models and Applications Sharing

The third use case is dedicated to sharing of results, models, and applications obtained from datasets and benchmarks. It is important to guarantee the sharing between research teams to allow cross-validation. This is particularly important to ensure the consistency of the results before they are sent to the authorities to inform them about their decision-making.

12.6 Constraints and Limitations

In addition to the physical limitations that are related to the hardware, the choice of encryption algorithms implies limitations in terms of amount of data encrypted with the same key and speed of encryption/decryption. The choice of file system impacts capabilities of storage and maximum file size that can be stored on it. In addition, network structure and bandwidth impact the data center replication and can limit them particularly when massive changes are operated on data.

12.6.1 Encryption Limitations

The size of the files or data package that can be protected by the same encryption key for XChaCha20Poly1305 algorithm is limited to 256 GB with a nonce of 192 bits, while AES-256-GCM algorithm is limited to 350 GB file with messages of 16KB with a same key. These maximum file sizes take time to be encrypted. A compromise is to split the files to be encrypted into a reasonable number of smaller files that can be encrypted fast and in parallel. In this scenario, we use a maximum file size of 50 GB offering a compromise between the number of files to be processed and the speed of encryption or decryption.

12.6.2 Storage Limitations

Our storage system uses Zettabyte File System (ZFS), which has the particularity of using an intermediate level of abstraction that has been added between the file system and the disks. It is the Volume Manager that allows the virtualization of a certain number of disks in a volume. Data integrity is ensured through the use of the SHA-256 algorithm that is used throughout the file system tree. Each data block is subject to a checksum, which is stored in the block pointer replicated throughout the system. This 128-bit file system is limited to a maximum number of snapshots and files limited to 2^{48}. The maximum size supported by the file system, and the maximum size of a single file, is 16 exbibytes.

12.6.3 Data Center Replication Limitations

The real-time replication of data between three data centers using Cross Data Center Replication (CDCR) implies to ensure an enough available bandwidth and to have a resilient network. Indeed, CDCR is not sufficient for overload scenarios where the rate of the update is increasing; in particular, in case of the bandwidth between and source and target is limited. Moreover, CDCR performs in more robust manner in terms of source and target collections.

12.7 Conclusion and Future Development

In this chapter, we provided a description and experimentation of our architecture allying the ease of managing of a cloud-based architecture, the robustness, and the resilience of a distributed architecture thanks to multisite replication. The novelty of our architecture is the integration of a Network Intrusion Detection and Prevention Systems (NIDS), an Intrusion Detection System (IDS), and an Intrusion Prevention System (IPS). The NIDS detects abnormal behavior caused by port scanning, malware, and security policy violation. The Intrusion Prevention System (IPS) proactively rejects packets of data at firewall level on the basis of a threats database regularly updated. The IDS/IPS protects against known threats, while the Network Intrusion Detection and Prevention System (NIDS) focuses on the identification of emerging threats inside the network.

Furthermore, our approach has the disadvantage of generating a lot of additional network traffics linked to multisite synchronization in real time and the need for more storage space than a solution distributed at the site level. Nevertheless, distributed solution performance stays conditioned by the network and storage capabilities of each partner and also the level of security implemented by each partner. In the case of the cloud-based, the network resilience is ensured by multiple peering points that allow to distribute traffic on several different networks, and the security is managed in one point.

From a perspective point of view, we aim to improve the possibility to monetize advanced models and applications in order to ease the valuation of researchers. Indeed, numerous research platforms have been developed to conduct longitudinal research and share large databases, benchmarks, and pipelines. However, the hosting and the direct usability of models and applications are rarely proposed. We will test our architecture proposition in other application domains to demonstrate its polyvalence.

Acknowledgement This work is partially funded by Infortech Research Institute. The authors would like to thank Meryem Elmoulat, PhD, for reviewing the English writing of this chapter.

References

1. T. Doel, D.I. Shakir, R. Pratt, M. Aertsen, J. Moggridge, E. Bellon, A.L. David, J. Deprest, T. Vercauteren, S. Ourselin, GIFT-Cloud: a data sharing and collaboration platform for medical imaging research. Comput. Methods Programs Biomed. **139**, 181–190 (2017)
2. X. Dong, R. Li, H. He, W. Zhou, Z. Xue, H. Wu, Secure sensitive data sharing on a big data platform. Tsinghua Sci. Technol. **20**(1), 72–80 (2015)
3. X. Niu, Y. Zhao, Research on big data platform security based on cloud computing, in *Security and Privacy in New Computing Environments. SPNCE 2019*, ed. by J. Li, Z. Liu, H. Peng. Lecture Notes of the Institute for Computer Sciences, Social Informatics and Telecommunications Engineering, vol. 284 (Springer, Cham, 2019), pp. 38–45
4. A. Scott, W. Courtney, D. Wood, R. De la Garza, S. Lane, R. Wang, J. Roberts, J.A. Turner, V.D. Calhoun, COINS: an innovative informatics and neuroimaging tool suite built for large heterogeneous datasets. Front. Neuroinf. **5**, Paper 33, 1–15 (2011). https://doi.org/10.1136/amiajnl-2010-000032
5. C.R. Jack Jr., M.A. Bernstein, N.C. Fox, P. Thompson, G. Alexander, D. Harvey, B. Borowski, P.J. Britson, J.L.Whitwell, C. Ward, A.M. Dale, J.P. Felmlee, J.L. Gunter, D.L. Hill, R. Killiany, N. Schuff, S. Fox-Bosetti, C. Lin, C. Studholme, C.S. DeCarli, G. Krueger, H.A. Ward, G.J. Metzger, K.T. Scott, R. Mallozzi, D. Blezek, J. Levy, J.P. Debbins, A.S. Fleisher, M. Albert, R. Green, G. Bartzokis, G. Glover, J. Mugler, M.W. Weiner, The Alzheimer's disease neuroimaging initiative (ADNI): MRI methods. J. Magn. Reson. Imaging **27**, 1685–691 (2008)
6. H.J. Bockholt, M. Scully, W. Courtney, S. Rachakonda, A. Scott, A. Caprihan, J. Fries, R. Kalyanam, J. Segall, R. De la Garza, S. Lane, V.D. Calhoun, Mining the mind research network: a novel framework for exploring large scale, heterogeneous translational neuroscience research data sources. Front. Neuroinf. **3**, 36 (2010). https://doi.org/10.3389/neuro.11.036.2009
7. R. Buccigrossi, M. Ellisman, J. Grethe, C. Haselgrove, D.N. Kennedy, M. Martone, N. Preuss, K. Reynolds, M. Sullivan, J. Turner, K. Wagner, The neuroimaging informatics tools and resources clearinghouse (NITRC). AMIA Annu. Symp. Proc. **2008**, 1000 (2008)
8. S. Das, A.P. Zijdenbos, D. Vins, J. Harlap, A.C. Evans, LORIS: a web-based data management system for multi-center studies. Front. Neuroinf. **5**(37), 1–11 (2012). https://doi.org/10.3389/fninf.2011.00037
9. K. Clark, B. Vendt, K. Smith, J. Freymann, J. Kirby, P. Koppel, S. Moore, P. Stanley, D. Maffit, M. Pingle, L. Tarbox, F. Prior, The cancer imaging archive (TCIA): maintaining and operating a public information repository. J. Digital Imaging **26**(6), 1045–1057 (2013). https://doi.org/10.1007/s10278-013-9622-7
10. D.S. Marcus, T.R. Olsen, M. Ramaratnam, R.L. Buckner, The extensible neuroimaging archive toolkit. An informatics platform for managing, exploring, and sharing neuroimaging data. Neuroinformatics **5**, 11–33 (2007). https://doi.org/10.1385/NI:5:1:11
11. J. Kalpathy-Cramer, J.B. Freymann, J.S. Kirby, P.E. Kinahan, F.W. Prior, Quantitative imaging network: data sharing and competitive algorithm validation leveraging the cancer imaging archive. Transl. Oncol. **7**(1), 147–152 (2014).

12. D.B. Keator, J.S. Grethe, D. Marcus, B. Ozyurt, S. Gadde, S. Murphy, S. Pieper, D. Greve, R. Notestine, H. Bockholt, P. Papadopoulos, A national human neuroimaging collaboratory enabled by the biomedical informatics research network (BIRN). IEEE Trans. Inf. Technol. Biomed. **12**(2), 162–172 (2008). https://doi.org/10.1109/TITB.2008.917893
13. K.G. Helmer, J.L. Ambite, J. Ames, R. Ananthakrishnan, G. Burns, A.L. Chervenak, I. Foster, L. Liming, D. Keator, F. Macciardi, R. Madduri, J.-P. Navarro, S. Potkin, B. Rosen, S. Ruffins, R. Schuler, J.A. Turner, A. Toga, C. Williams, C. Kesselman, for the biomedical informatics research network: enabling collaborative research using the biomedical informatics research network (BIRN). J. Amer. Med. Inf. Assoc. **18**(4), 416–422 (2011). https://doi.org/10.1136/amiajnl-2010-000032
14. I.B. Ozyurt, D.B. Keator, D. Wei, C. Fennema-Notestine, K.R. Pease, J. Bockholt, J.S. Grethe, Federated web-accessible clinical data management within an extensible neuroimaging database. Neuroinformatics **8**(4), 231–249 (2010). https://doi.org/10.1007/s12021-010-9078-6
15. A. Castiglione, R. Pizzolante, A. De Santis, B. Carpentieri, A. Castiglione, F. Palmieri, Cloud-based adaptive compression and secure management services for 3D healthcare data. Future Generation Comput. Syst. **43**, 120–134 (2015)
16. E. Birney, et al., Mining the draft human genome. Nature **409**(6822), 827–828 (2001)
17. D. Van Essen, et al., The human connectome project: a data acquisition perspective. Neuroimage **62**, 2222–2231 (2012)
18. D. Marcus, et al., Informatics and data mining tools and strategies for the human connectome project. Front Neuroinf. **5**, 4 (2011)
19. C. Hutter, J.C. Zenklusen, The cancer genome atlas: creating lasting value beyond its data. Cell **173**(2), 283–285 (2018). https://doi.org/10.1016/j.cell.2018.03.042
20. S. Paul, S. Saha, R.T. Goswami, testbeds, attacks, and dataset generation for big data cluster: A system application for big data platform security analysis, in *Progress in Computing, Analytics and Networking* (Springer, Singapore, 2020), pp. 545–554

Chapter 13
Artificial Intelligence Approaches for the COVID-19 Pandemic

Pilla Srinivas, Divya Midhun Chakkravarthy, and Debnath Battacharyya

13.1 Introduction

Novel coronavirus (n-CoV) or COVID-19 is a new virus that originated from the coronavirus family in 2019. It is originated during the early December 2019 in the provinces of Hubei, near Wuhan city in China [1]. Phylogenetic analysis has reported that this virus's main carrier is obtained from bats where these bats and other kinds of animals are sold in the Huanan Seafood Market. Later on, it started spreading from those animals to humans [2]. It also spreads among humans during direct or indirect transmission through the droplets of the affected person. When the infected person sneezes or coughs or exhales, there is a chance of releasing the droplets. The virus is heavier in nature and so cannot be in the air for a longer time; it reaches the ground or to the surfaces. These contaminated surfaces act as the carriers of the virus. When the intermediate persons come into close contact with these contaminated areas and then touch their eyes, nose, and mouth, these intermediate persons act as the carriers, resulting in the spread of the virus knowingly or unknowingly. The spread rate of this novel coronavirus is also higher

P. Srinivas (✉)
Department of Computer Science and Engineering, Dadi Institute of Engineering & Technology, Anakapalle, India

D. M. Chakkravarthy
Department of Computer Science and Multimedia, Lincoln University College, Petaling Jaya, Malaysia
e-mail: midhun@lincoln.edu.my

D. Battacharyya
Department of Computer Science and Engineering, K L Deemed to be University, KLEF, Guntur, India
e-mail: debnathb@kluniversity.in

L. Garg et al. (eds.), *Healthcare Informatics for Fighting COVID-19 and Future Epidemics*, EAI/Springer Innovations in Communication and Computing,
https://doi.org/10.1007/978-3-030-72752-9_13

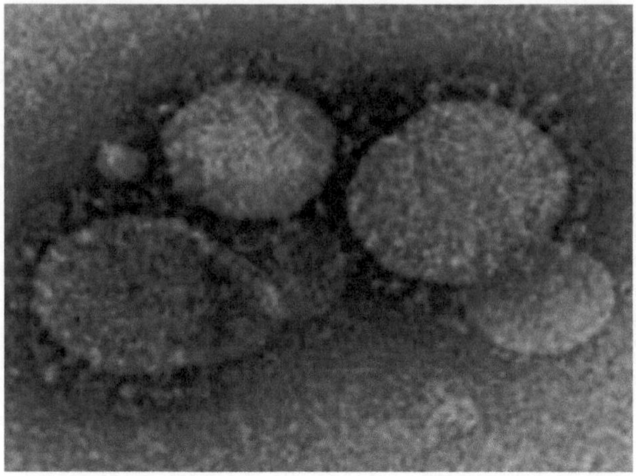

Fig. 13.1 Microscopic view of COVID-19

when compared to the other flus. The affected person experiences many symptoms, and among them, some of the main symptoms are high fever, dry cough, sore throat, and difficulty in breathing. The World Health Organization (WHO) has announced COVID-19 as a pandemic on March 11, 2020 [3].

The affected person may fall sick with a few of the symptoms. Some of the people experience mild to moderate symptoms like Middle East respiratory syndrome (MERS) and severe acute respiratory syndrome (SARS), and people act as carriers without any symptoms. COVID-19 is a highly infectious disease which has a main negative impact on respiratory tract infection. Generally, the virus has a particle size of 80–150 nm. The final stage of the severity of virus among the patients leads to difficulty in breathing, resulting in anaemia and finally leading to death. People with diabetes, respiratory tract infections, high blood pressure, cancer, and other diseases are at high risks and sometimes lead to death. Most people in the early stages and healthy persons with strong immunity recover from the virus without requiring hospital treatment. Early detection of this disease yields to early diagnosis. The person who is suffering from shortness of breath and chest pain needs to seek immediate medical attention. The conclusion of detecting the virus is also a time-consuming process, and sometimes the test results also furnish false results while testing the victims, increase in time results the number of cases day by day. (Fig. 13.1) [3].

Artificial intelligence (AI) is sometimes also realised as machine intelligence where machines demonstrate its intelligence rather than the human brains' natural intelligence. John McCarthy is the person who has first described the term artificial intelligence during 1956 when the computers are acting smarter in analysing and decision-making when compared to humans. AI plays a beneficial role in the field of healthcare systems in making smarter decisions compared to human intelligence. Artificial intelligence has practical purposes on dealing with clinical reports decision-making, assessment based on the clinical records, management of healthcare, and research on clinical records for better outcomes [4]. AI has proved its applications in many real-time applications like weather forecasting, detecting faces, fraud detection, and its positive medical benefits. AI is also applied in analysing images in radiology and pathology and thereby producing successful benefits in fast diagnosing and delivering accurate reports. It is advantageous when dealing with big data which is impossible for humans to create datasets and analyse the data. Natural language processing techniques help in analysing based on the patients' medical records [5].

Most artificial intelligence techniques such as artificial neural networks, Bayesian networks, and Fuzzy expert systems are used in healthcare systems. The Artifical Intelligence investments took place during 2016 were in healthcare systems compared to the other areas. After Matching Artificial Intelligence with Medicine, it can be dichotomised into virtual and physical. Virtual can be defined in analysing the clinical records by applying techniques like artificial neural networks to make decisions and diagnose. The physical parts are performing robotics in surgeries and for the disabled people [6]. We will take the medical records of the patients from the medical centre and thereby apply some of the artificial intelligence approaches to define the actual condition of the patients and help in diagnosing. The datasets are designed based on the collected database, containing the data such as the patients' symptoms and their conditions. As these symptoms are common like flu, it is also difficult to identify and differentiate the patients of normal flu and victims of COVID-19. The symptoms may not be the same for all the patients, and different data is collected, analysed, and integrated. Some of the artificial intelligence approaches like natural language processing techniques help understand the clinical records of data obtained from the clinical database of COVID-19 patients and provide better results. Artificial neural networks are also applied to identify the chest X-rays of some of the patients, making correct decisions in identifying the severity of the patients based on the chest radiographs. It helps in consuming less time and provides accurate results in specifying the presence of disease.

13.2 Artificial Intelligence

13.2.1 How Artificial Intelligence Is Related to Machine Learning

Machine learning works on the concept of machines should be able to learn and redesign through experience. Artificial intelligence (AI) works on the principle of making machines learn and execute the tasks smartly. Artificial intelligence applies machine learning concepts and deep learning concepts. Artificial intelligence and machine learning are not the same. Machine learning helps in learning from behaviour, examples, and definitions, whereas artificial intelligence helps in learning and analysing, reasoning, and solving problems [7]. Machine learning implements

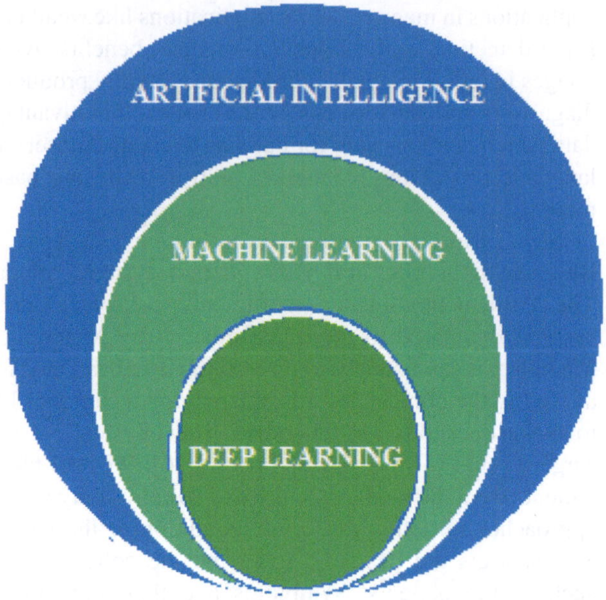

Fig. 13.2 Relation between artificial intelligence machine learning and deep learning

artificial building model. It makes use of neural networks, statistics, and research without implementing programming and learns from experience. In healthcare systems, AI provides better treatment efficiency which can be determined quickly. In case of online shopping, AI helps to add on items based on their purchase interest of items. In finance, AI helps to get rid of fraud instead of just detecting it. Artificial intelligence makes use of machine learning and deep learning concepts to solve problems. The relationship between artificial intelligence, machine learning, and deep learning can be explained in terms of deep learning which is a subset of machine learning. Machine learning is a subset of artificial intelligence (Fig. 13.2).

If we consider the algorithm's example, the math and the algorithm's logic imply machine learning, and math and the algorithm's code imply artificial intelligence. Artificial intelligence is incorporating human intelligence to machines. In AI, machines execute its tasks to solve the problems based upon some rules; this kind of intelligent behaviour is called AI. AI can be categorised into two categories: general and narrow. In general AI, machines can solve many problems and execute the tasks intelligently, whereas in narrow AI, machines can execute the task more intelligently than humans. In the case of machine learning, a lot of data is given to the machine, and the algorithm is trained based upon the given data. It learns how to make decisions while training the algorithm. Based on the data provided, it makes it easier for the machines to make accurate decisions. Machine learning is a simple procedure which helps in understanding AI.

AI and ML help in pattern recognition, advanced image processing in bioinformatics, medical imaging, and medical robotics [8].

13.2.2 Artificial Intelligence Techniques

AI technique is a method that should be represented so that the knowledge expresses generalisation where the properties need to be gathered and grouped together instead of taking them separately. In many AI domains, bulk data comes automatically for programming. The people must transfer the data to programs in an understandable form and in the program's format. The techniques can be easily modified to rectify errors and alter real-life condition changes [8]. The techniques can also be utilised even if it is incomplete and inaccurate, and it can be used in any kind of situations. There are many artificial intelligence techniques used in real-life applications. There are five major artificial intelligence techniques among numerous techniques: heuristics, support vector machines, artificial neural networks, Markov decision process, and natural language processing.

13.2.2.1 Heuristics

It is one of the best searching algorithms used in artificial intelligence. It solves problems to the solutions when compared to the other classic methods. It employs the technique of reducing the alternatives for the results. It is based on the concept of trial and error method; it learns from its mistakes. It is one of the best techniques used in AI, and it suits best for solving difficult problems. It is used to identify the best way among all the possible routes and the shortest route among different routes. In real-time applications, Google Maps [9] are used to mention the best shortest route from source to the destination. It is often used sometimes to calculate NP-complete problems and also decision problems. This algorithm may not find accurate results but finds the solution closer to the best one quickly and easily.

13.2.2.2 Support Vector Machine (SVM)

It is one of the best supervised machine learning algorithms used in classification problems and regression challenges. Artificial Intelligence deals with the classification problem it helps to classify among the based on some instances. The categories in email systems use vector machines to categorise the emails based on social, spam, and promotion. It is also used in detecting images, text recognition, and face recognition systems. Consider the graph in an n-dimensional space, n represents the number of features, and each coordinate represents different features. The points represented in the graph are data points. Vectors represent the coordinates of individual observation. By applying classification techniques, it separates the two classes based on their features (Fig. 13.3).

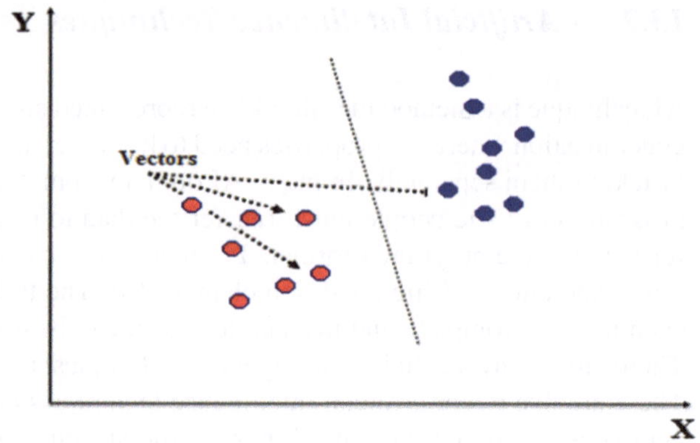

Fig. 13.3 Support vector machine classifier

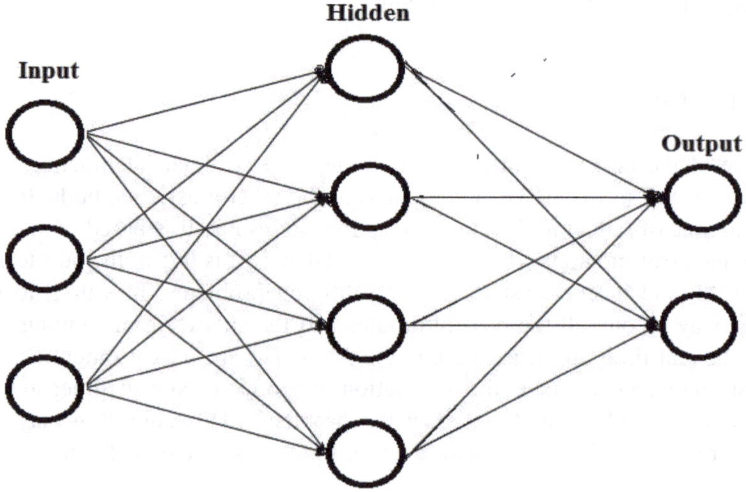

Fig. 13.4 Artificial neural networks

13.2.2.3 Artificial Neural Networks (ANN)

An artificial neural networks is a collection of interconnected nodes which resemble like neurons in a human brain. Each node represents an artificial neuron, and the connections represent the output of one neuron and input of another neuron. The outcome of each node is said to be node value. Each connection between the nodes has weights. If the network generates good outcomes, then there is no need to alter the weights (Fig. 13.4).

If the network generates bad outcomes, then the system alters its weights to generate the best results.

These weights control the signal between two neurons. Feedforward artificial neural network and feedback artificial neural networks are two types of artificial neural networks.

13.2.2.4 Markov Decision Processes (MDP)

It is used in modelling sequential decision problems and also reinforcement learning problems. Another advantage of the Markov decision process is optimised planning. Markov decision indicates to find the correct decision representing which decision results in which state. The MDP model consists of possible states, set of possible actions, transition probabilities, and rewards. Assume the scenario of Robot in which set of possible states represents the robots world, set of possible actions represents to the robot can take a right, left, front, back and transition probabilities represent robot moving from right to left and rewards represents. If the robot moves to the left to reach its destination where that is the actual destination, then that is the higher reward. It also has its advantages in solving stochastic, dynamic decisions to find optimal solutions [10].

13.2.2.5 Natural Language Processing (NLP)

It is used to deal with the interactions between human and computer languages. It allows computer how to program to process and to analyse a large amount of human language data. It is a technique used by the computer to understand, interpret, and manipulate the human language. It is also used in speech recognition. Markov decision is already in use by many multitude companies in real-life applications like Apple Siri, Microsoft Cortana, and Amazon Alexa. It also has its applications in parsing, text recognition, and part of speech. It is a technique from machine learning, and artificial intelligence reformats text for synthetic analysis. During text recognition, the text may be from medical prescription or medical records of the patient. NLP has provided successful medical decision-making results and tracking patient's records by identifying syndromes [11].

13.2.3 Artificial Neural Networks

Artificial neural networks takes multiple inputs and provide a single output. The computer code has several simple highly interconnected models meant for simulating and processing the information. It has one input and one output layer and at least one hidden layer. The main aim is to transfer from input to valuable output. Information flow happens between two ends in two ways, feedforward and feedback networks. The data flows only in one direction without having any loop from input to output in feedforward network. Feedforward is normally used in pattern recognition, and these may have zero or multiple hidden layers. In feedback network, data travels from input to output in both the directions with loops in the network. It can use its internal state to process a series of inputs (Fig. 13.5).

Neural networks make use of different algorithms to train neural networks. Feedforward algorithm, sigmoid, cost function, backpropagation, and gradient descent

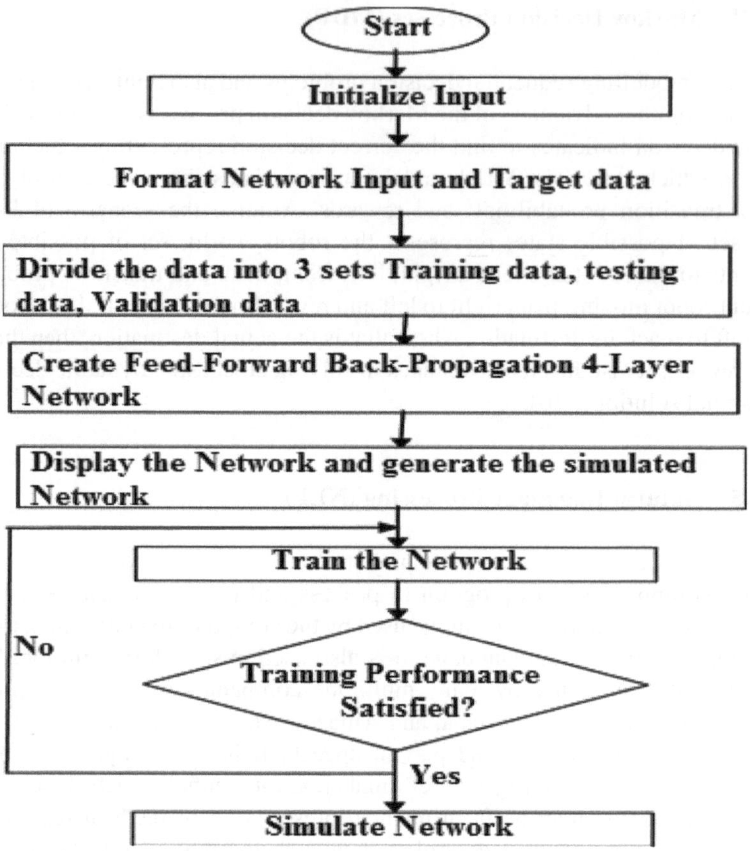

Fig. 13.5 Flowchart of artificial neural networks

are common algorithms used by neural networks. First, to start the algorithm, we need to assign the weights to all the links. Next, we need to find out the links of active hidden nodes by using the inputs and links. Next, we need to find the activation rate of output nodes and hidden nodes and link them to the output. Mean square errors found in the output node and to generate all the links between the output and hidden nodes. We need to pass these errors to hidden and output nodes using the errors at the output node. Generate the weights and repeat the process between the hidden and input nodes until the satisfactory criteria are met. The predicted value is output or the sum of all outputs of individual neurons in the output. Patterns of information are given to the network's input units, thereby travelling through hidden layers and finally obtained in output units.

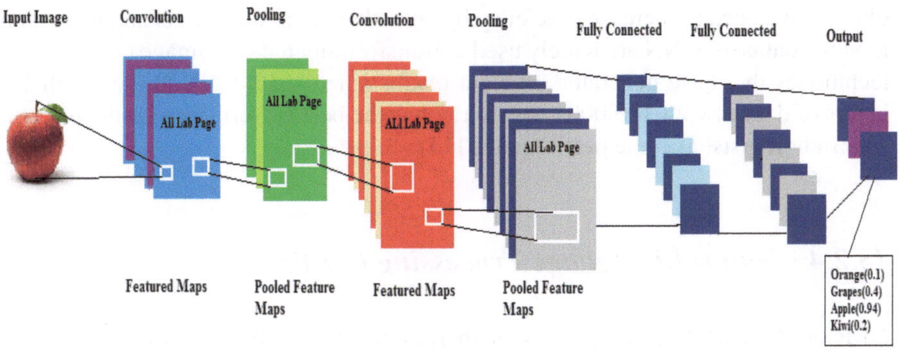

Fig. 13.6 Image processing of convolution neural network

13.2.3.1 Convolution Neural Network (CNN)

It belongs to the neural network class, which has proven its successful results in image recognition and image processing. This network has Multilayer Perceptron for processing and classification. It takes an image as inputs and puts weights and effectively differentiates images from one another. In artificial intelligence, it solves many solutions to real-life problems. It includes a special kind of operation called convolution. It is used in AI-based robots, virtual assistants, and self-driving cars. If we consider image processing, it scans the image to pass through the filter maps which are generated for each individual filter. We can add more and more filtering layers and feature maps to create deeper convolution neural network (CNN). CNN's real-life problems are image recognition, text recognition, gender recognition, and emotion recognition (Fig. 13.6).

It requires the models first to get trained and later tested. The input image is transferred through the series of Convolution layers using filters, pooling, fully connected layers and Softmax function is used to classify the object using the probabilities 0 or 1. Convolution and pooling layers act as extractors of the input image, and fully connected layers act as classifiers. The sum of all output layers is the convolution neural network comprise of some operations like convolution, nonlinearity, pooling, and classification. Many real-life business applications use convolution neural networks like Facebook automatic tagging algorithms, Google image search, and Amazon product recommendations. CNN has also proved its applications in healthcare systems like radiology [12].

Medical imaging also plays an important role in clinical care and diagnosing. CNN helps in medical image processing by using its methods. We have taken Chest X-rays CT scans for the best approach to diagnose the pneumonia. 50,000 patients die per year due to lack of classifying pneumonia from the normal Chest X-ray patients. Radiologists can identify which they were in lack in so regions because of rare and expensive resources. Normal classical methods like support vector machine (SVM) used in long years ago are time-consuming and vary according to different objects. We need to increase efficiency by considering small datasets and increasing it on big datasets. CNN are widely used in transforming medical image classification techniques that have generated efficient results since 2012. CNN trained with 121 layers of dataset with 100,000 chest X-ray has the best performance compared with four radiologists' average performance [13].

13.2.4 Natural Language Processing (NLP)

NLP used in healthcare systems is increasing rapidly because of its ability to search, analyse, and interpret large amounts of patient's datasets. NLP in healthcare provides the best results while dealing with unstructured data and providing better patient results. There are many difficulties for the doctors to maintain the chart notes of patient's records, but with increasing, modern technology, data is maintained in electronic health record (EHR) systems. NLP is the main source to understand the unstructured records to be understandable by the computer. NLP also uses some special engines to find previous records of the patient. The main advantage of NLP is it can scan and organise a large number of chart records of the patients into some important needs in the clinical reports. It is a very difficult process if it is treated manually by the hospital staff and identified per individual patient's personal information. The output of NLP and then EHR structured data is undergone through statistical analysis to identify the complications and the severity of COVID-19 patients. The risk factors associated with it help us to avoid the poor outcomes of the patients.

The data or the clinical prescription in unstructured format is taken and given as an input for the natural language processing. The available data is broken into paragraphs, words, and sentences. It helps identify and analyse the order of words in lexical analysis which is the first step in natural language processing. In syntactic analysis, it observes the words and the relation between them. It accepts only those sentences which are meaningful or else the analyser rejects it. This stage is also called parsing. In syntactic analysis, it uses two methods; they are context-free grammar and top-down parser. The semantic analysis checks for the meanings in the dictionary and checks for the meaningfulness and is rejected if it is not meaningful. It also checks the sentence, which is the succeeding sentence. The actual sentences are reinterpreted to know the real-world knowledge present in the database to derive the language's aspects. Finally, output data is obtained. NLP is also used in treating heart diseases and wound detections [14] (Fig. 13.7).

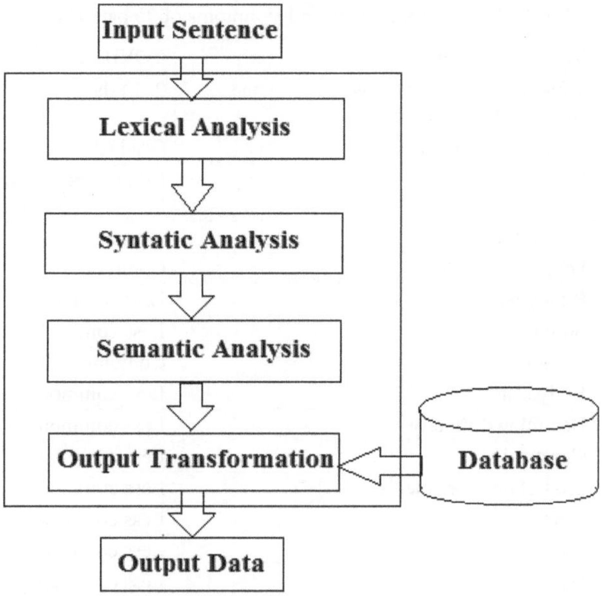

Fig. 13.7 Natural language processing

13.3 COVID-19

13.3.1 COVID-19 Clinical Records

Nowadays the world is suffering from the most dangerous virus which is named as COVID-19. The main risk factors of this disease are age factors and the underlying diseases of the patients. Many researchers are going on to treat the disease. However, apart from its diagnosis and vaccine trials, it is spreading widely within a few months. The main drawback or the time-consuming process takes place in identifying the disease. Since due to non availability of vaccine or medicine to cure this disease, we can only get rid of this disease to take the precautions to get rid of this disease or to diagnose in early stages once it is affected. Pneumonia is not treated seriously in the early stages, the main parts affected are the lungs and heart followed by the kidney and liver [15]. According to Xun Li's survey, they collected the clinical records of 25 patients died of COVID-19 the maximum patients who died are hypertension, diabetes and age are the maximum risk factors [15]. Some of the clinical records of the victims of COVID-19 are collected from the ICMR issued by the government district hospital, Anakapalle, Visakhapatnam. We have collected 25 clinical samples of patients like clinical records and their chest X-rays or computed tomography. Among the 25 patients, 10 were male, and 15 were female (Table 13.1).

For all those 25 patients, the symptoms started gradually and lasted within 2 weeks. Among those, only 10 patients have fever and cough, and the remaining has not experienced this. Only 5 patients have observed runny nose, sore throat, body

Table 13.1 Symptoms cycle and symptoms of 25 patients

Symptoms cycle	COVID-19	No. of patients
Time-lapse between virus catching and showing its symptoms	2–14 days	All
Symptoms starting	Gradual	All
Symptoms lasting	Minor cases: 2 weeks Severe: 3–6 weeks	All
Symptoms		
Fever	Common	10
Runny nose	Less common	5
Sore throat	Less common	5
Cough	Common	10
Body ache	Less common	5
Breathing difficulty	Less common	0
Chest pain	Less common	0
Loss of taste or smell	Less common	2
Diarrhoea	Less common	5
Tiredness	Less common	5
Headache	Less common	5

ache, tiredness, and headache. Only 2 people lost the sense of smell and taste. So, in our survey, the maximum symptoms which were observed are fever and cough. None of them was having severe symptoms among those 25 patients. A maximum people were of middle age, and 1 people died due to underlying disease (diabetes) at age 55. So, based on the majority of symptoms, we can say that people who experienced fever and cough are the main victims of COVID-19. The patients who been have recognised early are diagnosed early. Maximum risks are prone to people who have recognised the disease with serious symptoms. So, symptoms identified in the early stages have also helped the lives of many people or other adverse effects. Patients' maximum clinical records required less treatment as they were in early stages in diagnosing the disease; there were no complications held in treatment. Most of the patients were discharged within 2 weeks who have experienced fewer symptoms; they were discharged. Artificial Intelligence Techniques can apply these clinical records Approaches like Natural Language Processing Techniques to get better effective outcomes. Clinical records are meant to be the patient's prescription, and chest X-rays also help identify the disease severity levels. The external factors can be represented only through the behaviour of the patient's symptoms, but the right judgement can be made only by observing the internal factors like chest X-rays, also known as computed tomography. Chest X-ray of the patient with mild symptoms is taken and compared with the patient who is a severe victim (Fig. 13.8).

Chest X-rays' images are manually identified to spot out the difference between the healthy normal person and victim of COVID-19 patient. Still, it is difficult to find out manually as there are slight changes that can only be identified by the professional radiologists, which is a bit time-consuming process and a cost-effective

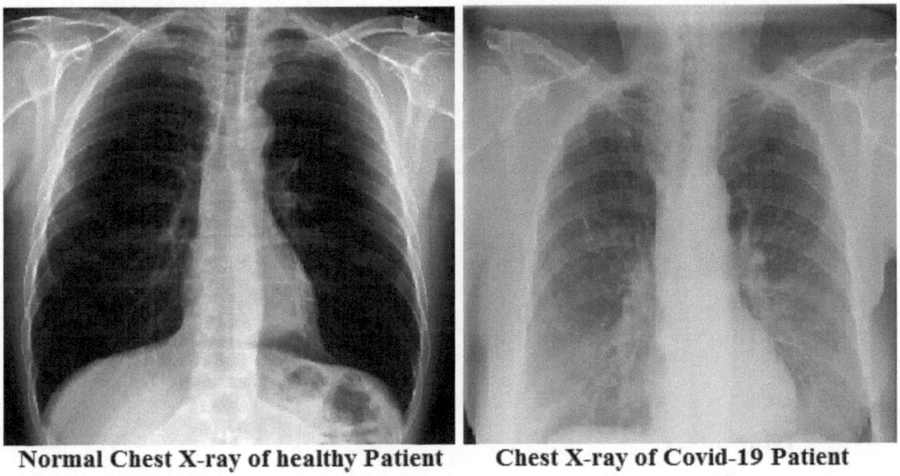

Fig. 13.8 Chest X-ray images of normal and COVID-19 patients

process that required resources. Artificial intelligence approaches like artificial neural networks help identify the victims' chest radiology, which is low cost and provides fast outcomes. In most of the places, people are not concentrating on taking the radiology by assuming to having mild symptoms as there were less professional available in some places to identify this radiology. The actual risk factors and severity of the disease can be identified through this radiology. As COVID-19 is a respiratory tract infection, it has significant effects first on the respiratory system.

So, it can only be observed through chest radiology. Apart from the clinical reports and the COVID-19 victims' records, these chest radiographs also play an essential role in researching the severity risks of COVID-19 [16]. These clinical records and these radiographs require a lot of time when we assume manually, and manual work may also have errors and false predictions, which may sometimes result in worse outcomes. In this modern world, using modern technology like artificial intelligence helps identify the exact outcomes with effective results and less time consumption. There are many techniques associated with artificial intelligence that anyone can use, which is relevant to our problem.

13.3.2 Artificial Intelligence Approaches for COVID-19

There are several techniques present in artificial intelligence topics to deal with healthcare systems. Mainly artificial neural networks and natural language processing play an essential role in identifying many diseases. These techniques have proven their results from past years. The convolution neural network, which is the

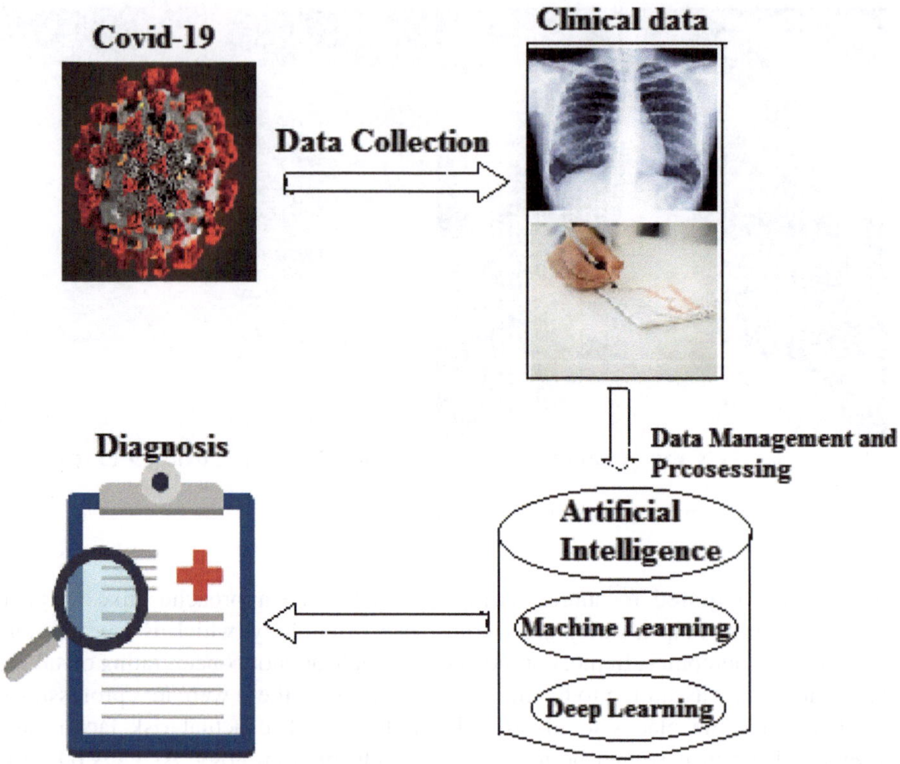

Fig. 13.9 Artificial intelligence approaches to COVID-19

artificial neural networks method, has proven its effective image recognition and analysis results (Fig. 13.9).

As the number of death and the spread rate of COVID-19 increases day by day, it is a serious topic to diagnose the victims from this virus. Artificial intelligence, machine learning, and deep learning have proven its advantages in medical diagnosis. These techniques also help in a few ways to recognise the disease earlier and to diagnose. Firstly, we are gathering the data regarding COVID-19 and the patients' health condition we are going to analyse and diagnose. Gathering of data includes large amounts of data like the physical prescription of the patient's data written by the physicians. The data is maintained in the form of electronic health record (EHR) systems. Clinical records for COVID-19 can also include chest radiographs which help a lot in examining the diseases. These clinical records are meant for data management and processing. We can apply many artificial intelligence techniques like artificial neural networks and some deep learning techniques like natural language processing techniques. By giving the clinical data as input to these techniques and based on the outcomes, we can diagnose the patients based on the patients' actual condition. If all these are done in manual, it requires a lot of time consumption to process the data, and the prediction analysis can be false sometimes and inadequate. Artificial Intelligence technique provides the best results with accurate results and less time consuming, which is one of the best advantages that let the world use it from last past years.

13.3.2.1 Artificial Neural Networks for COVID-19

Artificial neural networks comprise of many methods like multilayer perception (MLP), radial basis function network (RBFN), and convolution neural network (CNN). Convolution Neural Network is one of the best ANN methods that have proved its efficiency in dealing with image analysis and recognition. Convolution neural networks have already proved its results in generating the best results in identifying COVID-19 [13]. Firstly the medical images of COVID-19 victims have been taken and applied to convolution neural networks. CNN is based on convolution, nonlinearity, pooling, and classification process. The input image which we need to find out has been given to the network. We have trained the dataset by adding all the clinical chest radiology of all the patients and mentioned the images' values based upon the dissimilarities present in the images. Based on the datasets, the input images go through featured maps and pooled feature maps and finally generate an outcome, showing whether the image belongs to which disease is based upon the values. After creating the datasets, we need to train the datasets based upon some criteria. Synthesis of Dataset were done manually containing the patients' ID, patients' records, and patients' radiology (Fig. 13.10).

CNN uses the most powerful networks like VGG, ResNet, DenseNet, Inception, and Xception. Xception is one of the best convolution neural networks which has added more number of inception layers. It uses depth-wise convolution layers and also point-wise convolution layers. ResNet50V2 is the better version of ResNet50. ResNEt50V2 and Xception have achieved better results in ImageNet dataset [17].

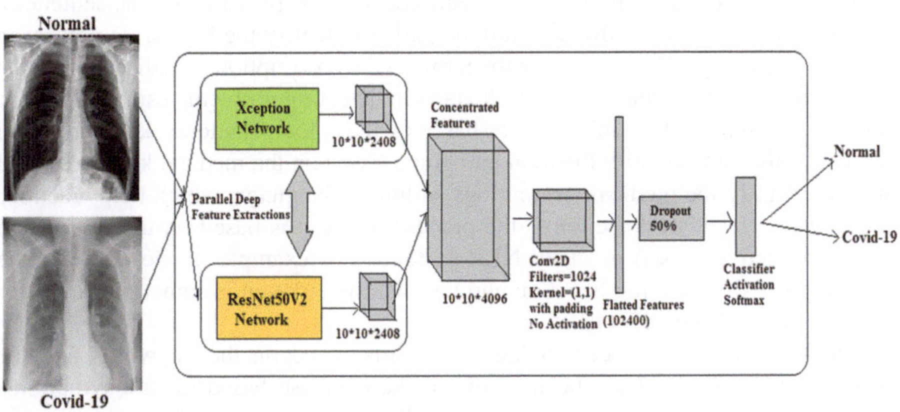

Fig. 13.10 Artificial neural network approach to COVID-19 chest radiography

To create a dataset, it involves some step-by-step procedures. Firstly we need to gather the data of COVID-19 patients, and we need to handle the missing values if they are present. The next step is to take the data for the feature extraction process. We need to decide the key factors in creating the dataset, which is important with regard to creating the dataset—based upon the gathered data, we need to classify the data into a training set and testing set. Here we have taken 25 sample clinical records of the patients based upon the records, and we need to classify them into training sets and testing sets. Training dataset is assigned by assigning some values, and later on, we need to compare them with testing values.

We have taken the image of 300 × 300 pixels. Based on the input image, Xception generates 10 × 10 × 2048 feature map on its last feature. ResNEt50V2 also produces the same feature map on its final layer. As these networks both produced the same feature maps, they both use inception-based layers and residual-based layers. The quality of semantic features is enhanced. The features are connected to a convolution layer, and later they are connected to the classifier. The feature's kernel size was added when 1 × 1 with 1024 filters and no activation function. Each channel is a feature map, and it acts as a spatial point between all the channels.

13.3.2.2 Natural Language Processing for COVID-19

NLP is also one of the best AI techniques used in healthcare systems. It has proven its results in many multitude companies like test recognition and image recognition. NLP Technique work by taking image as an input and performing lexical analysis, syntactic analysis, semantic analysis, and output transformation and finally providing its output. Here in treating COVID-19, we will take the medical prescription of the COVID-19 patient and give the image of this clinical record as an input to the NLP technique. Next, the preprocessing stage is where the classification and detection of paragraphs in the prescription take place. Here section detection, sentence detection, and ambiguity are reduced, which is presented in the sentences. The total image has been divided into the parts to identify the key terms present in medical technology. By identifying the terms in the prescription, it is discovered that the patient has a fever but no cough. It starts in detecting problems using mind map transfer technique, which makes notes based on the colours, patterns, keywords, and images. This helps identify the total paragraph based on the medical keywords, and we can identify the medical terminology in human language, which helps identify the disease. Negation detection is the process where it is based on the rule which is very effectively used in many NLP systems. For example, if we consider the NegEx process by finding negation and termination terms, it is sometimes used for termination [18] (Fig. 13.11).

The total image has been divided into parts based on the keywords and the medical terms. Codes have been given on the database based on the symptoms. Ambiguity has been removed, which made disturbances in identifying the disease. During the post-processing process, the ambiguity issues have been resolved and

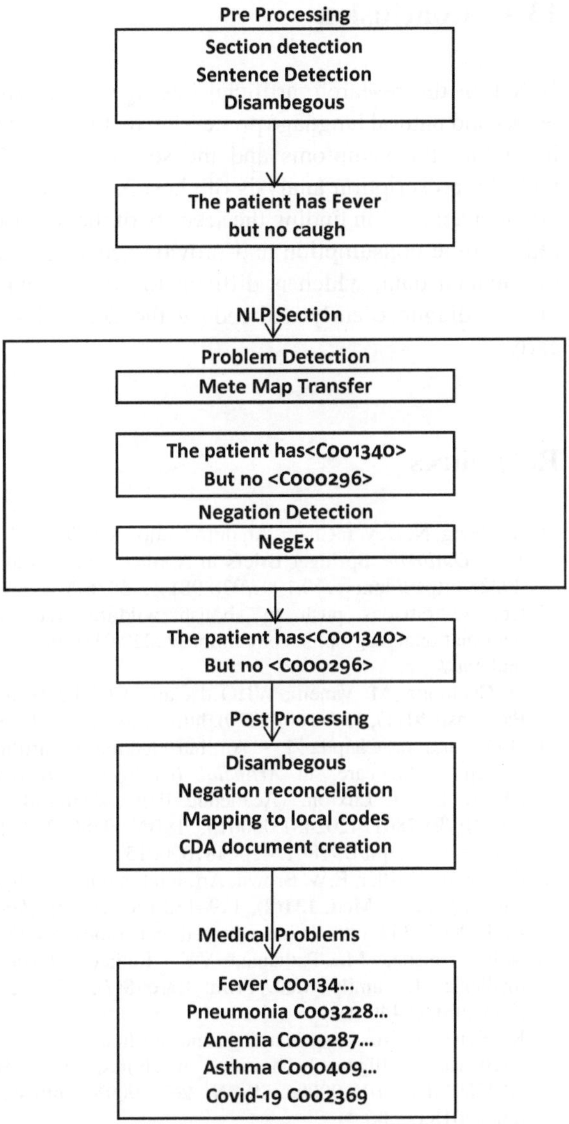

Fig. 13.11 Natural language processing approach for COVID-19

maintain compatibility with other sentences. The mapping process is done based on the codes of the medical terminology terms and processing. Finally, clinical data analysis (CDA) has been created based on the analysis based on the processing techniques. Finally, an electronic report of the prescription of the COVID-19 patient has been obtained as an outcome. When we applied patient records to NLP, one patient's symptoms are different from another, and it differs from person to person. Still, in maximum cases of patients, the main symptom they have experienced is fever.

13.4 Conclusion

Based on the research, artificial intelligence approaches like artificial neural networks and natural language processing techniques have generated its efficient results in finding the symptoms and the severeness of COVID-19 patients. Compared with the prescription analysis of chest X-ray images, it has provided accurate and efficient analysis in finding the severity of the disease and its risks. These techniques reduce time consumption and provide accurate data electronically compared with the manual data, which is difficult to process manually. These findings help the victims diagnose early and reduce the death risks that help the patients recover early.

References

1. S.J. Fong, N. Dey, J. Chaki, An introduction to COVID-19, in *Artificial Intelligence for Corona Virus Outbreak*, Springer Briefs in Applied Sciences and Technology, (Springer, Singapore, 2022). https://doi.org/10.1007/978-981-15-5936-5_1
2. Chinese citizens push to abolish wildlife trade as corona virus persists, https://www.nationalgeographic.com/animals/2020/01/china-bans-wildlife-trade-after corona virus-outbreak/
3. D. Cucinotta, M. Vanelli, WHO declares COVID-19 a pandemic. Acta Bio medica Atenei Parmensis **91**(1), 157–160 (2020). https://doi.org/10.23750/abm.v91i1.9397
4. D.D. Luxton, Chapter 1 - An introduction to artificial intelligence in behavioral and mental health care, in *Artificial Intelligence in Behavioral and Mental HealthCare*, ed. by D. D. Luxton, (Academic Press, Cambridge, 2016), pp. 1–26. https://doi.org/10.1016/B9780124202481.000015. ISBN 9780124202481. http://www.sciencedirect.com/science/article/pii/B9780124202481000015
5. D. Douglas Miller, E.W. Brown, Artificial intelligence in medical practice: The question to the answer? Am. J. Med. **131**(2), 129–133 (2018). https://doi.org/10.1016/j.amjmed.2017.10.03. ISSN 00029343. http://www.sciencedirect.com/science/article/pii/S0002934317311178
6. M.P. Amisha, M. Pathania, V.K. Rathaur, Overview of artificial intelligence in medicine. J. Family Med. Prim. Care **8**(7), 2328–2331 (2019). https://doi.org/10.4103/jfmpc.jfmpc_440_19
7. K. Kristian, Machine learning and artificial intelligence: Two fellow travelers on the quest for intelligent behavior in machines. Front. Big Data **1** (2018). https://doi.org/10.3389/fdata.2018.00006. ISSN 2624-909X. https://www.frontiersin.org/article/10.3389/fdata.2018.00006
8. S.L. Goldenberg, G. Nir, S.E. Salcudean, A new era: Artificial intelligence and machine learning in prostate cancer. Nat. Rev. Urol. **16**, 391–403 (2019). https://doi.org/10.1038/s41585-019-0193-3
9. S.H. Chen, A.J. Jakeman, J.P. Norton, Artificial intelligence techniques: An introduction to their use for modelling environmental systems. Math. Comput. Simul. **78**(2–3), 379–400 (2008). https://doi.org/10.1016/j.matcom.2008.01.028. ISSN 0378-4754. http://www.sciencedirect.com/science/article/pii/S0378475408000505
10. A.J. Schaefer, M.D. Bailey, S.M. Shechter, M.S. Roberts, Modeling medical treatment using Markov decision processes, in *Operations Research and Health Care*, International Series in Operations Research & Management Science, ed. by M. L. Brandeau, F. Sainfort, W. P. Pierskalla, vol. 70, (Springer, Boston, MA, 2005). https://doi.org/10.1007/1-4020-8066-2_23

11. M. Chary, S. Parikh, A.F. Manini, E.W. Boyer, M. Radeos, A review of natural language processing in medical education. West. J. Emerg. Med. **20**(1), 78–86 (2019). https://doi.org/10.5811/westjem.2018.11.39725
12. R. Yamashita, M. Nishio, R. Do, K. Togluenashi, Convolutional neural networks: An overview and application in radiology. Insights Imag. **9**(4), 611–629 (2018). https://doi.org/10.1007/s13244-018-0639-9
13. S.S. Yadav, S.M. Jadhav, Deep convolutional neural network based medical image classification for disease diagnosis. J. Big Data (2019). https://doi.org/10.1186/s40537-019-0276-2
14. M. Topaz, K. Lai, D. Dowding, V.J. Lei, A. Zisberg, K.H. Bowles, L. Zhou, Automated identification of wound information in clinical notes of patients with heart diseases: Developing and validating a natural language processing application. Int. J. Nurs. Stud. **64**, 25–31 (2016). https://doi.org/10.1016/j.ijnurstu.2016.09.013. ISSN 0020-7489. http://www.sciencedirect.com/science/article/pii/S0020748916301602
15. X. Li et al., Clinical characteristics of 25 death cases with COVID-19: A retrospective review of medical records in a single medical center, Wuhan, China. Int. J. Infect. Dis **94**, 128–132 (2020). https://doi.org/10.1016/j.ijid.2020.03.053
16. A. Jacobi, M. Chung, A. Bernheim, C. Eber, Portable chest X-ray in coronavirus disease-19 (COVID-19): A pictorial review. Clin. Imag. **64**, 35–42 (2020). https://doi.org/10.1016/j.clinimag.2020.04.001
17. M. Luengo-Oroz, K. Hoffmann Pham, J. Bullock, et al., Artificial intelligence cooperation to support the global response to COVID-19. Nat. Mach. Intell. **2**, 295–297 (2020). https://doi.org/10.1038/s42256-020-0184-3
18. S. Meystre, P.J. Haug, Natural language processing to extract medical problems from electronic clinical documents: Performance evaluation. J. Biomed. Informatics **39**(6), 589–599 (2006). https://doi.org/10.1016/j.jbi.2005.11.004. ISSN 1532-0464. http://www.sciencedirect.com/science/article/pii/S1532046405001140

Chapter 14
Towards the Development of Triboelectricity-Based Virus Killer Face Mask for COVID-19: Role of Different Inputs

Sanjay Banerjee, Barnali Ghatak, Sk. Babar Ali, Krittish Roy, Kuntal Maity, Nityananda Das, Rajib Bandyopadhyay, Dipankar Mandal, and Bipan Tudu

14.1 Introduction

The rapid evolution of technology is dragging towards miniaturization of electronic gadgets. The new era has stepped into the world of miniaturization of cell phone and other gadgets to make these very handy.

These small-sized electronics consume minute power, making it practicable to be driven by the natural source of energy [1]. To be environment-friendly, these low-power nano-sized devices have been so designed to operate using environmental energy. Therefore, the chances of getting health hazards become very less. In this

S. Banerjee
Department of Applied Electronics and Instrumentation Engineering, Future Institute of Engineering and Management, Kolkata, India

B. Ghatak · B. Tudu (✉)
Department of Instrumentation and Electronics Engineering, Jadavpur University, Kolkata, West Bengal, India

S. B. Ali
Department of Electronics and Communication Engineering, Future Institute of Engineering and Management, Kolkata, West Bengal, India

K. Roy · K. Maity
Department of Physics, Jadavpur University, Kolkata, India

N. Das
Department of Physics, Jagannath Kishore College, Purulia, West Bengal, India

R. Bandyopadhyay
Department of Instrumentation and Electronics Engineering, Jadavpur University, Kolkata, West Bengal, India

D. Mandal
Institute of Nano Science and Technology (INST), Habitat Centre, Mohali, India

L. Garg et al. (eds.), *Healthcare Informatics for Fighting COVID-19 and Future Epidemics*, EAI/Springer Innovations in Communication and Computing,
https://doi.org/10.1007/978-3-030-72752-9_14

regard, Wang et al. have constructed self-powered nanogenerators (NGs) by utilizing piezoelectric and triboelectric effect. Piezoelectric effect and related applications were extensively studied in different review articles and book chapters [2, 3]. The present book chapter would bring light into the importance of triboelectricity in smart electronics, applying triboelectric nanogenerators (TENGs) in different health monitoring sectors. Mainly, two differently polarized tribo materials come into play in order to generate static electricity. TENG's array of advantages makes it a good choice as a self-powered and environmentally friendly [4–16]. Moreover, TENG gets activated through different mechanical motions because of its capability to generate electricity through frictional energy including touching [17, 18], impact [19, 20], linear sliding [21, 22], rotation [10, 23], vibration [24, 25], and so on.

14.1.1 Fundamentals of Triboelectricity and Triboelectric Material

The frictional motion drives two oppositely charged tribo-series materials (TSM) which leads to contact electrification. The conventional electrostatics in our daily life deals with triboelectricity. Based on the relative polarity of the tribo materials adjacent to each other, the sign of the charges of TSMs varies. Triboelectric effect can be considered as an effect that has been acknowledged for decades. In view of some shortcomings of triboelectric effect, air friction on the airframe is likely to interfere with radio frequency communication during the take-off aircraft. Electrostatic charges can cause an explosion and ignite flammable vapors. To avoid a fire in carts/cars, the flammable and explosive gases have to be removed properly. In this book chapter, the positive insights and applications of triboelectrification such as converting mechanical energy to electrical energy and active sensor in health monitoring are emphasized.

The actual mechanism of triboelectrification is still under research with contradictory explanations [26, 27]. The transferred charges can either be ions/molecules or electrons. During separation, some bonded atoms either keep extra electrons or push them away. And hence, triboelectric charges generated on surfaces.

14.1.2 Triboelectric Material

Triboelectric materials are mainly less conductive in nature. The materials transfer the electrostatic capture charges produced by some mechanical action for a longer period. Almost all existing material such as metal, silk, wood, the polymer has triboelectric properties, which can be used to fabricate TENGs. In 1957, Johan Carl Wilcke first published triboelectric series of some conventional materials based on their static charges [28, 29]. The materials placed at the top of the series will attain more charge when it touched with materials at the end of the series. Thus more charge will be transferred if the materials are placed far away with each other.

14.1.2.1 Triboelectric Nanogenerators (TENG)

The concept of TENG [5] is first introduced by F.R. Fan et al. in early 2012. The concept was implemented in microelectronics system [20] to generate "blue power" in the bulk amount [30]. The basic principle of TENG is lying on static electricity and contact electrification. So, the current generated on a contact surface by vertical or horizontal movement of triboelectric layers of opposite charges [31, 32]. So, the material gets electrically charged during contact with different materials [33–35]. The external mechanical motions can trigger the triboelectrically charged surface; in turn, two electrodes accounted for the induced potential difference. The free electrons maintain equilibrium between two electrodes by flow back and forth motion in the surface. In this way, TENG is capable of converting applied mechanical energy into electricity. The increasing contact area and proper charging material can generate more triboelectric charge density. Different interfacial structures include the use of a silicon template-based process [6, 36, 37], nanoparticle dispersion process [8, 38], chemical growth process [20, 39], plasma treatment process [7, 40, 41], block copolymer patterning process [24, 42], sponge-based process [43], and nature replication process [44]. The interfacial structure engineering is a rapidly growing technology to maximize output performance compared with other innovative technology.

14.1.3 Mode 1: Vertical Contact-Separation Mode

As the name suggests, two differently polarized tribo materials are placed with each other in a stacked configuration [7, 45]. In this configuration, one of the films must be dielectric. The effective switching between the fully separated state and the intimate contact state is required to activate the electricity generation process. Based on those innovative nano-structured devices like the arched structure [20], the spring-based structure [24] has been designed. The specific configuration is effective for short-range cyclic motion, viz., vibrations and periodic impacts [9, 25, 41, 46–48].

14.1.4 Lateral Sliding Mode

The sequential contact and separation between the two triboelectric faces generate electrical charges [10, 22]. Sliding between two layers produces triboelectric charges between these surfaces. Therefore, AC output is generated due to the back and forth sliding, which will drive the electrons on the top and bottom electrodes. This phenomenon can be obtained from planar-based motions [22, 49], disc-like rotation [21], or cylindrical rotation [15]. This lateral sliding mode is likely to be advantageous than vertical contact separation mode since the charge generation due to sliding process is very effective.

14.1.5 Single-Electrode Mode

In nature, some moving objects are often get charged naturally due to their contact with air or other objects available in nature. The objects can be considered as a triboelectric layer in the electricity generation process. In the case of single-electrode TENG [50–52], one electrode directly interacts with the moving triboelectric layer. Another electrode is considered a reference electrode. In the case of finite-sized TENG, the local electric field distribution can be varied by the electrode itself.

The relative motion between the layers can have both the contact mode (vertical and lateral) [50, 51] and the fusion of the two modes as well [11]. Due to the reason, single-electrode mode TENG gains its effectiveness for acting as a self-powered active sensor to detect any charged particles.

14.2 TENG in Health Monitoring Application

Sometimes we need to monitor our health such as temperature, rate of respiration, heartbeat, etc. to know about our health. Periodically monitoring health can help us treat, diagnose, or prevent several diseases like cardiovascular diseases, strokes, diabetes, etc. Therefore in recent years, health monitoring needs more attention for a human being. There are two approaches in which TENGs are useful for continuous health monitoring applications. The first approach is to generate electrical signals from different stimuli generated from our body and used it as a medical purpose that does not need external power.

14.2.1 TENG as Self-Powered Health Monitors

Intending to measure the abdominal respiration as a function of anti-electromagnetic radiation, Zhang et al. have designed a textile supported hybrid nanogenerator (HNG) [53, 54].

Human's sleep behavior was observed by using a textile TENG array [55]. The textile TENG is constructed by using conductive fibers sandwiched between wavy-structured polyethylene terephthalate (PET) films. The experiment is done using a textile TENG-based smart mattress, which measures body position of sleeping person, pressure, and posture in real time.

Yi et al. have reported a rubber-based TENG that can measure bending frequency, bending angle of the knee, amplitude, and abdominal respiration frequency [56]. An interesting approach of devising gait monitoring wearable sensor has been explored by Lin et al. [57]. A TENG-based real-time gait monitoring device was reported by Lin et al. [58]. A membrane-based TENG was developed by Bai et al. It can detect the chest's heartbeat by inducing air pressure on the device [59]. Ouyang et al. developed a TENG-based pulse sensor which can obtain a voltage signal without complex circuit designs and mathematical operations [60]. Yang et al. developed a TENG-based multifunctional sensor which can detect voice by a microphone [61].

14.2.2 Self-Powered Health Monitoring Sensor Integrated with TENG

Zhang et al. designed an active wireless temperature monitoring system that harvests energy from mechanical motion [23]. The TENG was constructed using carbon nanotube as an electrode and cotton thread as a substrate, which measures body temperature when it was placed on the wrist. Chen et al. have explored a TENG by a polymer sensor which can detect the lactate concentration in human perspiration [62].

14.2.3 Different Input Signals in TENG

Basically, TENG depends on the mechanical movement exerted by any physiological or environmental signal and the strength of the signal electrical output. In this proposed chapter, few important physiological input signals will be discussed, which have a predominant impact in generating the output signal. The following signals are very important to trigger any TENG.

14.2.3.1 Body Movement

TENG can sense the number of fingers. For instance, the movements of the joint can be monitored continuously after attaching it to an elbow joint. The regular electrical output is being generated upon properly bending and releasing the arm. One of the body movements includes eyeball motion [1]. The involuntary eye movements of nystagmus are mainly due to the brain's abnormal function, which subsequently controls eye movements. These nerve movements can start up TENG to generate electricity in the system.

Another important movement can be tracked from a sleeping body movement. In addition, movements during sleeping are mainly caused by sleep apnea. Generally, kids are spending huge time on sleeping; in those cases, input signals get very high. During sleeping, mainly shoulder and leg are found to highly movable [63]. On the other side, joint movements (bending angle and frequency of the knee) of a human body also come under this category.

14.2.3.2 Expiration and Inspiration

Inspiration occurs via active contraction diaphragm resulting in inspiration, whereas expiration is passive unless forced. In the breathing process, breathing pressure plays a key role in inducing power in TENG. The breathing pressure depends on the user's type of work, viz., talking, laughing, singing, shouting, different breathing rhythms, different active states, etc. The more the pressure, the more will be the output signal. If the TENG is subjected by ample pressure, the positive and negative tribo-series materials (TSM) come closer to each other, which causes static electricity. Electric potential difference is induced by mechanical agitation through physical contact.

14.2.3.3 Triboelectric Nanogenerator (TENG)

As the possible inputs for the TENG have already been discussed, TENG works as a self-powered mode. Hair, acrylic, glass, and nylon are in the top of the positive series, whereas polypropylene and polyurethane belong to the extreme negative series. Interestingly, steel and wood share no charge; therefore, these materials are triboelectrically inactive. Based on the combination of positive and negative triboelectric materials, different varieties of NG can be designed. Fig. 14.1 highlighted the list of some important and widely used triboseries materials.

14.2.4 Different Energy Harvesting Circuits for Nanogenerator

Energy harvesting is a technique in which a very small amount of energy (kinetic energy, thermal energy, RF energy, etc.) is acquired and then changed to equivalent electrical energy. So, this unstable electrical energy is then accumulated and stored for various small power applications. This is an alternative source of power than the high-cost establishment of non-conventional energy sources like a solar panel or wind turbines. Batteries operate low-powered electronic devices like embedded controllers, sensors, etc. with limited life span. So, these batteries should be replaced, which become expensive in remote locations. Energy harvesting technology is ideal

Fig. 14.1 List of TSMs

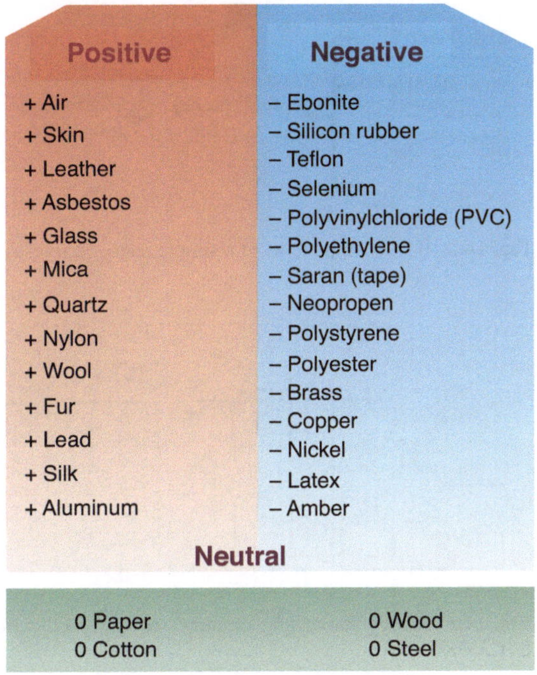

in such cases, which provides power for these devices' whole life span. Therefore, the technology offers a low-cost solution. The energy is generated nearer to the devices, so there is no requirement of using a long cable, thus no transmission loss.

These micro-energy sources are mainly thermal or kinetic energy, which converts to electrical energy by some physical changes known as nanogenerator. Nanogenerators are generally three types: piezoelectric, pyroelectric, and triboelectric. Triboelectric nanogenerator converts applied mechanical energy into an electrical signal by using triboelectric materials. The electricity is produced here by electrostatic induction due to the frictional energy [64, 65]. The triboelectricity can be generated by harvesting any mechanical energy type like human motion (walking), vibration, wind, flowing water, etc. [66]. A nano-structured pyroelectric material converts external thermal energy into thermal energy in the pyroelectric nanogenerator harvesting system. The electrical energy is produced here by Seebeck effect, in which a diffusion charge drives the electrical energy due to the temperature difference at two ends of the pyroelectric device [67, 68].

The energy harvesting process seems to be specific to its source, and the type of energy to be converted to electrical ennergy, etc. Basically, techniques of designing NG seem to be dependent on the type of energy sources and related circuitry. A simple energy harvesting required NG, interfacing circuit and energy storage and power management. The simplest block diagram is shown in Fig. 14.2. The NGs may be triboelectric, piezoelectric, pyroelectric, or RF depending on their kinetic, thermal, or RF energy sources. The signal from NG is AC in nature, so an interfacing

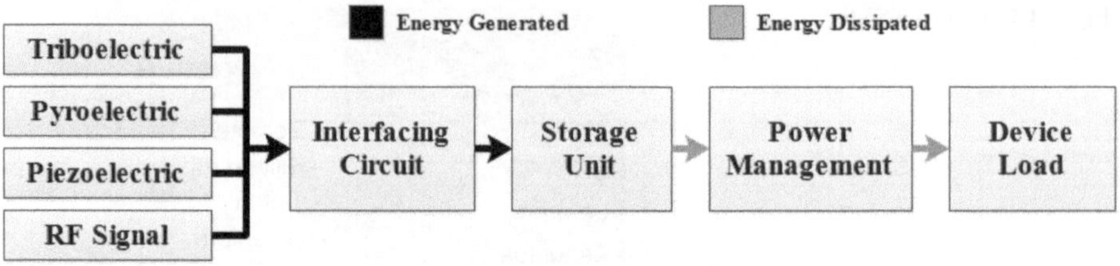

Fig. 14.2 Basic components of a simple energy harvesting system

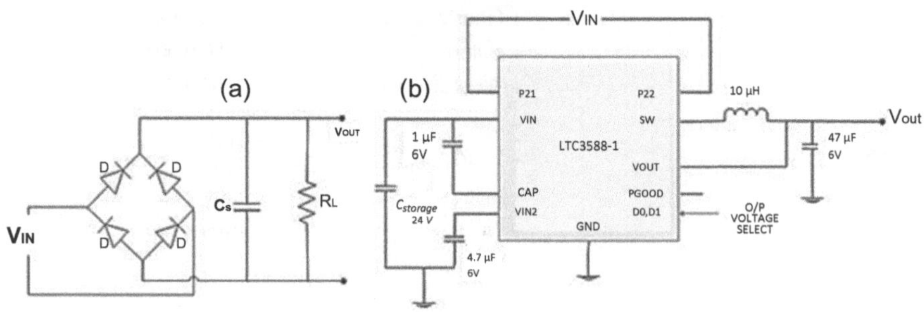

Fig. 14.3 Energy harvesting circuits: (**a**) designed with a bridge rectifier; (**b**) designed with LTC3588-1

circuit is required for signal conditioning for the further storage operation. A battery or a supercapacitor is used to power the management block to regulate the voltage required for applicable devices like embedded controllers, sensors, etc. by storing this electrical energy.

Our focus is on various energy harvesting circuits for powering the small powered devices or appliances in our present study. A lot of research has been done on energy harvesting system. Zhoua et al. [69] have reported an energy harvesting system that produces electric energy by converting mechanical energy. The output AC generated by PNBJ is capable of driving only a small powered AC device but not DC electronics appliances. The authors have designed two energy harvesting circuits. First one is a simple rectifier circuit (Fig. 14.3a) designed with four diodes followed by a capacitor to get filtered and storage purposes. In another approach, LTC3588-1 (Fig. 14.3b) IC can be used as an energy harvesting circuit developed by Linear Technology. The buck converter produces 100 mA continuous current output by producing 1.8, 2.5, 3.3, and 3.6 V selectable output by turning on and off the buck converter to maintain regulation.

Mustapha et al. [70] developed a high-efficiency piezoelectric energy harvesting system, which involves a series of stages (Fig. 14.4) to extract the electrical energy from applied kinetic energy. The AC output generated was initially in the rage of few volts with a current rating of few μA, which is rectified and then regulated through a DC/DC step-down process. The bridge rectifier's output is investigated using BAT754L low drop Schottky diode, which has a very low voltage drop

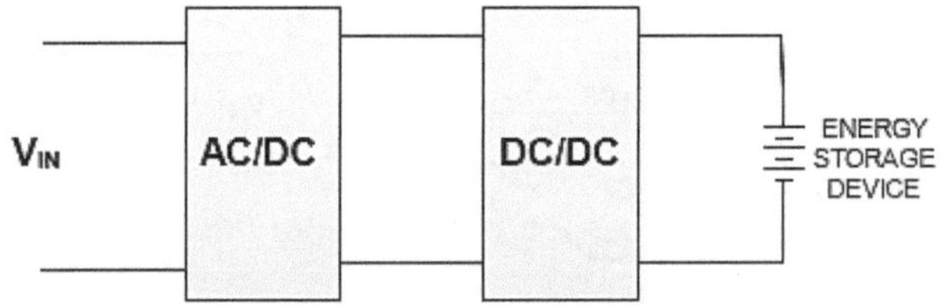

Fig. 14.4 Stages of energy harvesting system

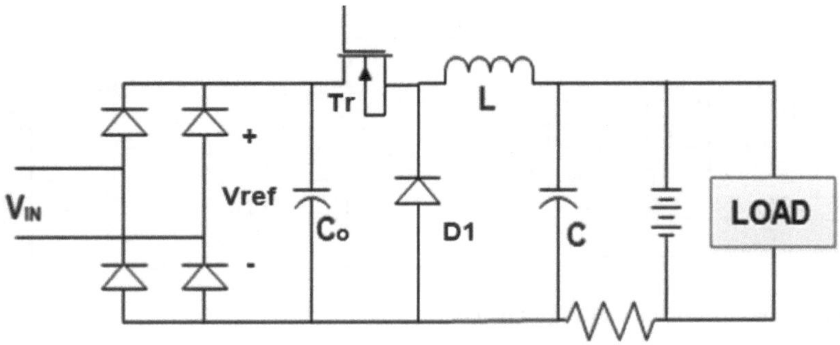

Fig. 14.5 Energy harvesting circuit: two-stage

compared with a normal diode of voltage drop. The rectifier's output is fed to the high-efficiency 5 V, 50 mA step-down DC/DC converter LTC3642.

Guan et al. [71] experimentally compared between one-stage energy harvesting circuits and two-stage energy harvesting circuits. The major drawback of energy harvesting circuits is their average power, which is very low. So a capacitor is used to accumulate and store the energy for further use. A day's higher density storage device is also used to accumulate harvesting energy, so a series of batteries or supercapacitors are the alternative choice to store more energy in terms of voltage. The author has compared one-stage energy harvesting circuits and two-stage energy harvesting circuits in their different storage voltages. The one-stage harvesting circuits (Fig. 14.2) are simple bridge rectifier circuits with a storage device's capacitor. Ottman et al. [72] developed a bridge rectifier (Fig. 14.5) followed by a buck DC/DC converter. After comparing several parameters, the one-stage energy harvesting system is more efficient than the two-stage energy harvesting system because of the internal energy loss of the DC/DC converter circuit's electronic components.

Tran et al. [5] have described different voltage multiplier circuits. In some applications where a simple bridge rectifier is inadequate to develop voltage, a voltage multiplier is used by stacking DC in series using a single rectifier. Several voltage multiplier circuits are shown in Fig. 14.6. The Cockcroft-Walton voltage multiplier is the mostly used voltage multiplier as harvesting circuit. Figure 14.6a shows a three-stage voltage multiplier but has more stage for more voltage gain. Figure 14.6b shows a Dickson multiplier, which is the modification of Cockcroft-Walton voltage multiplier. The stage capacitors are shunted in Dickson multiplier to

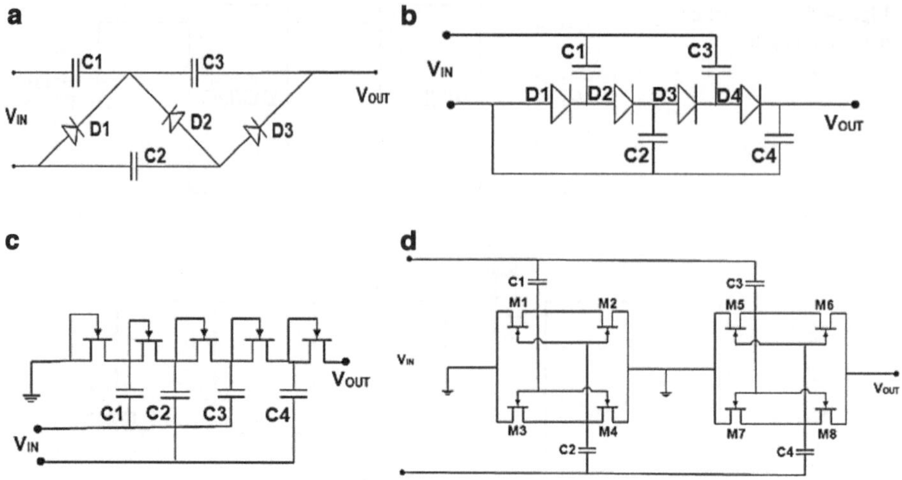

Fig. 14.6 Various voltage multiplier circuits

reduce the parasitic effects of Cockcroft-Walton voltage multiplier, thus preferable for low-voltage appliances. In voltage multiplier, the efficiency will reduce if the stages are increased due to the diode's leakage current and high resistive load. Recently, the MOSFET technology became an alternate solution for voltage multiplier circuits as it overcame diodes' limitation. Figure 14.6c shows a Dickson charge pump circuit in which the diode is replaced with NMOS and integrated within an IC.

Gollakota et al. have designed a power harvesting circuit utilizing a rectified steady current as shown in Fig. 14.7 [73]. The circuit is composed of diodes and capacitors, which boost the output voltage at multiple stages. The capacitor is used to store the charge, which is used to supply the stable voltage to run low-powered devices.

Research interest in harvesting energy from non-conventional sources has increased over the past few years to find an alternative energy source for powering low-power devices. The original harvested power from nanogenerators is in the range of few milliwatts. However, it can be accumulated and stored using proper energy harvesting circuit, power small powered devices like sensors or embedded controllers, etc.

TENG (triboelectric nanogenerator) is an energy harvesting fertilizer that generates energy through static electricity as it does with external mechanical energy [68]. When positive charge density and negative charge density triboelectric materials come with mechanical friction, according to charge affinity, both of them create a huge charge and transfer the produced charge to the proper electrode attached with them. Hence, it is a self-potential energy harvesting system [68–72]. TENG electric potential level bust-up by a harvesting circuit increases the produced voltage for

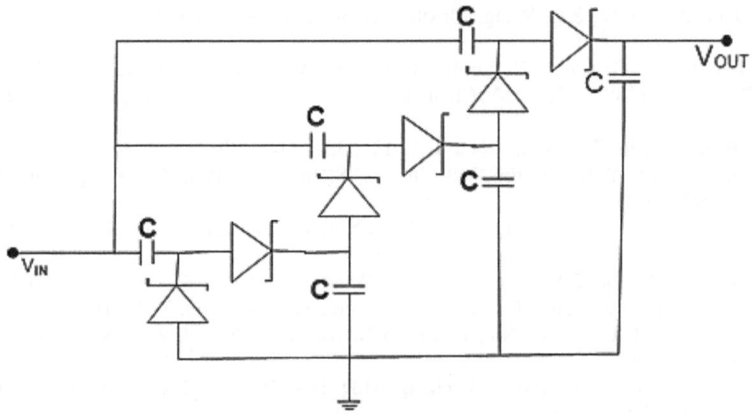

Fig. 14.7 Power harvesting circuit with diode and capacitors

different applications [74–77]. The following advantage and disadvantages of self-powered TENG are listed below [78–91].

The advantage of self-powered TENG:

1. Generates electricity without any application of electrical power.
2. Simple household materials are used as TENG.
3. Application of renewable energy source and environmentally friendly.
4. Ease of simplicity, reliability, and accuracy.
5. Used in a remote place to generate electric power due to the source of non-conventional energy.

The disadvantage of self-powered TENG:

1. Difficult to collect the generated charge of TENG materials.
2. The developed potential is very low in a few volts.
3. Multistage harvesting circuit is essential to enhance its voltage level.
4. The rigidity of TENG materials is quite complex when mechanical friction acts.
5. Electrode life span is less due to mechanical friction.
6. System output affected by moisture.

References

1. Z.L. Wang, J.H. Song, Piezoelectric nanogenerators based on zinc oxide nanowire arrays. Science **312**, 242–246 (2006). https://doi.org/10.1126/science.1124005
2. C. Wan, C.R. Bowen, Multiscale-structuring of polyvinylidene fluoride for energy harvesting: The impact of molecular-, micro- and macro-structure. J. Mater. Chem. A **5**, 3091 (2017)
3. S.K. Ghosh, D. Mandal, Piezoelectricity of 2D materials and its applications toward mechanical energy harvesting, in *2D Nanomaterials for Energy Applications*, (Elsevier, Amsterdam, 2020), pp. 1–38
4. Z.L. Wang, ACS Nano **7**(11), 9533–9557 (2013)

5. F.R. Fan, Z.Q. Tian, Z.L. Wang, Flexible triboelectric generator. Nano Energy **1**, 328–334 (2012)
6. F.R. Fan, L. Lin, G. Zhu, W.Z. Wu, R. Zhang, Z.L. Wang, Nano Lett. **12**, 3109–3114 (2012)
7. G. Zhu, C.F. Pan, W.X. Guo, C.Y. Chen, Y.S. Zhou, R.M. Yu, Z.L. Wang, Nano Lett. **12**, 4960–4965 (2012)
8. S.H. Wang, L. Lin, Z.L. Wang, Nano Lett. **12**, 6339–6346 (2012)
9. G. Zhu, J. Chen, Y. Liu, P. Bai, Y.S. Zhou, Q.S. Jing, C.F. Pan, Z.L. Wang, Nano Lett. **13**, 2282–2289 (2013)
10. L. Lin, S.H. Wang, Y.N. Xie, Q.S. Jing, S.M. Niu, Y.F. Hu, Z.L. Wang, Nano Lett. **13**, 2916–2923 (2013)
11. S.H. Wang, Y.N. Xie, S.M. Niu, L. Lin, Z.L. Wang, Adv. Mater. **26**, 2818–2824 (2014)
12. G. Zhu, J. Chen, T.J. Zhang, Q.S. Jing, Z.L. Wang, Nat. Commun. **5** (2014)
13. S.H. Wang, Z.H. Lin, S.M. Niu, L. Lin, Y.N. Xie, K.C. Pradel, Z.L. Wang, ACS Nano **7**, 11263–11271 (2013)
14. B. Meng, W. Tang, Z.H. Too, X.S. Zhang, M.D. Han, W. Liu, H.X. Zhang, Energy Environ. Sci. **6**, 3235–3240 (2013)
15. Y. Yang, Y.S. Zhou, H.L. Zhang, Y. Liu, S.M. Lee, Z.L. Wang, Adv. Mater. **25**, 6594–6601 (2013)
16. S.H. Wang, Y.N. Xie, S.M. Niu, L. Lin, C. Liu, Y.S. Zhou, Z.L. Wang, Adv. Mater. (2014). https://doi.org/10.1002/adma.201402491
17. G. Zhu, W.Q. Yang, T.J. Zhang, Q.S. Jing, J. Chen, Y.S. Zhou, P. Bai, Z.L. Wang, Nano Lett. **14**, 3208–3213 (2014)
18. Y. Yang, H.L. Zhang, Z.H. Lin, Y.S. Zhou, Q.S. Jing, Y.J. Su, J. Yang, J. Chen, C.G. Hu, Z.L. Wang, ACS Nano **7**, 9213–9222 (2013)
19. L. Lin, Y.N. Xie, S.H. Wang, W.Z. Wu, S.M. Niu, X.N. Wen, Z.L. Wang, ACS Nano **7**, 8266–8274 (2013)
20. G. Zhu, Z.-H. Lin, Q.S. Jing, P. Bai, C.F. Pan, Y. Yang, Y.S. Zhou, Z.L. Wang, Toward large-scale energy harvesting by a nanoparticle-enhanced triboelectric nanogenerator. Nano Lett. **13**, 847–853 (2013)
21. S.H. Wang, L. Lin, Y.N. Xie, Q.S. Jing, S.M. Niu, Z.L. Wang, Nano Lett. **13**, 2226–2233 (2013)
22. G. Zhu, Y.S. Zhou, P. Bai, X.S. Meng, Q.S. Jing, J. Chen, Z.L. Wang, Adv. Mater. **26**, 3788–3796 (2014)
23. L. Lin, S.H. Wang, S.M. Niu, C. Liu, Y.N. Xie, Z.L. Wang, ACS Appl. Mater. Inter. **6**, 3038–3045 (2014)
24. J. Chen, G. Zhu, W.Q. Yang, Q.S. Jing, P. Bai, Y. Yang, T.C. Hou, Z.L. Wang, Adv. Mater. **25**, 6094–6099 (2013)
25. J. Yang, J. Chen, Y. Liu, W.Q. Yang, Y.J. Su, Z.L. Wang, ACS Nano **8**, 2649–2657 (2014)
26. J. Henniker, Triboelectricity in polymers. Nature **196**, 474 (1962)
27. D.K. Davies, Charge generation on dielectric surfaces. J. Phys. D. Appl. Phys. **2**, 1533–1537 (1969)
28. http://owlsmag.wordpress.com/2010/01/20/a-naturalhistory-devin-corbin/
29. Disputatio Physica Experimentalis, De Electricitatibus Contrariis. Typis Ioannis Iacobi Adleri (1757)
30. Z.L. Wang, On Maxwell's displacement current for energy and sensors: The origin of nanogenerators. Mater. Today **20**, 74–82 (2017)
31. R.D.I.G. Dharmasena, K.D.G.I. Jayawardena, C.A. Mills, J.H.B. Deane, J.V. Anguita, R.A. Dorey, S.R.P. Silva, Triboelectric nanogenerators: Providing a fundamental framework. Energy Environ. Sci. **10**, 1801–1811 (2017)
32. G.S.P. Castle, J. Electrost. **40-1**, 13–20 (1997)
33. A.F. Diaz, R.M. Felix-Navarro, J. Electrost. **62**, 277–290 (2004)
34. L.S. McCarty, G.M. Whitesides, Angew. Chem. Int. Edit. **47**, 2188–2207 (2008)
35. H.T. Baytekin, A.Z. Patashinski, M. Branicki, B. Baytekin, S. Soh, B.A. Grzybowski, Science **333**, 308–312 (2011)

36. J.A. Wiles, B.A. Grzybowski, A. Winkleman, G.M. Whitesides, Anal. Chem. **75**, 4859–4867 (2003)
37. M.-L. Seol, J.-H. Woo, S.-B. Jeon, D. Kim, S.-J. Park, J. Hur, Y.K. Choi, Nano Energy **14**, 201 (2015)
38. G. Cheng, Z.H. Lin, L. Lin, Z.L. Du, Z.L. Wang, ACS Nano **7**, 7383 (2013)
39. Z.H. Lin, Y. Xie, Y. Yang, S. Wang, G. Zhu, Z.L. Wang, ACS Nano **7**, 4554 (2013)
40. Z.H. Lin, G. Cheng, Y. Yang, Y.S. Zhou, S. Lee, Z.L. Wang, Adv. Funct. Mater. **24**, 2810 (2014)
41. W. Yang, J. Chen, G. Zhu, J. Yang, P. Bai, Y. Su, Q. Jing, X. Cao, Z.L. Wang, ACS Nano **7**, 11317 (2013)
42. C.K. Jeong, K.M. Baek, S. Niu, T.W. Nam, Y.H. Hur, D.Y. Park, G. Hwang, M. Byun, Z.L. Wang, Y.S. Jung, K.J. Lee, Nano Lett. **14**, 7091 (2014)
43. D. Kim, S. Jeon, J.Y. Kim, M. Seol, S.O. Kim, Y. Choi, Nano Energy **12**, 331 (2015)
44. K.Y. Lee, J. Chun, J.H. Lee, K.N. Kim, N.R. Kang, J.Y. Kim, M.H. Kim, K.S. Shin, M.K. Gupta, J.M. Baik, S.W. Kim, Adv. Mater. **26**, 5037 (2014)
45. M.-L. Seol, J.-H. Woo, D.-I. Lee, H. Im, J. Hur, Y.-K. Choi, Small **10**, 3887 (2014)
46. Y.F. Hu, J. Yang, Q.S. Jing, S.M. Niu, W.Z. Wu, Z.L. Wang, ACS Nano **7**, 10424–10432 (2013)
47. J. Yang, J. Chen, Y. Yang, H.L. Zhang, W.Q. Yang, P. Bai, Y.J. Su, Z.L. Wang, Adv. Energy Mater. **4** (2014)
48. X.N. Wen, W.Q. Yang, Q.S. Jing, Z.L. Wang, ACS Nano **8**, 7405–7412 (2014)
49. P. Bai, G. Zhu, Y. Liu, J. Chen, Q.S. Jing, W.Q. Yang, J.S. Ma, G. Zhang, Z.L. Wang, ACS Nano **7**, 6361–6366 (2013)
50. Y. Yang, H.L. Zhang, J. Chen, Q.S. Jing, Y.S. Zhou, X.N. Wen, Z.L. Wang, ACS Nano **7**, 7342–7351 (2013)
51. S.M. Niu, Y. Liu, S.H. Wang, L. Lin, Y.S. Zhou, Y.F. Hu, Z.L. Wang, Adv. Funct. Mater. **25**(43), 6184–6193 (2013)
52. H.L. Zhang, Y. Yang, X.D. Zhong, Y.J. Su, Y.S. Zhou, C.G. Hu, Z.L. Wang, ACS Nano **8**, 680–689 (2014)
53. Z. Lin, J. Yang, X. Li, Y. Wu, W. Wei, J. Liu, J. Chen, J. Yang, Adv. Funct. Mater. **28**, 1704112 (2018)
54. F. Yi, L. Lin, S. Niu, P.K. Yang, Z. Wang, J. Chen, Y. Zhou, Y. Zi, J. Wang, Q. Liao, Y. Zhang, Z.L. Wang, Adv. Funct. Mater. **25**, 3688 (2015)
55. X. Zhao, Z. Kang, Q. Liao, Z. Zhang, M. Ma, Q. Zhang, Y. Zhang, Nano Energy **48**, 312 (2018)
56. Z. Lin, Z. Wu, B. Zhang, Y.-C. Wang, H. Guo, G. Liu, C. Chen, Y. Chen, J. Yang, Z.L. Wang, Adv. Mater. Technol. **2018**, 1800360 (2018)
57. P. Bai, G. Zhu, Q. Jing, J. Yang, J. Chen, Y. Su, J. Ma, G. Zhang, Z.L. Wang, Adv. Funct. Mater. **24**, 5807 (2014)
58. H. Ouyang, J. Tian, G. Sun, Y. Zou, Z. Liu, H. Li, L. Zhao, B. Shi, Y. Fan, Y. Fan, Z.L. Wang, Z. Li, Adv. Mater. **29**, 1703456 (2017)
59. J. Yang, J. Chen, Y. Su, Q. Jing, Z. Li, F. Yi, X. Wen, Z. Wang, Z.L. Wang, Adv. Mater. **27**, 1316 (2015)
60. J. Zhong, Y. Zhang, Q. Zhong, Q. Hu, B. Hu, Z.L. Wang, J. Zhou, ACS Nano **8**, 6273 (2014)
61. C.-H. Chen, P.-W. Lee, Y.-H. Tsao, Z.-H. Lin, Nano Energy **42**, 241 (2017)
62. Y.N. Xie, S.H. Wang, S.M. Niu, L. Lin, Q.S. Jing, J. Yang, Z.Y. Wu, Z.L. Wang, Adv. Mater. (2014)
63. F.R. Fan, Z.Q. Tian, Z. Lin Wang, Flexible triboelectric generator. Nano Energy **1**(2), 328–334 (2012). https://doi.org/10.1016/j.nanoen.2012.01.004
64. Z.L. Wang, Triboelectric nanogenerators as new energy technology for self-powered systems and as active mechanical and chemical sensors. ACS Nano **7**(11), 9533–9557 (2013). https://doi.org/10.1021/nn404614z
65. Y. Yang, K.C. Pradel, Q. Jing, J.M. Wu, F. Zhang, Y. Zhou, Y. Zhang, Z.L. Wang, Thermoelectric nanogenerators based on single Sb-doped ZnO micro/nanobelts. ACS Nano **6**(8), 6984–6989 (2012). https://doi.org/10.1021/nn302481p

66. Y. Yang, W. Guo, K.C. Pradel, G. Zhu, Y. Zhou, Y. Zhang, Y. Hu, L. Lin, Z.L. Wang, Pyroelectric nano-generators for harvesting thermoelectric energy. Nano Lett. **12**(6), 2833–2838 (2012). https://doi.org/10.1021/nl3003039
67. Y. Zhoua, S.X. Zhanga, G.P. Lia, Piezoelectric nuclear battery driven by the jet-flow, Proceedings of the 2017 25th International Conference on Nuclear Engineering, ICONE25, July 2–6 2017, Shanghai, China, https://doi.org/10.1115/ICONE25-66981
68. A.A. Mustapha, N.M. Ali, K.S. Leong, Experimental comparison of piezoelectric rectifying circuits for energy harvesting. IEEE Student Conf. Res. Dev. (2013). https://doi.org/10.1109/SCOReD.2013.7002653
69. M.J. Guan, W.H. Liao, On the efficiencies of piezoelectric energy harvesting circuits towards storage device voltages. Smart Mater. Struct. **16**, 498–505 (2007). https://doi.org/10.1088/0964-1726/16/2/031
70. G.K. Ottman, H.F. Hofmann, G.A. Lesieutre, Optimized piezoelectric energy circuit using step-down converter in discontinuous conduction mode. IEEE Trans. Power Electron. **18**, 696–703 (2003)
71. L.G. Tran, H.K. Cha, W.T. Park, RF power harvesting: A review on designing methodologies and applications. Micro Nano Syst. Lett. (2017). https://doi.org/10.1186/s40486-017-0051-0
72. S. Gollakota, M.S. Reynolds, J.R. Smith, D.J. Wetherall, The emergence of RF-powered computing. IEEE Comput. Soc., 32–39 (2014). https://doi.org/10.1109/MC.2013.404
73. K.Y. Lee, J. Chun, J.H. Lee, Hydrophobic sponge structure-based triboelectric nano-generator. Adv. Mater. **26**(29), 5037–5042 (2014)
74. G. Zhu, C. Pan, W. Guo, Triboelectric-generator-driven pulse electrode position for micropatterning. Nano Lett. **12**(9), 4960–4965 (2012)
75. G. Zhu, Z.-H. Lin, Q. Jing, Toward large-scale energy harvesting by a nanoparticle-enhanced triboelectric nano-generator. Nano Lett. **13**(2), 847–853 (2013)
76. J. Yang, J. Chen, Y. Yang, Broadband vibration energy harvesting based on a triboelectric nano-generator. Adv. Energy Mater. **4**(6), 1301322 (2014)
77. S. Kim, M.K. Gupta, K.Y. Lee, Transparent flexible graphene triboelectric nano-generators. Adv. Mater. **26**(23), 3918–3925 (2014)
78. S. Niu, Z.L. Wang, Theoretical systems of triboelectric nano-generators. Nano Energy (2014). https://doi.org/10.1016/j.nanoen.2014.11.034
79. J. Wang, C. Wu, Y. Dai, Z. Zhao, A. Wang, T. Zhang, Z.L. Wang, Achieving ultrahigh triboelectric charge density for efficient energy harvesting. Nat. Commun. https://doi.org/10.1038/s41467-017-00131-4
80. S. Xu, W. Ding, H. Guo, X. Wang, Z.L. Wang, Boost the performance of triboelectric nanogenerators through circuit oscillation. Adv. Energy Mater. **2019**, 1900772 (2019)
81. S. Niu, Y. Liu, Y.S. Zhou, S. Wang, L. Lin, Z.L. Wang, Optimization of triboelectric nanogenerator charging systems for efficient energy harvesting and storage. IEEE Trans. Electron Devices **62**(2), 641–647 (2015)
82. Renewables in Global Energy Supply: An IEA facts sheet (2007)
83. Z. Lin, J. Chen, J. Yang, Recent progress in triboelectric nanogenerators as a renewable and sustainable power source. J. Nanomater. **2016**, 5651613 (2016)
84. X. Fan, J. Chen, J. Yang, P. Bai, Z. Li, Z.L. Wang, Ultrathin, rollable, paper-based triboelectric nanogenerator for acoustic energy harvesting and self-powered sound recording. ACS Nano **9**(4), 4236–4243 (2015)
85. X. Pu, M. Liu, X. Chen, J. Sun, C. Du, Y. Zhang, J. Zhai, W. Hu, Z.L. Wang, Ultra stretchable, transparent triboelectric nano-generator as electronic skin for biomechanical energy harvesting and tactile sensing. Sci. Adv. **3**(5) (2017)
86. S. Wang, X. Mu, X. Wang, A.Y. Gu, Z.L. Wang, Y. Yang, Elasto-aerodynamics-driven triboelectric nanogenerator for scavenging air-flow energy. ACS Nano **9**(10), 9554–9563 (2015)
87. L. Lin, S. Wang, S. Niu, C. Liu, Y. Xie, Z.L. Wang, Noncontact free-rotating disk triboelectric nanogenerator as a sustainable energy harvester and self-powered mechanical sensor. ACS Appl. Mater. Inter. **6**(4), 3031–3038 (2014)

88. Y. Yang, H. Zhang, X. Zhong, F. Yi, R. Yu, Y. Zhang, Z.L. Wang, Electret film-enhanced triboelectric nanogenerator matrix for self-powered instantaneous tactile imaging. ACS Appl. Mater. Inter. **6**(5), 3680–3688 (2014)
89. L. Hongbin Lina, H. Minghui, J. Qingshen, Y. Weifeng, W. Shutang, L. Ying, Z. Yaoli, L. Jing, L. Ning, M. Yanwen, W. Lianhui, X. Yannan, Angle-shaped triboelectric nano-generator for harvesting environmental wind energy. Nano Energy **56**, 269–276 (2019)
90. A. Pandey, P. Badoniya, J. George, Rotary triboelectric nanogenerators as a wind energy harvester. Int. J. Recent Technol. Eng. **8**, 2277–3878 (2019)
91. H. Zou, Y. Zhang, L. Guo, P. Wang, X. He, G. Dai, H. Zheng, C. Chen, A.C. Wang, C. Xu, Z.L. Wang, Quantifying the triboelectric series. Nat. Commun.. https://doi.org/10.1038/s41467-019-09461-x

Chapter 15
SmartCovSens: A Multimodal Approach for Detection of COVID-19

Sanjoy Banerjee, Debangana Das, Anwesha Sengupta, Nilava Debabhuti, Barnali Ghatak, Prolay Sharma, Sk. Babar Ali, Saurabh Pal, Nityananda Das, Prabal Patra, Chitresh Kundu, Arunangshu Ghosh, Rajib Bandyopadhyay, Dipankar Mandal, and Bipan Tudu

15.1 Introduction

The outbreak of COVID-19 has shown an almost uncontrolled spread worldwide and has posed a challenge to existing healthcare systems to handle the sudden public emergency. The outbreak has also caused an unprecedented shutdown of social life and commerce worldwide, resulting in an economic depression and acute suffering for millions of people [1].

S. Banerjee
Department of Applied Electronics and Instrumentation Engineering, Future Institute of Engineering and Management, Kolkata, India

D. Das · N. Debabhuti · B. Ghatak · P. Sharma · R. Bandyopadhyay · B. Tudu
Department of Instrumentation and Electronics Engineering, Jadavpur University, Kolkata, West Bengal, India

A. Sengupta
Department of Electrical Engineering, National Institute of Technology Rourkela, Rourkela, Odisha, India
e-mail: Senguptaan@nitrkl.ac.in

S. B. Ali
Department of Electronics and Communication Engineering, Future Institute of Engineering and Management, Kolkata, West Bengal, India

S. Pal
Department of Applied Physics, University of Calcutta, Kolkata, West Bengal, India

N. Das
Department of Physics, Jagannath Kishore College, Purulia, West Bengal, India

P. Patra · C. Kundu
Automation Division, Tata Steel Jamshedpur, Jamshedpur, Jharkhand, India
e-mail: prabal.patra@tatasteel.com

L. Garg et al. (eds.), *Healthcare Informatics for Fighting COVID-19 and Future Epidemics*, EAI/Springer Innovations in Communication and Computing,
https://doi.org/10.1007/978-3-030-72752-9_15

An essential step towards controlling the disease is the early identification of infected individuals to adopt appropriate measures. The management of the disease is further complicated due to its high spreading rate, limited information about the nature of symptoms, restricted-availability of medicines and vaccines, the relatively high mortality rate for patients with comorbidities especially for older people, and difficulty in screening for large population due to lack of testing kit and trained workforce.

With the vaccination drive yet to reach the entire population, early diagnosis and subsequent management are indispensable for containing the outbreak. Extensive testing for the identification of potential carriers is essential for disease diagnosis, the virus spread confinement, and contact tracing. Thus, the need for the development of noncontact and unobtrusive methods for quick screening of potential carriers to stall the spread of the virus is of utmost importance [2].

The limited availability of data is a deterrent in studying dynamics of an emerging and rapidly growing disease as COVID-19. Data-based estimates of the outbreak's growth are further confounded by non-availability of diagnostic reagents early in the outbreak, changes in the intensity of surveillance and case definitions, and overworked healthcare systems [3]. One of the efficient complementary approaches for mitigation and managing pandemics such as COVID-19 is automated digital contact tracing. Garg et al. [4] categorizes current approaches for contact tracing and design of a novel privacy anonymous IoT model and presentation of an RFID proof of concept for the model. The model solution would allow moving objects to receive or send notifications when close to a probable or confirmed diseased case.

The proposed chapter will describe a multimodal approach for rapid screening of potential COVID-19 carriers based on symptomatic sensing using a combination of sensors. The proposed system would be suitable for screening purposes at areas that record high footfall throughout the day, such as ATMs, airports, train/metro stations, smart gates, shopping malls, etc.

15.2 The COVID-19 Pandemic: Symptoms and Markers

Till date, body temperature has been identified as the most significant parameter for rapid screening of potential carriers. It has also been observed that persistent dry cough is a predominant indicator. Fatigue may also be considered a mild marker of the infection, especially for asymptomatic carriers. Hence thermoscan systems and cough and/or sneeze detection may be used to screen potential patients. The

A. Ghosh
Department of Electrical Engineering, National Institute of Technology Patna, Patna, Bihar, India
e-mail: arunangshu.ghosh@nitp.ac.in

D. Mandal
Institute of Nanoscience and Technology (INST), Habitat Center, Mohali, Punjab, India
e-mail: dmandal@inst.ac.in

detection mechanism must be suitable for mass screening in various locations, equipped with adequate internet connectivity, and should preferably be mobile.

15.3 Detection Systems

The current state-of-the-art methods available for detection of COVID-19 will be discussed in this section. The detection methods may be broadly divided into two types: biotechnology-based instrumental detection and rapid screening-based testing systems. The instrumental methods are accurate, mostly rely on lab-based setup, and require higher detection time, whereas the rapid detection methods are more suitable for large-scale screening and testing purposes. The conventional open-ended reverse transcription polymerase chain reaction (RT-PCR) is considered the "gold standard" for detecting COVID-19 mainly due to its high accuracy of detection. The system produces results with high rates of true positive (high sensitivity) and a moderate rate of a true negative (moderate specificity). This method requires the costly RT-PCR instrument and skilled lab technicians who need to follow elaborate biosafety and biosecurity norms. Testing samples usually takes around 4–5 h, excluding the sample transportation time to labs. A batch of 90 samples may be tested in a single run. Availability of this instrument is thus limited to sophisticated virology laboratories. The above limitations regarding this system hinder its widespread penetration in hospitals and health centres for mass testing situations.

The cartridge-based systems like TrueNAT and CB-NAT had been widely used for the diagnosis of tuberculosis. These systems also proved their efficacy when they were used for the detection of COVID-19. Their response is typically characterized by moderate sensitivity and high specificity. The automated sequence of sample preparation steps that are followed in this method, as opposed to RT-PCR test, facilitates the conformance of biosafety norms, aids portability, and access to testing at a grass-root level in a significant manner. However, RT-PCR is still required, but analysis time is greatly reduced to 30–60 min, due to the presence of cartridge-based sample preprocessing step. The TrueNAT, being a battery-operated device, possesses more portability than a CB-NAT system that requires air conditioning systems and an uninterrupted power supply.

The mechanisms mentioned earlier employed the PCR amplification process to increase the number of viral RNA, thus facilitating the sensitivity of detection even if the viral load is of less quantity in the nasopharyngeal/oropharyngeal samples. As a result, RT-PCR-based methods have good sensitivity. However, high detection time and low throughput remain a concern for these accurate methods. In this situation, the Rapid Point-of-Care (PoC) Antigen Detection Test with moderate sensitivity, very high specificity, independence from specialized instruments, and low result declaration time of 15–30 min becomes an ideal point-of-care solution for early detection of the virus. This technique's principle of operation is based on a chromatographic immunoassay of antigens specific to the spike protein of SARS-

CoV-2 virus that coated on a test strip. Samples from the subject are collected in a nasopharyngeal swab, and viral particles are extracted in a buffer solution that inactivates the virus. After that, two to three drops of a sample with a buffer solution are put on a test strip coated with antigen molecules. The presence of viral particles is indicated by the appearance of test lines on the strip. The technique is characterized as high specificity, which means that a positive result can be considered a true positive. However, a negative result may not always indicate a true negative as the system has been observed to be of low to moderate sensitivity. The sensitivity of detection improves with the amount of viral load in collected samples. RT-PCR is thus required to ensure the authenticity of negative results for the antigen test.

Nevertheless, the antigen test ensures true positives at a high probability, provides rapid results, is portable, and is very useful for mass testing activities.

Rapid antibody tests for COVID-19 are carried out to assess the spread disease in the population. Antibodies are proteins that are developed in the body against an agent for infection in the human body. This test can be carried out using well-known ELISA enzyme-linked immunosorbent assay) or CIA (chemiluminescent immunoassay). The antibody tests help monitor the spread of the disease and are also useful in planning vaccination drives and identifying potential volunteers for convalescent plasma therapy.

Recently, high-resolution computerized tomography of chest (HRCT chest) has been proven as a rapid and useful tool to screen COVID-19. Studies have indicated that CT and HRCT of COVID-19 patients typically display multiple ground-glass opacity (GCO) regions, septal thickening, vascular enlargement, and air bronchogram signatures. Most of the COVID-19 infections were shown to be correctly detected. However, these imaging techniques could not be used to distinguish between similar viruses, that elicit overlapping symptoms and indications.

The ML-based methodologies mainly rely on the quality and severity of symptoms to predict the probability of infection within a concise time. ML-based methods are therefore very much suitable for screening purposes and are the upcoming technologies. No technology developed so far has been found to be accurate, and this chapter attempts to improve on such conceptual systems.

15.4 Proposed System

The proposed system consists of a sensor array for simultaneous recording of signals for rapid screening of potential COVID-19 carriers, followed by a module for processing of data and communication of the results for surveillance and tracking.

15.4.1 *Sensing Module*

The sensing module would consist of an infrared temperature sensor, optical imaging camera, a microphone, and a gas sensor to analyse breath samples of the subject being screened. Section 15.4.2 will review the sensors currently in use.

15.4.2 *Sensors: The Current State of the Art*

In the conceptual system, the subject's body temperature will be captured by the IR thermal detector. If the recording temperature (T) of the human subject is above 100 °F, the optical imager module will be activated. A face recognition framework will be developed to extract the image of the face (FP) of the subject by use of segmentation algorithms, followed by a fatigue detection (FD) procedure using ocular features. The microphone module is activated in case of a cough or sneezing sound (CS), and the nature of cough will be detected. The presence of persistent dry cough (PDC) will affect the value of SI significantly. Gas sensors of high sensitivity are employed to detect concentration of nitric oxide (NO) (CONO) that may be produced as a result of inflammation of lung cells in COVID-19-infested subjects. The use of novel functionalized triboelectric gas sensors may be envisaged for sensing purposes and generating operating power for the proposed system.

15.4.2.1 Thermal Sensors

The normal temperature (normothermia) in the human body varies from 36.5 to 37.5 °C, from 97.7 to 99.5 °F [5]. Human body controls the body temperature by using homeostatic mechanism and controls the average body temperature about 37.0 °C (98.6 °F) with a variation of 0.5–1.0 °C. However, human body temperature differs depending on their sex, time of the measurement, age, health (illness), emotions, and many others. When the human body produces more heat than it can dissipate, then it is called hyperthermia (fever), in which the body temperature rises about 40 °C (104 °F) or above. There are various measurement techniques in use to measure the body temperature like oral thermometer in which a traditional glass thermometer is placed in the mouth, tympanic thermometer [6] which is a cone-type thermometer placed inside the ear canal, forehead thermometer which is typically an IR radiation thermometer used to scan heat over the forehead, basal thermometer [7] which is used for high accuracy body temperature measurement, pacifier thermometer [8] which is used to measure the temperature of the young child, etc.

Thermal images are amenable to digital storage and processing using readily available software packages. Anomalous body temperature may be considered a common indicator of illness. Development of advanced infrared sensors has established infrared thermal imaging (IRT) as an alternative to clinical thermometers to measure abnormal temperatures. IRT is devoid of side effects, is a noncontact method, and has the advantages of improved temperature sensitivity and spatial resolution. IRT can also be used to map body temperature from a distance. IRT has been employed for fever screening, diagnosis of vascular disorders, analysis of neonatal physiology, kidney transplantation, dermatology, and heart and brain imaging.

Studies have revealed fever to be the most significant indication in patients with SARS, and SARS may be transmitted only by patients with fever. Pitman et al. [9] reported that an epidemic of SARS or influenza might be effectively prevented by screening at airports' entry. Considering the large number of visitors entering the airport daily, it is essential to devise a consistent method for temperature screening which is also less time-consuming.

The high-resolution infrared thermography digital infrared thermal imaging (IRTDITI) reported in [10] can be used for contactless and noninvasive screening of a huge volume of visitors. However, the effectiveness of IRT is subject to the following primary concerns [11]:

- Precision of the relationship between deep body temperature and infrared thermal images of chosen skin zones on the head.
- Poor ability to recognize or detect affected people during any phase of fever development.
- Camera quality and/or utilization in fever screening installations.

The recent data demonstrates that the temperature of the inward canthus of the eye is reliably the hottest zone on the head and the most reasonable site for use in fever recognition [12]. In any case, it is significant that there must be a satisfactory number of pixels here to enlist temperature and record difference between an ordinary and febrile individual. The methodology requires accurate positioning so that the face fills the larger part (zone) of the picture. It additionally needs an insignificant number of pixels in that certain zone. Application of thermal imaging techniques to the clinical field by Jones and Plassmann [13] revealed that commotion in infrared images could originate from numerous sources such as intrinsic thermal noise, white noise, etc. It was found that such issues can be minimized by enhanced techniques like median filtering and morphological processes. The infrared camera performs an examination of a specific pixel's temperature level against the normal temperature of the scene. Images captured by the camcorder are further represented by grey pixels on a scale of 0–255. A grey level of 0 represents the least temperature in the image, and the temperature increases with the increase in level. The infrared picture thus resembles a distribution map of temperatures of the items whose images have been captured. To acquire the accurate temperature, calibration of the grey levels as per the actual temperatures is of utmost importance. This should be done so that the relation between the two, i.e. grey level and actual temperature, can be easily derived. Budzan et al. [14] developed an algorithm based on randomized Hough transform [RHT] for detecting and locating the face and eyes in thermal images by specific measurement of the body temperature using the temperature of the eye corner [inner canthus]. The developed algorithm reduces the complexity of inner canthus localization, and a good correlation has been reported between actual and predicted axilla temperature. Selent et al. [15] compared the work of three infrared thermal detection systems (ITDS), namely, FLIR ThermoVision 360, OptoTherm Thermoscreen, and Thermofocus 0800H3, for mass screening of body temperature during fever in children (<18 years age). The observed results were compared with standard results based on the appropriate temperature measurement of the patients (confirmed fever defined as >38 °C (oral or rectal), >38 °C (axillary)). The experimental study of the body temperature showed good correlation with traditional thermometry. It results in 0.78 (OptoTherm) and 0.75 (FLIR) for detecting fever in children and is found helpful for noninvasive fever detection in paediatric age groups. Ring et al. [16] also performed a series of studies to detect fever in children using FLIR infrared camera SC640. The study involved examining 402 children from 2006 to 2011, where the subject was photographed. The face would occupy at least 75% of the image concerning the regions of inner canthi. The forehead temperature was also recorded as a suitable area of interest. The thermograms were correlated with the patients' axilla recordings, and it was found that the eye and the axilla measurements showed better consistency (reliability coefficient alpha of 0.724).

An automated thermal imaging system was proposed in [17] to segregate frontal face views from non-frontal ones. The system has been built successfully and is important in many areas, such as measuring a human face's temperature, face recognition, etc. Distance from the centroid (DFC) of the human face to the lower part of the face outline is termed as boundary signature and is employed to detect the face's position. However, this method had a low accuracy rate. More exploration on the left lower head outline and right lower head outline needs to be done to improve the detection rate. Techniques have been normally used in pattern recognition, such as Fisher's Linear Discriminant Analysis (FLDA).

Mohammed et al. [18] designed an IoT-based smart helmet to detect COVID-19 patients using body temperature. Three segments are incorporated within a helmet. The first segment includes the sensor module, which consists of a thermal and an optical camera. The second segment refers to the microcontroller for performing an image processing operation. The third segment consists of a GPS module and a smart GSM module for IoT application. The thermal camera is used to detect a person with high temperature, and the optical camera is used to recognize the person. Arduino IDE is used here for image processing application with a suitable detecting algorithm. Whenever a person is identified, then the data related to that person like the current position (indicated by GPS module), temperature, and facial image are sent to the operator for further analysis using the IoT application.

Somboonkaew et al. [19] employed a 2D thermal imaging device to develop a mobile, efficient, noncontact temperature screening system. The system consists of an RGB camera and an IR camera. The RGB image from the RGB camera is used to target the measurement area, and then the maximum temperature is measured within that area using thermal imaging. Two images are then mapped with each other by using image alignment, which is achieved using image cropping and scaling operation. A built-in RGB face detection algorithm is used here to detect the human position for target allocation. The temperature of the subject is taken from the forehead.

Fever screening dependent on infrared (IR) thermographs (IRTs) is a methodology that has been actualized during infectious and communicable pandemics, for example, Ebola and severe acute respiratory syndrome. Various researches on noncontact thermal imaging possess a wide impact for easy and effective detection of fever estimating the body temperature and employing effective facial recognition and image processing algorithms. The modern advent of microcontrollers and microcomputers can be effectively coupled with thermal imaging cameras and image processing algorithms to develop user-friendly and cost-effective instruments for crucial situations like pandemic at public places like airports and railway stations, shopping malls, restaurants, etc. In this way, the quick identification of asymptomatic patients can be made.

15.4.2.2 Optical Sensors

The optical sensing system consists of a face detection framework, followed by the ocular region's detection and detection of fatigue using ocular parameters.

Face Detection

Facial feature detection encompasses numerous techniques, all of which transfer the original data into a space that highlights the face's specific features. Yang et al. [20] have defined face detection as the determination of the presence or absence of any faces in an image by the face detection algorithm and location of all faces in the image in case faces are present. According to Yang et al. [20] based on the approach, face detection methods may be knowledge-based, feature invariant, template matching, or appearance based. Rules that encode a face define the knowledge-based methods and are mostly used for localization of the face. This approach was utilized by Yang and Huang [21] for locating a human face against a complex background by means of three knowledge-based levels. Level 1 comprises scanning the whole image and locating all the faces. Level 2 locates faces obtained in the first level through 8×8 cell window screens. In level 3, more screening is done by matching the eye and mouth regions with the established characteristics, whereafter presence of a face is established if the matching is complete. Structural features are used to identify faces in an image in case of feature-invariant approach thereby making this approach robust to changes in ambient lighting conditions or to variations in viewpoint, scale, translation, rotation, or pose. Leung et al. [22] used this approach to locate faces in cluttered scenes. A set of local feature detectors coupled with a statistical model of the mutual distances between them formed the basis of their work. Yow and Cipolla [23] devised a feature-based algorithm to detect feature points from the image by using spatial filters. Thereafter, using geometric and grey level constraints, they grouped them into faces (using a probabilistic framework).

Dai and Nakano [24] developed a method to detect faces in cluttered colour scenes by forming a face texture model based on the feature parameters present in space grey-level dependence (SGLD) matrix by deriving a set of inequalities to help define the location of the face. A real-time face tracker was developed by Yang and Waibel [25] wherein using a skin colour model in chromatic colour space, human faces were characterized. Additionally, a camera model to predict camera motion and a motion model to track head motion was devised. McKenna et al. [26] used Gaussian mixture models to detect human faces. Template matching approach correlates an image against pre-stored patterns for both face detection and localization. Craw et al. [27] presented a method to locate individual face features like the eyes and mouth in a greyscale face image.

Face detection comprises two steps: first being the general localization of the faces in an image and second further assessment and refinement for face-finding. Lanitis et al. [28] present a model-based representation of the grey-level appearance and shape of human faces. The models as mentioned earlier have been used to classify images. Appearance-based methods, primarily modelled for face detection, focus on the variability of the images. Turk and Pentland [29] performed face recognition and identification using principal component analysis, which is utilized to generate subspace-spanning Eigenfaces. These images are clustered, after being projected to the subspace. The non-face images appear differently when projected to the subspace than the face images, which do not show radical changes. The distance of the face space from each location in the image is computed to detect the presence of a face. This distance, used as a measure of closeness to a face, is a face map. The local minima of the face map help detect the particular face. Sung and Poggio [30] presented a system to learn about a class's image patterns from the positive and negative examples of that class. They used a two-component approach to distinguish faces from non-faces: the first component consisting of distribution-based models for face/non-face patterns. The second is a multilayer perceptron classifier.

The most significant work in face detection using neural networks has been done by Rowley et al. [31]. They have used a multilayer neural network to differentiate between non-face and face patterns from the non-face and face images. The only drawback of this approach is that it is suitable only for detecting upright frontal faces.

Osuna et al. [32] utilized an SVM for face detection for the first time, the novelty of low error rates and fast recognition. Schneiderman and Kanade [33] devised an approach employing a naive Bayes classifier to compute the joint probability of local appearance and position of the subregions of the face at different resolutions. The focus on sub-regions or local patterns is significant as they contain distinctive information. For instance, a clear distinction exists between the patterns around the cheeks and those around the eyes. This approach essentially divides the face into four subregions at each scale, subsequently projected onto a lower-dimensional space using PCA. After that, it is quantized into a finite set of patterns. Local appearance is encoded using the statistics from each subregion. Hence, a face's presence is reported when the likelihood ratio is higher than the ratio of prior probabilities. This method can detect a few rotated and profile faces. Schneiderman and Kanade [34] later extended this work using wavelet representations to detect cars and profile faces. A couple of probabilistic methods for face detection have been proposed by Rajagopalan et al. [35]. Higher-order statistics have been employed by the first method for density estimation, whereas in the second method, the hidden Markov model (HMM) is used for defining faces and non-faces in an image. In spite of these approaches having a high detection rate, there are also some false positives. Lew [36] carried out face detection by associating different probability functions to the template's events being a face and not being a face. The face distribution is computed using a face training database consisting of 9 views of 100 individuals, while the non-face probability distribution density function is estimated using a set of 143,000 non-face templates.

Extraction of Ocular Region

Extraction of facial features is a significant factor in automatic interpretation and recognition of human faces. Many face recognition systems require facial features in addition to holistic face as suggested by psychology studies. Literature suggests that holistic matching methods such as Eigenfaces [29] and Fisherfaces [37] need accurate locations of key facial features such as the eyes, nose, and mouth for normalizing the detected face. Various types of facial features are region [38, 39], key point (landmark) [40, 41], and contour [42, 43].

Key point features have lower computational burden and complexity than contour feature extraction and provide more consistent and accurate representation for alignment than region-based features. Feature extraction processes may be classified into three major types:

1. Generic methods (based on edges, lines, and curves).
2. Feature template-based methods (for detection of facial features such as the eyes).
3. Structural matching methods (based on geometrical constraints on features).

Early attempts at facial recognition, such as the template-based approach introduced by Hallinan for detection and subsequent recognition of the eye in a frontal face [44], stressed upon individual features. These methods have obvious drawbacks of not recognizing the subject when the feature changes, viz. closed eyes, open mouth, etc. Various methods have also been conceptualized by researchers for locating facial features such as the eyes and mouth. Lam and Yan [45] have developed a snake model, corner detection, and cost functions to detect the eyes. However, the model could handle images with a bland/plain background or with a single person, and the snake had to be initialized manually. Eye detection using three indicators, namely, the orientation of the line joining two eye centres, relatively low intensity of eye regions, and response obtained due to the convolution of the eye variance filter with the face image, had been proposed by Feng and Yuen [46].

Radial basis function neural networks (RBFNN) and optimal wavelet packets for eye representation had been proposed by Huang and Wechsler [47] for eye classification. Template matching was used in [48] to locate the eyes and mouths. Wavelet decomposition for facial feature detection and three-layer backpropagation neural networks for classification of the eyes were applied by Wang and Yuan [49]. You et al. [50] devised a method of representation of the face using non-tensor product wavelets. The technique developed by Heisele et al. [51] evaluates the part of the image cantered in correspondence to each pixel in a multi-resolution way. Squares of (58 × 58) pixels, obtained from the image at the different scales, are fed as input to SVMs trained to detect specific features. This method can work on images of face ranging in dimensions from 80 × 80 to 130 × 130 pixels and handles face rotation even for a bespectacled image. A method devised by Nikolaidis et al. [52–54] detects the features (like eyes) by projecting the grey levels on both axes after having localized the face region. A Hough-like technique then searches for the eyes by looking for the most probable circles and confirms through a template that represents two eyes side by side. The technique developed by Hsu et al. [55] uses a colour combination and a morphological characterization to select hypothetical eyes and mouths; each possible triplet has to be validated according to the knowledge of the distances among them. In addition to being independent of pose and being on a scale, the technique is very efficient for skin region detection.

The transformation proposed by Herpers et al. [56] applied a bank of high-pass filters to obtain a saliency map. The maxima in the saliency map have a high probability of correspondence to features. The maxima are extracted, and deformable templates verify the corresponding portions of images to be a feature. Smeraldi and Bigun have adopted a different characterization based on the Gabor wavelet transform in [57]. The work presented in Hamouz et al. [58] involves the localization of features by the extraction of corner points of the eye using the Harris method [59], followed by acceptance or rejection of corresponding image portions following evaluation through PCA. This technique makes use of an energy function to match eye components to previously designed templates. Ren et al. [60] employs a method for eye localization with rotation invariance for face processing algorithm to increase face recognition accuracy. Heat map with pyramid-like detecting method is used to locate the eye centres in eye localization method.

Fatigue Detection Using Ocular Features

A study of features for study of fatigue and drowsiness such as eye closure and/or yawning has been employed for assessment of driver states and to avert vehicular accidents [61]. Eye movement signals (such as face detection, eye positioning, detection of pupil, and eye angles) have been used in conjunction with EEG, and ECG signal analysis for real-time monitoring of drivers' mental state and generation of decision signals decide whether or not the driver is fatigued. The relation between operator fatigue and blink-based, pupil-based, and saccade-based eye metrics has been explored in [62, 63].

PERCLOS has been used as a metric and approximate entropy for detecting fatigue due to sleepiness in military aviation operators [64]. The metric ocular aspect ratio has been devised based on the eye's shape to detect eye closure in drivers due to fatigue [65]. An eye tracking method has been developed to detect eye closure to detect driver fatigue in [66]. A scheme for detection of onset of fatigue due to drowsiness in car drivers in [67] incorporates a system for eye tracking with an aim to measure eyelid separation. A system for real-time detection of driver fatigue based on vision has been developed in [68]. Eye region is located from the driver's face (located from facial images captured in the car) using edge detection techniques. The derived eye images are used for fatigue detection and development of an alarm system to ensure fatigued drivers' safety.

A real-time drowsiness detection system using a combination of PERCLOS and greyscale image processing has been developed to establish a fatigue model for vehicle drivers and monitor the driver's state of alertness continuously. The approximate position of the face in the greyscale images is calculated, and eye positions are analysed therefrom. Information about eye positions and PERCLOS is used to develop a fatigue model. The model is used to monitor the driver's state and alert the driver at the onset of fatigue [69]. A combination of eyelid movements and pose face (extracted from images captured using an active IR illuminator) has been used to develop a non-intrusive system for real-time monitoring of driver vigilance levels [70]. PERCLOS was used to measure the drop in vigilance levels in professional drivers due to sleep deprivation during a simulated driving task.

The study in [71] examines the changes in ocular parameters to sleep deprivation and explores the correspondence between changes in PERCLOS with the drop-in performance levels in a simulated driving task under fatigue due to loss of sleep. A framework for detection of the effects of sleep deprivation during a simulated driving task in conjunction with psychomotor vigilance task (PVT) and the Karolinska sleepiness scale (KSS) has been developed using eyelid closure as a metric in [72]. A correspondence has been established between an increase in drowsiness and a slowing of eyelid closure and an increase in eye closure duration and frequency.

The development of warning systems to enable detection of reduced vigilance levels using ocular measures has been discussed in [73]. The performance of eye-tracking based in-vehicle fatigue prediction measures has been evaluated. Eye blink and eye closure (eyelid movement parameters) have been combined with principal facial features to generate a framework to measure drivers' vigilance levels in [74]. A system for analysis of visual attention in human drivers has been developed in [75] through robust tracking of subjects' head and facial features by estimating global motion and colour statistics. Rotation is classified in all viewing directions along with detection of occlusion of the eye and mouth, eye blinking, and eye closure. The three-dimensional gaze of the eyes is also detected. The system can also track occlusion due to eye blinking, eye closure, large mouth movement and rotation.

A system for analysis and monitoring alertness in drivers using robust tracking of head and facial features developed in [76] classifies rotation in different viewing directions, detects occlusion of the eye and mouth and eye blinking, and recovers

3D gaze of the eyes. A computer vision-based system for non-intrusive real-time monitoring of driver vigilance involving the recording of visual parameters such as eyelid movement, face orientation, and gaze movement (pupil movement) was found to be robust under various illumination conditions as well [77]. Changes in blink behaviour from EOG data have been combined with subjective assessments and an EEG-based scoring scale to devise a drowsiness detection scheme to detect the early onset of fatigue in drivers [78]. The relation between blink amplitude and frequency obtained from EOG signal was employed to detect drowsiness stages, along with a subjective assessment of alertness [79].

PERCLOS was used to indicate the drop-in performance in a simulated driving task under fatigue due to sleep deprivation [80]. PERCLOS is used along with greyscale image processing to develop a real-time system to detect fatigue in drivers [69]. The possibility of use of an eye tracker for detection of changes in vigilance levels in military operations was explored in [81]. Changes in blink frequency, blink duration, PERCLOS, pupil diameter, pupil eccentricity, and pupil velocity were observed during a 40-min vigilance task.

15.4.2.3 Sound Sensor

A forceful discharge of air mainly characterizes coughing through mouth accompanied by an unpleasant sound meant for clearing of air passages. Although cough may not necessarily imply an underlying disease, physicians have been using cough for centuries to diagnose diseases. This is because the cough is one of the most common markers for many diseases such as asthma, chronic obstructive pulmonary disease, pulmonary fibrosis, bronchiectasis, etc. [82]. The available detection methods are highly subjective and mostly dependent on the patient's self-reported history. Lately, several studies and literature have attempted to address this issue using advanced machine learning algorithms combined with sophisticated recording devices.

Extraction of time, frequency, and entropy features of cough by Martinek et al. [83] for useful segregation of cough have resulted in a differentiation between speech and voluntary cough sounds using a decision tree. The study used 46 coughs from each of 20 subjects to yield a median sensitivity and specificity of 100% and 85%, respectively. Tracey et al. [84] put to use an interesting algorithm for monitoring patients recovering from tuberculosis. Using a combination of support vector machine (SVM) and artificial neural networks (ANN) as classifiers, MFCCs extracted from audio signals of ten subjects were used to detect coughs, yielding an overall sensitivity of 81%.

However, automatic counting was still extremely essential for efficient recording of cough signals. To address this issue, Barry et al. [85] devised an automatic cough counting tool called Hull Automatic Cough Counter (HACC) using Mel-frequency cepstral coefficients and linear predictive coding (LPC) coefficients with a probabilistic neural network (PNN) classifier. The HACC was sensitive enough to discriminate between a cough and non-cough event in 33 subjects with sensitivity and specificity values of 93% and 94%, respectively. The method required subjects to perform the last count to handle false positives and multiple coughs overlapping into a single classification. For recognition of sound analysis, Swarnkar et al. [86] used Mel-frequency cepstral coefficient (MFCC) features with other spectral features such as format frequencies, kurtosis, and *B*-score. A dataset consisting of 342 coughs from 3 subjects was fed into a neural network resulting in a specificity of 94% and a sensitivity of 93%, and hence ensuring high reliability of the technique used. Martos et al. [87] extracted 13 MFCCs from a dataset of 2155 coughs from 9 subjects with a sensitivity of 82%. To determine the cough location, the dataset was classified using the hidden Markov model (HMM). It would be interesting to note that the finite state machine represented by the HMM could learn about the structure of cough sounds with only the knowledge of the number of sub-states with the cough state.

Carrying the work of Martos forward, Birring et al. [88] designed the Leicester cough monitor. The portable recorder and the microphone recorded the patients' coughs for six hours while the patients performed their daily chores. In comparison with the study by Martos, this study has led to a large increase in the number of coughs and variety of sounds recorded compared to Martos. Barton et al. [89, 90] published a two-channel recording device involving both contact and noncontact microphones to simplify the challenge of processing disambiguating cough sound signals. The system captures the signal regions with high energy and high spectral centre of gravity, followed by manual counting of the coughs. To build a cough detector with the help of a noncontact recording system for use in paediatric wards, Amrulloh et al. [91] used ANN classification consisting of a dataset of over 1400 cough sounds from 14 subjects and achieved a sensitivity and specificity of 93% and 98%, respectively. Cough frequency and duration can also be measured by recording the start and the end times of coughs. Monge-Alvarez et al. used Hu moments with a KNN classifier to detect cough and employed the analysis to demonstrate the efficacy of Hu moments as a basis of cough detection in spite of their computational complexity [92]. Hu moments that have been calculated have been implemented as robust feature sets for automatic segregation of cough events [93, 94]. Their method achieved a sensitivity and specificity of 88% and 96%, respectively.

You et al. [95] detected cough using spectral subbands fed into linear SVMs with 78% sensitivity and 88% specificity. Their study focussed on the performance of their adopted classifiers in the presence of noise and synthesizing noise. This work involved the collection of data with intentionally created noisy backgrounds. The deep learning system developed by Amoh et al. [96] used convolutional networks to achieve 82% sensitivity and specificity of 93%. The authors also utilized a recurrent neural architecture for variable-length segmentation which yielded 84% sensitivity and 75% specificity. Liu et al. [97] used Gammatone cepstral coefficient (GMCC) features along with SVM classification to achieve 91% sensitivity and 85% specificity from a dataset containing 903 coughs from 4 subjects. Larson et al. [98] used eigenvalue decompositions on cough sounds fed into random forest classifiers with a maximum of 500 decision trees to detect cough on over 2500 cough sounds from 17 individuals. The algorithm has a privacy-preserving feature to transform the raw audio data through the eigenvector matrix built during training. This method renders the speech parts unintelligible and retains only the cough sounds and has 92% sensitivity.

Studies described above aim to create devices like cough monitors, cough counters, and partial automatic cough detection using machine learning. However, there is still a research gap in the practical detection and diagnosis of cough. The study by Charles N. John [99] attempts to bridge the gap by proposing and analysing a machine learning-based method to detect cough automatically in presence of background noise. The author implemented ResNet and XGBoost to detect and diagnose cough sounds of asthma, bronchitis, bronchiolitis, normal, and pertussis with the different sample size [18]. Using ResNet, this model can achieve an impressive accuracy of 99% by just using the cough sound, without the subject having to wear any extra equipment. Successful cough detection is followed by investigating the possibility of preliminary differential diagnosis by distinguishing coughs associated with asthma/bronchitis/bronchiolitis/pertussis patients and healthy people.

15.4.2.4 Gas Sensor

A self-powered, highly sensitive triboelectric gas sensor was proposed in [100] to detect CO_2 at room temperature using threshold concentration detection and continuous detection modes of sensing and utilizing gas discharge induced by the triboelectric nanogenerator (TENG) as the major sensing parameter. The sensor involves a change in discharge characteristics because of the obstruction of plasma formation by the negative CO_2 ion. The detectable threshold concentrations lie in the range of 1000–200,000 ppm. The study in [101] involves the synthesis of polyaniline-based triboelectrodes to detect ammonia in self-powered mode. The output voltage of the developed TENG was found to decrease with increase in the concentration of NH_3. The nanosensor offers good selectivity and sensitivity with the limit detection of 500 ppm at room temperature. A chemoresistive gas sensor based on zinc oxide-reduced graphene oxide (ZnO-RGO) hybrid films has been introduced in [102]. The voltage drop across the interdigital electrodes (IDE) was found to change proportionally with the concentration of NO_2. A promising response of 16.8–100 ppm of NO_2 was obtained using the sensor. The work also describes developing a self-powered NO_2 gas alert system for real-time monitoring of ambient NO_2 concentration through a signal processing circuit. A system for converting mechanical energy to electrical energy through triboelectric effect has been presented in [103]. The work describes the synthesis of a surface-modified polydimethylsiloxane (PDMS) (micropyramids) film to make and break contacts with Pd nanoparticles decorated 1D ZnO nanorods array (Pd NPs/ZnO NRs). The open-circuit voltage and short-circuit current were found to be around 5.2 V and 80 nA, respectively, in ambient air. A variation in output voltages was obtained with various concentrations of H_2 gas. The sensor's output voltage and response were approximately recorded as 1.1 V and 373% at 10,000 ppm H_2, respectively, and the response time of the sensor is 100 s. Design of a triboelectric ammonia sensor (TEAS) based on PANI-MWCNTs composite thin film has been presented in [104]. The TEAS@PANI-MWCNT sensor was found to exhibit a good response of 255% at 100 ppm NH_3, in addition, fast response with good recovery time, excellent long-term stability, satisfactory selectivity, and good anti-bending ability. A preliminary test of human exhaled NH_3 concentration has also been carried out to validate the practical application of the developed TEAS. A blow-driven triboelectric nanogenerator introduced by Wen et al. in [105] recorded a fast response time of 11 s and a fast recovery of 20 s. The induced voltage across the sensor was found to be proportional to the breathed-out alcohol concentration by using the electricity generated via the blowing of the mouth, irrespective of the blow speed and quality of airflow. Development of a polyamide 6,6 (PA) film or polytetrafluoroethylene (PTFE) film-based self-powered active sensor for detecting water or ethanol in gas or liquid phase was described in [106]. Performance of the developed sensor was measured by the level of wettability of solid polymer surfaces. A scheme for scalable nanomanufacturing and assembly of tellurium (Te) nanowires with chiral chain structure into the wearable piezoelectric device has been described in [107]. The feasibility of such devices for self-powered sensing applications such as cardiovascular monitoring has also been explored. A self-powered implantable skin-like glucometer based on the piezo-enzymatic-reaction coupling effect of GOx@ZnO nanowire has been developed [108] for real-time detection of blood glucose level.

15.4.3 Sensor Arrangement

As discussed in the earlier sections, the following sensors shall be utilized for the proposed system:

- An optical camera
- An acoustic microphone
- IR temperature detector/IR camera
- Gas sensor

The arrangement of sensors will be decided by the form of the detection system. The detection system may be envisaged as a distributed sensing arrangement inside a walk-through tunnel, sensing kiosk, and wearables. In a tunnel-based walk-through distributed sensing arrangement, the subject walks inside the sensing enclosure fitted with an IR camera at the exit point. The sensing tunnel will also contain one or more microphone pickups for detecting the number of coughs for a given amount time. An optical camera will be useful to detect the fatigue level from the facial expression and gait of the walking subject. Mounting a gas sensor-based arrangement will be technically challenging in this configuration and may result into low sensitivity of detection. However, signals from IR camera and microphone pickups will offer maximum feasibility in terms of technical implementation. This sort of system arrangement will be typically suitable for large-scale screening and detection purposes. A schematic of the arrangement is provided in Fig. 15.1.

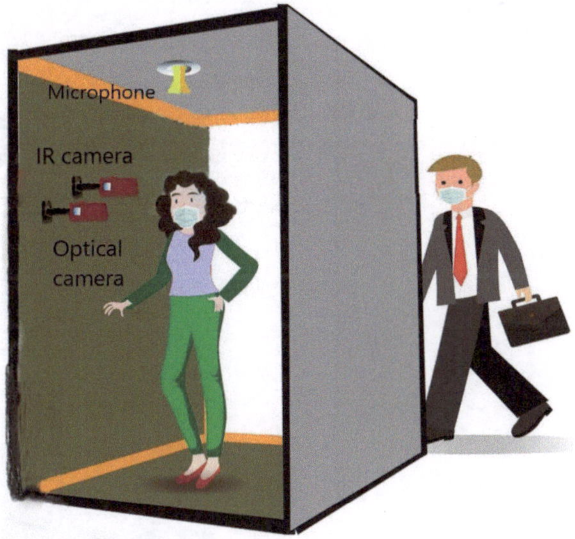

Fig. 15.1 Placement of sensors in the proposed sanitization tunnel

If a higher sensitivity of detection is required, a testing kiosk-based solution may be adopted. In this configuration, the subject will be required to stand in front of an automated testing panel. The optical camera will be utilized to capture a face picture of the subject which will be instructed to look into a specific point. At the same time, the subject's temperature will be measured using the IR camera/IR gun. The subject will be instructed to hold the breath for 15 s, and the resulting cough if any will be recorded and tested for the type of cough. The subject will then be instructed to breathe out into a suction tube in a noncontact fashion. The breath samples will be carried into TENG-based self-powered gas sensors to detect NO in breath samples. The schematic of such a setup is presented in Fig. 15.2.

The wearable sensing arrangement is desirable when a mobile testing cum surveillance mechanism becomes crucial. The testing methods remain the same as described earlier, except that the whole unit will be portable and will be operated under the control of a human operator who is wearing the sensor assembly. Such an assembly as shown may be mounted on a helmet worn by an individual who wants to carry out the surveillance. In this case, again, the IR camera, optical camera, and acoustic microphone may be used for sensing purpose. The sensing assembly has been shown in Fig. 15.3.

15.4.4 Information Processing and Decision Module

The output of different modules will be subjected to information processing and decision module (IPDM) to generate a metric indicating severity of COVID-19-related symptoms; Severity Index (SI). An IoT system may be used thereafter to

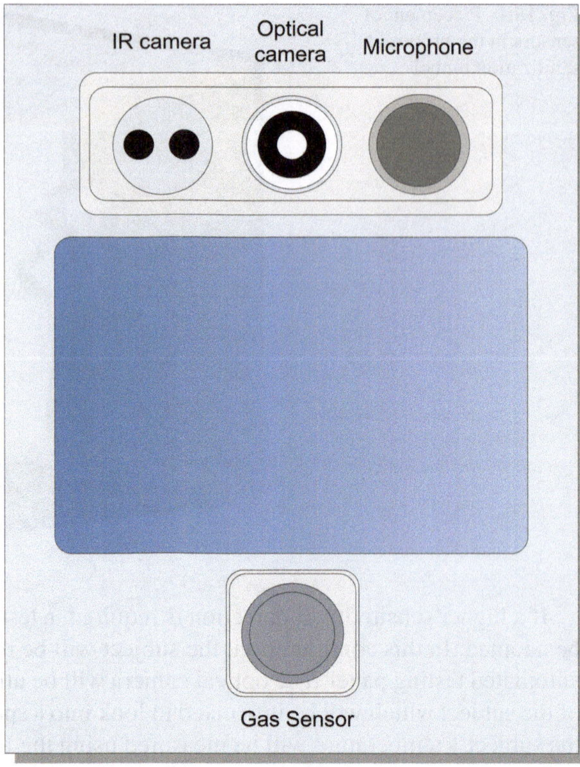

Fig. 15.2 Instrument arrangement

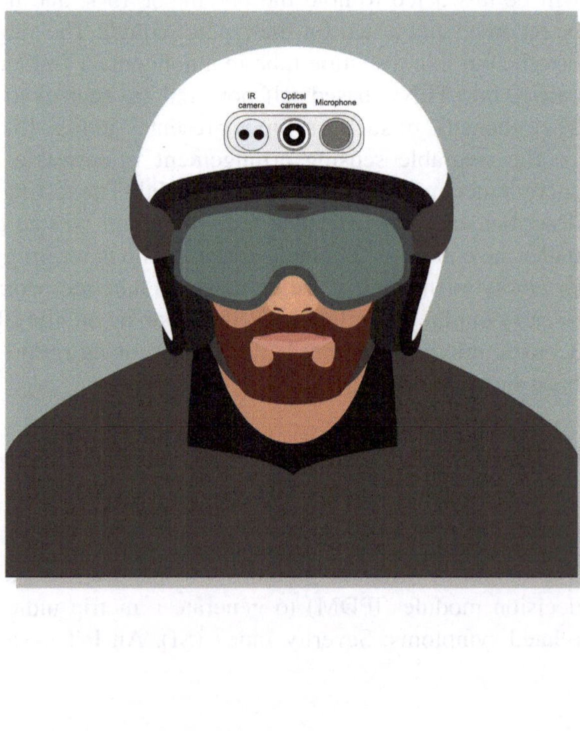

Fig. 15.3 Wearable sensing assembly

communicate the condition of the person screened to the nearby health officer for surveillance and tracking purposes. The data processing task may be carried out on an embedded platform, preferably on a single board computer system. The severity index of individual systems may be calculated based on the frequency of occurrence of a symptom. For example, suppose the cough intensity is high and accompanied by appreciable energy content in the cough waveform. In that case, a higher SI value may be deduced to reflect the intensity of cough. Moreover, the temperature detected by an IR sensor may be directly correlated with the severity of fever if it crosses 98 °F. Fatigue detection tasks are challenging to execute. In such a scenario, slow blinks and percentage of eye opened (to detect droopy eyes) may be utilized to infer a subject's fatigue level. The SI value for fatigue detection may also be correlated directly with the level of fatigue in a person. For gas sensors, the level of volatiles like CO_2 and NO produced due to infection or stress on cardiovascular system may be estimated to indicate the severity of the disease on an individual's cardiovascular system. The overall severity index $SI_{Overall}$ values may be calculated from the severity metrics for each sensing system SI_x, as shown in Eq. (15.1).

$$SI_{Overall} = \frac{(W_{IR} \times SI_{IR} + W_{OC} \times SI_{OC} + W_{AM} \times SI_{AM} + W_{GS} \times SI_{GS})}{W_{IR} + W_{OC} + W_{AM} + W_{GS}} \tag{15.1}$$

All threshold values will be assumed to be positive so that the effect of conflicting severity index values may be handled. The overall SI value may be calculated from the component SI values using a weighted average rule. The weight values may be decided from the dominance of a particular symptom for COVID-19.

To declare the patient's condition, a threshold-based mechanism may be used, and the value of the threshold may be decided from experiment. Different regression techniques like logistic regression, robust regressions, or even nonlinear regression models like neural networks may also be used towards this end. Figure 15.4 presents a connected conceptual system that may be implemented on a suitable hardware platform.

15.4.5 Uses and Recommendations

One of the most important aspects regarding the containment of COVID-19 infection is a rapid screening of the disease, particularly in a country like India, where population density is a factor of concern. The proposed system will be ideal for places with compulsory footfall such as ATMs, airports, train/metro stations, smart gates, shopping malls, etc. The screening tunnel shall be ideal for entry to airports, railways, and shopping complexes where a huge volume of individuals can be screened. Rapid screening gates may be installed in places to avoid possible contact. The screening kiosks will be suitable for conducting elaborate and comparatively more accurate automated tests. Such installations will be useful to screen an

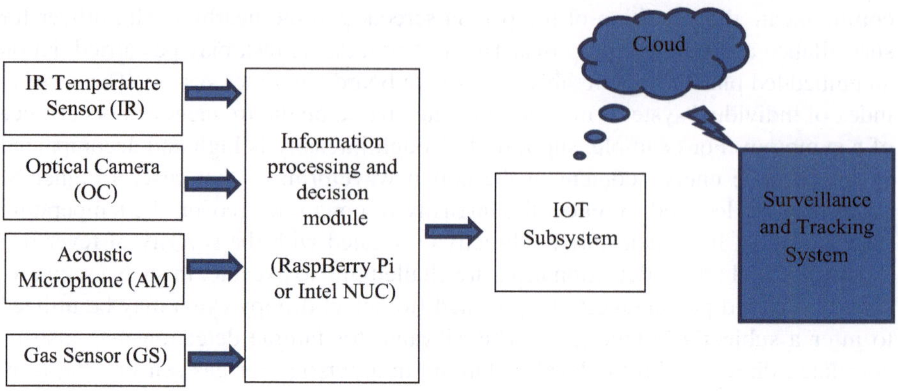

Fig. 15.4 Information processing and decision module

incoming patient at the hospital entry gate. The form factor of such devices can be varied to satisfy a variety of localized screening requirements. This will be a portable and a cloud-connected instrument that will screen and transmit the patient's condition to the nearby health centre. The individual's location history may be then tracked to identify possible contacts and suggest appropriate directives for adopting necessary precautions to ensure required isolation protocols and social distancing. The wearable sensing system shall be more appropriate for conducting quiet surveillance and identification of mobile subjects. The system may be mounted on a helmet connected with internet and working under the supervision of the person wearing the device. This system may be utilized in any location and thus should provide rapid indications of the disease.

With the advent of good quality sensors at a reasonable cost and easy availability of efficient computing platforms, the concepts discussed may be effectively implemented. The effective use of easily available machine learning techniques shall bolster the sensitivity and specificity of detection. However, research is needed to improve novel sensing methodologies, using gas sensors and fatigue detection from ocular features. The novel concepts discussed in this chapter are expected to improve the penetration of automation technologies powered by sensors and artificial intelligence (AI) for rapid detection of possible COVID-19-infected individuals and help contain the disease.

15.5 Conclusion

The present chapter proposes a multimodal system for capturing signals that would help identify potential COVID-19 carriers in densely populated areas when combined. The system would aim to be suitable for real-time detection of potential carriers and is likely to be a significant addition to the research for identification of carriers, which would go a long way in stalling the spread of COVID-19.

References

1. M. Cascella, M. Rajnik, A. Cuomo, S.C. Dulebohn, R. Di Napoli, Features, evaluation and treatment coronavirus (covid-19), in *Statpearls [internet]*, (StatPearls Publishing, Treasure Island, FL, 2020)
2. B. Chen, S. Marvin, A. While, Containing covid-19 in china: AI and the robotic restructuring of future cities. Dialog. Hum. Geogr. **10**, 2043820620934267 (2020)
3. M.C. Read, Eid: High contagiousness and rapid spread of severe acute respiratory syndrome coronavirus 2. Emerg. Infect. Dis. **26** (2020)
4. L. Garg, E. Chukwu, N. Nasser, C. Chakraborty, G. Garg, Anonymity preserving IoT-based covid-19 and other infectious disease contact tracing model. IEEE Access **8**, 159402–159414 (2020)
5. J.S. Hutchison, R.E. Ward, J. Lacroix, P.C. Hébert, M.A. Barnes, D.J. Bohn, P.B. Dirks, S. Doucette, D. Fergusson, R. Gottesman, et al., Hypothermia therapy after traumatic brain injury in children. N. Engl. J. Med. **358**(23), 2447–2456 (2008)
6. G.I. Gasim, I.R. Musa, M.T. Abdien, I. Adam, Accuracy of tympanic temperature measurement using an infrared tympanic membrane thermometer. BMC Res. Notes **6**(1), 194 (2013)
7. P. Händel, J. Wahlström, Digital contraceptives based on basal body temperature measurements. Biomed. Signal Process. Cont. **52**, 141–151 (2019)
8. H. Zeindler, Pacifier thermometer, US Patent 5,534,013, 9 Jul 1996
9. R. Pitman, B. Cooper, C. Trotter, N. Gay, W. Edmunds, Entry screening for severe acute respiratory syndrome (SARS) or influenza: Policy evaluation. BMJ **331**(7527), 1242–1243 (2005)
10. M.-F. Chiang, P.-W. Lin, L.-F. Lin, H.-Y. Chiou, C.-W. Chien, S.-F. Chu, W.-T. Chiu, Mass screening of suspected febrile patients with remote-sensing infrared thermography: Alarm temperature and optimal distance. J. Formos. Med. Assoc. **107**(12), 937–944 (2008)
11. J.B. Mercer, E.F.J. Ring, Fever screening and infrared thermal imaging: Concerns and guidelines. Thermol. Int. **19**(3), 67–69 (2009)
12. F. Ring, Pandemic: Thermography for fever screening of airport passengers. Thermol. Int. **17**(2), 67 (2007)
13. B.F. Jones, P. Plassmann, Digital infrared thermal imaging of human skin. IEEE Eng. Med. Biol. Mag. **21**(6), 41–48 (2002)
14. S. Budzan, R. Wyżgolik, Face and eyes localization algorithm in thermal images for temperature measurement of the inner canthus of the eyes. Infrared Phys. Technol. **60**, 225–234 (2013)
15. M.U. Selent, N.M. Molinari, A. Baxter, A.V. Nguyen, H. Siegelson, C.M. Brown, A. Plummer, A. Higgins, S. Podolsky, P. Spandorfer, et al., Mass screening for fever in children: A comparison of 3 infrared thermal detection systems. Pediatr. Emerg. Care **29**(3), 305–313 (2013)
16. E. Ring, A. Jung, B. Kalicki, J. Zuber, A. Rustecka, R. Vardasca, Infrared thermal imaging for fever detection in children, in *Medical Infrared Imaging Principles and Practices*, ed. by M. Diakides, J. B. Bronzino, D. R. Peterson, (CRC Press, Boca Raton, FL, 2013)
17. L. Jiang, A. Yeo, J. Nursalim, S. Wu, X. Jiang, Z. Lu, Frontal infrared human face detection by distance from centroid method, in *Proceedings of 2004 International Symposium on Intelligent Multimedia, Video and Speech Processing*, (IEEE, New York, 2004), pp. 41–44
18. M. Mohammed, H. Syamsudin, S. Al-Zubaidi, R.R. AKS, E. Yusuf, Novel COVID-19 detection and diagnosis system using IoT based smart helmet. Int. J. Psychosoc. Rehabilit. **24**(7) (2020)

19. A. Somboonkaew, P. Prempree, S. Vuttivong, J. Wetcharungsri, S. Porntheeraphat, S. Chanhorm, P. Pongsoon, R. Amarit, Y. Intaravanne, K. Chaitavon, et al., Mobile-platform for automatic fever screening system based on infrared forehead temperature, in *2017 OptoElectronics and Communications Conference (OECC) and Photonics Global Conference (PGC)*, (IEEE, New York, 2017), pp. 1–4
20. M.-H. Yang, D.J. Kriegman, N. Ahuja, Detecting faces in images: A survey. IEEE Trans. Pattern Anal. Mach. Intell. **24**(1), 34–58 (2002)
21. G. Yang, T.S. Huang, Human face detection in a complex background. Pattern Recogn. **27**(1), 53–63 (1994)
22. T.K. Leung, M.C. Burl, P. Perona, Finding faces in cluttered scenes using random labeled graph matching, in *Proceedings of IEEE International Conference on Computer Vision*, (IEEE, New York, 1995), pp. 637–644
23. K.C. Yow, R. Cipolla, Feature-based human face detection. Image Vis. Comput. **15**(9), 713–735 (1997)
24. Y. Dai, Y. Nakano, Face-texture model based on SGLD and its application in face detection in a color scene. Pattern Recogn. **29**(6), 1007–1017 (1996)
25. J. Yang, A. Waibel, A real-time face tracker, in *Proceedings Third IEEE Workshop on Applications of Computer Vision. WACV'96*, (IEEE, New York, 1996), pp. 142–147
26. S.J. McKenna, S. Gong, Y. Raja, Modelling facial colour and identity with Gaussian mixtures. Pattern Recogn. **31**(12), 1883–1892 (1998)
27. I. Craw, D. Tock, A. Bennett, Finding face features, in *European Conference on Computer Vision*, (Springer, New York, 1992), pp. 92–96
28. C. Lanitis, J. Taylor, T.F. Cootes, Automatic face identification system using flexible appearance models. Image Vis. Comput. **13**(5), 393–401 (1995)
29. M. Turk, A. Pentland, Eigenfaces for recognition. J. Cogn. Neurosci. **3**(1), 71–86 (1991)
30. K.-K. Sung, T. Poggio, Example-based learning for view-based human face detection. IEEE Trans. Pattern Anal. Mach. Intell. **20**(1), 39–51 (1998)
31. H.A. Rowley, S. Baluja, T. Kanade, Neural network-based face detection. IEEE Trans. Pattern Anal. Mach. Intell. **20**(1), 23–38 (1998)
32. E. Osuna, R. Freund, F. Girosit, Training support vector machines: An application to face detection, in *Proceedings of IEEE Computer Society Conference on Computer Vision and Pattern Recognition*, (IEEE, New York, 1997), pp. 130–136
33. H. Schneiderman, T. Kanade, Probabilistic modeling of local appearance and spatial relationships for object recognition, in *Proceedings. 1998 IEEE Computer Society Conference on Computer Vision and Pattern Recognition (Cat. No. 98CB36231)*, (IEEE, New York, 1998), pp. 45–51
34. H. Schneiderman, T. Kanade, A statistical method for 3d object detection applied to faces and cars, in *Proceedings IEEE Conference on Computer Vision and Pattern Recognition. CVPR 2000 (Cat. No. PR00662)*, vol. 1, (IEEE, New York, 2000), pp. 746–751
35. K. Rajagopalan, S. Kumar, J. Karlekar, R. Manivasakan, M.M. Patil, U.B. Desai, P. Poonacha, S. Chaudhuri, Finding faces in photographs, in *Sixth International Conference on Computer Vision (IEEE Cat. No. 98CH36271)*, (IEEE, New York, 1998), pp. 640–645
36. M.S. Lew, Information theoretic view-based and modular face detection, in *Proceedings of the Second International Conference on Automatic Face and Gesture Recognition*, (IEEE, New York, 1996), pp. 198–203
37. P.N. Belhumeur, J.P. Hespanha, D.J. Kriegman, Eigenfaces vs. Fisherfaces: Recognition using class specific linear projection, in *European Conference on Computer Vision*, (Springer, New York, 1996), pp. 43–58
38. Y.-S. Ryu, S.-Y. Oh, Automatic extraction of eye and mouth fields from a face image using eigenfeatures and multilayer perceptrons. Pattern Recogn. **34**(12), 2459–2466 (2001)
39. D. Cristinacce, T.F. Cootes, Facial feature detection using AdaBoost with shape constraints, in *Proc. British Machine Vision Conf.*, (2003), pp. 1–10
40. L. Wiskott, N. Krüger, N. Kuiger, C. Von Der Malsburg, Face recognition by elastic bunch graph matching. IEEE Trans. Pattern Anal. Mach. Intell. **19**(7), 775–779 (1997)

41. R.S. Feris, J. Gemmell, K. Toyama, V. Kruger, Hierarchical wavelet networks for facial feature localization, in *Proceedings of Fifth IEEE International Conference on Automatic Face Gesture Recognition*, (IEEE, New York, 2002), pp. 125–130
42. T.F. Cootes, G.J. Edwards, C.J. Taylor, Active appearance models, in *European Conference on Computer Vision*, (Springer, New York, 1998), pp. 484–498
43. J. Xiao, S. Baker, I. Matthews, T. Kanade, et al., Real-time combined 2d + 3d active appearance models. CVPR (2), 535–542 (2004)
44. L. Yuille, P.W. Hallinan, D.S. Cohen, Feature extraction from faces using deformable templates. Int. J. Comput. Vis. **8**(2), 99–111 (1992)
45. K.-M. Lam, H. Yan, Locating and extracting the eye in human face images. Pattern Recogn. **29**(5), 771–779 (1996)
46. G.C. Feng, P.C. Yuen, Multi-cues eye detection on gray intensity image. Pattern Recogn. **34**(5), 1033–1046 (2001)
47. J. Huang, H. Wechsler, Eye detection using optimal wavelet packets and radial basis functions (RBFS). Int. J. Pattern Recognit. Artif. Intell. **13**(07), 1009–1025 (1999)
48. M.H. Yang, N. Ahuja, Detecting human faces in color images, in *Proceedings of International Conference on Image Processing. ICIP98 (Cat. No. 98CB36269)*, vol. 1, (IEEE, New York, 1998), pp. 127–130
49. Y. Wang, B. Yuan, A novel approach for human face detection from color images under complex background. Pattern Recogn. **34**(10), 1983–1992 (2001)
50. X. You, D. Zhang, Q. Chen, P. Wang, Y.Y. Tang, Face representation by using non-tensor product wavelets, in *18th International Conference on Pattern Recognition (ICPR'06)*, vol. 1, (IEEE, New York, 2006), pp. 503–506
51. B. Heisele, P. Ho, T. Poggio, Face recognition with support vector machines: Global versus component-based approach, in *Proceedings Eighth IEEE International Conference on Computer Vision. ICCV 2001*, vol. 2, (IEEE, New York, 2001), pp. 688–694
52. A. Nikolaidis, I. Pitas, Facial feature extraction and pose determination. Pattern Recogn. **33**(11), 1783–1791 (2000)
53. S. Tsekeridou, I. Pitas, Facial feature extraction in frontal views using biometric analogies, in *9th European Signal Processing Conference (EUSIPCO 1998)*, (IEEE, New York, 1998), pp. 1–4
54. L. Rujie, Y. Baozong, Automatic eye feature extraction in human face images. Comput. Informatics **20**(3), 289–301 (2012)
55. R.-L. Hsu, A.K. Jain, Face modeling for recognition, in *Proceedings 2001 International Conference on Image Processing (Cat. No. 01CH37205)*, vol. 2, (IEEE, New York, 2001), pp. 693–696
56. R. Herpers, G. Sommer, An attentive processing strategy for the analysis of facial features, in *Face Recognition*, (Springer, New York, 1998), pp. 457–468
57. F. Smeraldi, J. Bigun, Retinal vision applied to facial features detection and face authentication. Pattern Recogn. Lett. **23**(4), 463–475 (2002)
58. M. Hamouz, J. Kittler, J.-K. Kamarainen, H. Kälviäinen, Hypotheses-driven affine invariant localization of faces in verification systems, in *International Conference on Audio and Video-Based Biometric Person Authentication*, (Springer, New York, 2003), pp. 276–284
59. C.G. Harris, M. Stephens, et al., A combined corner and edge detector, in *Alvey Vision Conference*, vol. 15(50), (Citeseer, Manchester, UK, 1988), pp. 10–5244
60. Y. Ren, S. Wang, B. Hou, J. Ma, A novel eye localization method with rotation invariance. IEEE Trans. Image Process. **23**(1), 226–239 (2013)
61. A.I. Gaidar, P. Yakimov, Real-time fatigue features detection. J. Phys. Conf. Ser. **1368**(5), 052017 (2019)
62. W. Xiao-yu, C. Nai-meng, Y. Wan-jun, W. Zi-chen, Z. Huai-lin, L. Jia-lan, Driver's EEG eye movement fatigue detection based on CMAC, in *2019 International Conference on Intelligent Informatics and Biomedical Sciences (ICIIBMS)*, (IEEE, New York, 2019), pp. 57–63

63. X. Hu, G. Lodewijks, Detecting fatigue in car drivers and aircraft pilots by using noninvasive measures: The value of differentiation of sleepiness and mental fatigue. J. Saf. Res. **72**, 173–187 (2020)
64. R.A. McKinley, L.K. McIntire, R. Schmidt, D.W. Repperger, J.A. Caldwell, Evaluation of eye metrics as a detector of fatigue. Hum. Factors **53**(4), 403–414 (2011)
65. R. Galindo, W.G. Aguilar, R.P.R. Ch, Landmark based eye ratio estimation for driver fatigue detection, in *International Conference on Intelligent Robotics and Applications*, (Springer, New York, 2019), pp. 565–576
66. M. Eriksson, N.P. Papanikotopoulos, Eye-tracking for detection of driver fatigue, in *Proceedings of Conference on Intelligent Transportation Systems*, (IEEE, New York, 1997), pp. 314–319
67. D. Tock, I. Craw, Tracking and measuring drivers' eyes. Image Vis. Comput. **14**(8), 541–547 (1996)
68. W.-B. Horng, C.-Y. Chen, Y. Chang, C.-H. Fan, Driver fatigue detection based on eye tracking and dynamic template matching, in *IEEE International Conference on Networking, Sensing and Control, 2004*, vol. 1, (IEEE, New York, 2004), pp. 7–12
69. J.-J. Yan, H.-H. Kuo, Y.-F. Lin, T.-L. Liao, Real-time driver drowsiness detection system based on PERCLOS and grayscale image processing, in *2016 International Symposium on Computer, Consumer and Control (IS3C)*, (IEEE, New York, 2016), pp. 243–246
70. L.M. Bergasa, J. Nuevo, M.A. Sotelo, R. Barea, M.E. Lopez, Real-time system for monitoring driver vigilance. IEEE Trans. Intell. Transp. Syst. **7**(1), 63–77 (2006)
71. M.L. Jackson, S. Raj, R.J. Croft, A.C. Hayley, L.A. Downey, G.A. Kennedy, M.E. Howard, Slow eyelid closure as a measure of driver drowsiness and its relationship to performance. Traffic Inj. Prev. **17**(3), 251–257 (2016)
72. M.L. Jackson, G.A. Kennedy, C. Clarke, M. Gullo, P. Swann, L.A. Downey, A.C. Hayley, R.J. Pierce, M.E. Howard, The utility of automated measures of ocular metrics for detecting driver drowsiness during extended wakefulness. Accid. Anal. Prev. **87**, 127–133 (2016)
73. F. Friedrichs, B. Yang, Camera-based drowsiness reference for driver state classification under real driving conditions, in *2010 IEEE Intelligent Vehicles Symposium*, (IEEE, New York, 2010), pp. 101–106
74. J. Batista, A drowsiness and point of attention monitoring system for driver vigilance, in *2007 IEEE Intelligent Transportation Systems Conference*, (IEEE, New York, 2007), pp. 702–708
75. P. Smith, M. Shah, N. da Vitoria Lobo, Determining driver visual attention with one camera. IEEE Trans. Intell. Transp. Syst. **4**(4), 205–218 (2003)
76. P. Smith, M. Shah, N. da Vitoria Lobo, Monitoring head/eye motion for driver alertness with one camera, in *Proceedings 15th International Conference on Pattern Recognition. ICPR-2000*, vol. 4, (IEEE, New York, 2000), pp. 636–642
77. Q. Ji, X. Yang, Real-time eye, gaze, and face pose tracking for monitoring driver vigilance. Real-Time Imag. **8**(5), 357–377 (2002)
78. U. Svensson, *Blink Behaviour Based Drowsiness Detection: Method Development and Validation* (Statens väg- och transportforskningsinstitut, Linköping, Sweden, 2004)
79. B. Thorslund, *Electrooculogram Analysis and Development of a System for Defining Stages of Drowsiness* (Statens väg- och transportforskningsinstitut, Linköping, Sweden, 2004)
80. R. Grace, S. Steward, *Drowsy Driver Monitor and Warning System* (University of Iowa, Iowa, 2001)
81. L. McIntire, R.A. McKinley, J. McIntire, C. Goodyear, J. Nelson, Eye metrics: An alternative vigilance detector for military operators. Mil. Psychol. **25**(5), 502–513 (2013)
82. R. Jorge, Effects of the transcutaneous synchronous diaphragmatic pacing in moderate and severe chronic obstructive pulmonary disease (COPD) [Thesis], Pontificia Universidade Católica do Paraná, Curitiba, 2009
83. J. Martinek, M. Tatar, M. Javorka, Distinction between voluntary cough sound and speech in volunteers by spectral and complexity analysis. J. Physiol. Pharmacol. **59**(6), 433–440 (2008)

84. B.H. Tracey, G. Comina, S. Larson, M. Bravard, J.W. López, R.H. Gilman, Cough detection algorithm for monitoring patient recovery from pulmonary tuberculosis, in *2011 Annual International Conference of the IEEE Engineering in Medicine and Biology Society*, (IEEE, New York, 2011), pp. 6017–6020
85. S.J. Barry, A.D. Dane, A.H. Morice, A.D. Walmsley, The automatic recognition and counting of cough. Cough **2**(1), 1–9 (2006)
86. V. Swarnkar, U.R. Abeyratne, Y. Amrulloh, C. Hukins, R. Triasih, A. Setyati, Neural network based algorithm for automatic identification of cough sounds, in *2013 35th Annual International Conference of the IEEE Engineering in Medicine and Biology Society (EMBC)*, (IEEE, New York, 2013), pp. 1764–1767
87. S. Matos, S.S. Birring, I.D. Pavord, H. Evans, Detection of cough signals in continuous audio recordings using hidden Markov models. IEEE Trans. Biomed. Eng. **53**(6), 1078–1083 (2006)
88. S. Birring, T. Fleming, S. Matos, A. Raj, D. Evans, I. Pavord, The Leicester cough monitor: Preliminary validation of an automated cough detection system in chronic cough. Eur. Respir. J. **31**(5), 1013–1018 (2008)
89. A. Barton, P. Gaydecki, K. Holt, J.A. Smith, Data reduction for cough studies using distribution of audio frequency content. Cough **8**(1), 12 (2012)
90. A.J. Barton, *Signal Processing Techniques for Data Reduction and Event Recognition in Cough Counting* (The University of Manchester, UK, 2013)
91. Y.A. Amrulloh, U.R. Abeyratne, V. Swarnkar, R. Triasih, A. Setyati, Automatic cough segmentation from non-contact sound recordings in pediatric wards. Biomed. Signal Process. Control **21**, 126–136 (2015)
92. J. Monge-Álvarez, C. Hoyos-Barceló, P. Lesso, P. Casaseca-de-la Higuera, Robust detection of audio-cough events using local HU moments. IEEE J. Biomed. Health Inform. **23**(1), 184–196 (2018)
93. J. Monge-Álvarez, C. Hoyos-Barceló, P. Lesso, J. Escudero, K. Dahal, P. Casaseca-de-la Higuera, Effect of importance sampling on robust segmentation of audio-cough events in noisy environments, in *2016 38th Annual International Conference of the IEEE Engineering in Medicine and Biology Society (EMBC)*, (IEEE, New York, 2016), pp. 3740–3744
94. Y. Sun, G. Wen, J. Wang, Weighted spectral features based on local HU moments for speech emotion recognition. Biomed. Signal Process. control **18**, 80–90 (2015)
95. M. You, Z. Liu, C. Chen, J. Liu, X.-H. Xu, Z.-M. Qiu, Cough detection by ensembling multiple frequency subband features. Biomed. Signal Process. Control **33**, 132–140 (2017)
96. J. Amoh, K. Odame, Deep neural networks for identifying cough sounds. IEEE Trans. Biomed. Circuits Syst. **10**(5), 1003–1011 (2016)
97. J.-M. Liu, M. You, G.-Z. Li, Z. Wang, X. Xu, Z. Qiu, W. Xie, C. An, S. Chen, Cough signal recognition with Gammatone cepstral coefficients, in *2013 IEEE China Summit and International Conference on Signal and Information Processing*, (IEEE, New York, 2013), pp. 160–164
98. E.C. Larson, T. Lee, S. Liu, M. Rosenfeld, S.N. Patel, Accurate and privacy preserving cough sensing using a low-cost microphone, in *Proceedings of the 13th International Conference on Ubiquitous Computing*, (2011), pp. 375–384
99. C. John, Practical cough detection in presence of background noise and preliminary differential diagnosis from cough sound using artificial intelligence, a thesis submitted to the graduate faculty in partial fulfillment of the requirements for the Degree of Master of Science in Electrical and Computer Engineering, Norman, Oklahoma, 2020
100. K. Zhao, G. Gu, Y. Zhang, B. Zhang, F. Yang, L. Zhao, M. Zheng, G. Cheng, Z. Du, The self-powered CO_2 gas sensor based on gas discharge induced by triboelectric nanogenerator. Nano Energy **53**, 898–905 (2018)
101. S. Cui, Y. Zheng, T. Zhang, D. Wang, F. Zhou, W. Liu, Self-powered ammonia nanosensor based on the integration of the gas sensor and triboelectric nanogenerator. Nano Energy **49**, 31–39 (2018)

102. Y. Su, G. Xie, H. Tai, S. Li, B. Yang, S. Wang, Q. Zhang, H. Du, H. Zhang, X. Du, et al., Self-powered room temperature NO_2 detection driven by triboelectric nanogenerator under UV illumination. Nano Energy **47**, 316–324 (2018)
103. I. Uddin, G.-S. Chung, A self-powered active hydrogen gas sensor with fast response at room temperature based on triboelectric effect. Sensors Actuators B Chem. **231**, 601–608 (2016)
104. S. Wang, G. Xie, H. Tai, Y. Su, B. Yang, Q. Zhang, X. Du, Y. Jiang, Ultrasensitive flexible self-powered ammonia sensor based on triboelectric nanogenerator at room temperature. Nano Energy **51**, 231–240 (2018)
105. Z. Wen, J. Chen, M.-H. Yeh, H. Guo, Z. Li, X. Fan, T. Zhang, L. Zhu, Z.L. Wang, Blow-driven triboelectric nanogenerator as an active alcohol breath analyzer. Nano Energy **16**, 38–46 (2015)
106. H. Zhang, Y. Yang, Y. Su, J. Chen, C. Hu, Z. Wu, Y. Liu, C.P. Wong, Y. Bando, Z.L. Wang, Triboelectric nanogenerator as self-powered active sensors for detecting liquid/gaseous water/ethanol. Nano Energy **2**(5), 693–701 (2013)
107. Y. Wang, R. Wang, S. Wan, Q. Wang, M.J. Kim, D. Ding, W. Wu, Scalable nanomanufacturing and assembly of chiral-chain piezoelectric tellurium nanowires for wearable self-powered cardiovascular monitoring. Nano Futures **3**(1), 011001 (2019)
108. W. Zhang, L. Zhang, H. Gao, W. Yang, S. Wang, L. Xing, X. Xue, Self-powered implantable skin-like glucometer for real-time detection of blood glucose level in vivo. Nano-Micro Lett. **10**(2), 32 (2018)

Chapter 16
Explainable Deep Learning for Covid-19 Detection Using Chest X-ray and CT-Scan Images

Sidi Ahmed Mahmoudi, Sédrick Stassin, Mostafa El Habib Daho, Xavier Lessage, and Saïd Mahmoudi

16.1 Introduction

The advances in AI have got a significant influence in our daily lives within several domains such as computer vision [1, 2], features extraction [3], medical imaging [4, 5], medicine, robotics, etc. If we follow the history of Artificial Intelligence, we can distinguish two forms of AI: symbolic programming and machine learning. The symbolic approach allows to represent the human knowledge in a declarative and sequential form using facts, rules, and conditions (such as if-so rule) allowing to illustrate all situations. The Machine Learning (ML) approach consists of developing models that are able to mime and learn information from data and examples in order to offer a generalized solution for unknown examples. In this context, DL presents one of the main branches of ML, which proposes deep neural networks, composed of multiple layers, allowing to transform input data into a model. In computer vision and medical imaging domains, the first layer (input data) is presented by a grid (2D or 3D) of pixels. The intermediate layers allow to extract features (corners, edges, faces, etc.) in order to classify images, localize objects, or segment images. We note that CNNs (convolutional neural networks) [6] are particularly used in the above-mentioned domains (computer vision and medical imaging), where the features are computed after applying several convolutions. The success of DL is mainly due to the advances of the domains of high-performance computing (HPC) [7, 8] and the high availability of massive volumes of data

S. A. Mahmoudi (✉) · S. Stassin · X. Lessage · S. Mahmoudi
University of Mons, Mons, Belgium
e-mail: sidi.mahmoudi@umons.ac.be; said.mahmoudi@umons.ac.be

M. E. H. Daho
University of Tlemcen, Chetouane, Algeria
e-mail: mostafa.elhabibdaho@univ-tlemcen.dz

L. Garg et al. (eds.), *Healthcare Informatics for Fighting COVID-19 and Future Epidemics*, EAI/Springer Innovations in Communication and Computing,
https://doi.org/10.1007/978-3-030-72752-9_16

(Big Data) [9]. This allowed to execute deep neural networks that are composed of tens or even hundreds of layers with a huge number of connections between neurons, increasing the number of adjustable parameters to hundreds of millions. In terms of precision and accuracy, these networks solved and even outperformed human in several tasks such as video games, images classification and retrieval, car driving, etc. However, these AI and DL algorithms are considered as black boxes since they cannot be easily explainable and interpretable. In fact, the neural network solution leads us to ask questions about the features and rules that were taken into acount to achieve this result. This is commonly called the black-box problem of neural networks. Even if we create a network using training, validation, and test datasets, we have no idea what the network detects exactly, and what makes it ultimately choose. So, do we trust the DL model decisions? In this context, model interpretation allows to understand and explain these decisions by the response function, i.e., what, why, and how? In this book chapter, we propose an approach for explaining DL algorithms when applied to images classification and segmentation such as required in the problem of Covid-19 detection using medical images. Our approach allows to provide the most appropriate explanation method (perturbation-based approach, gradient-based approach, relevance-based approach, and proxy models) and the most accurate and explainable DL model by following three main steps: (1) analysis and comparison between XAI visualization methods for the predicted class only; (2) comparison and analysis of XAI visualization methods between all the existing classes; (3) non-visual evaluation of XAI methods according to noise injection. As a use case, we applied our explanation approach for Covid-19 image classification and segmentation using two modalities: X-ray and CT-scan images. Experimental results showed the interest of our explanation approach within three facts: (1) identification of the most interpretable DL model; (2) measurement of positive and negative contributions of input parameters (image pixels) in the decision of DL models; and (3) detection of data (training and validation datasets) biases, where the deep neural networks are focusing on less important regions.

The remainder of the book chapter is structured as follows: Sect. 16.2 outlines the related works in the domain of explainable Deep Learning and more particularly those applied for image classification and Covid-19 detection and segmentation. In Sect. 16.3, we describe our DL approach for Covid-19 detection and segmentation using X-ray and CT-scan images. The fourth section is devoted to present our DL explanation approach, while Sect. 16.5 presents experimental results. Conclusions and perspectives are discussed in Sect. 16.6.

16.2 Related Work

In the literature, two types of related works can be identified when treating the problem of explaining image classification DL models that are used for Covid-

19 detection: Deep Learning explanation approaches and Covid-19 Deep Learning detection models.

16.2.1 Deep Learning Explanation Approaches

The explanation of DNNs (deep neural networks) is necessary to solve the black-box problem, and it is also necessary to have a complete and correct explanation.

Gilpin et al. [10] presented two possible ways to evaluate an explanation: interpretability and completeness, where interpretability is defined by "the ability to explain in comprehensive terms to a human" [11]. On the other hand, the completeness allows to present, accurately, the working mechanism of a system. The most complete explanation of a DNN can always be the description of its mathematical functioning, which is not easily interpretable, and will not be a good explanation for everyone. On the contrary, the easiest explanation will never be complete.

In the literature, one can find several methods, published recently, that trend to explain deep neural networks. Our research is focused on DNN classification models in order to provide an adapted explanation for our use case problem: Covid-19 detection and classification using X-ray and CT-scan images. The main related works in this area are focusing on explaining CNNs only since they are mainly used for computer vision and medical imaging applications. We can categorize four main explanation approaches: perturbation-based methods, gradient-based methods, relevance-based methods, and proxy models.

16.2.1.1 Perturbation-Based Methods

1. **Feature ablation:** involves the replacement of each feature (or a group of features) by a baseline value in order to compute the output difference. A low difference means that the replaced features are less important and vice versa.
2. **Feature permutation:** Molnar [12] presented a similar approach to the ablation one, where features are switched between them within a batch. A feature is considered as important if the shuffling causes an increase of model error and vice versa.
3. **Occlusion:** is mainly used in image classification and developed by Zeiler and Fergus [13], which is proposed to replace a square of input pixels by a grey square. The occluded pixels are important if the class probability drops significantly. This method can be seen as an application of feature ablation to image classification.

The drawback of the perturbation-based approaches is present in the highly intensive computation since the output needs to be recomputed after each new applied perturbation. The computation gets more intensive as the input image gets larger.

16.2.1.2 Gradient-Based Methods

1. **Deconvolutional networks:** Zeiler and Fergus [13] proposed an approach using a deconvolutional network to visualize the most discriminating parts of an image. The deconvolutional layer is created for each convolutional layer, providing a path back. This approach is based on the following five steps (Fig. 16.1):
   - An image is fed to the trained model.
   - The model computes the forward pass up to the last convolutional layer (or another chosen convolutional layer).
   - The strongest activation (or a selected activation) of this layer is left non-zero.
   - The reverse order of the operations carried out during the forward pass is executed by unpooling, rectifying, and filtering until the input of the model is reached.
   - A reconstructed image shows what strongly activates the input image with the current model.

   We note that the network extracts firstly basic features such as lines, circles, points of interest, edges, etc. Then, it extracts general shapes and ends with the recognition of objects to be classified.
2. **Gradient (or backpropagation):** Based on the deconvolutional method from Zeiler and Fergus [13], Simonyan et al. [15] proposed a new approach that can be described as follows:
   We consider I_0 as a given image, c as a class and $S_c(I)$ as a class score function

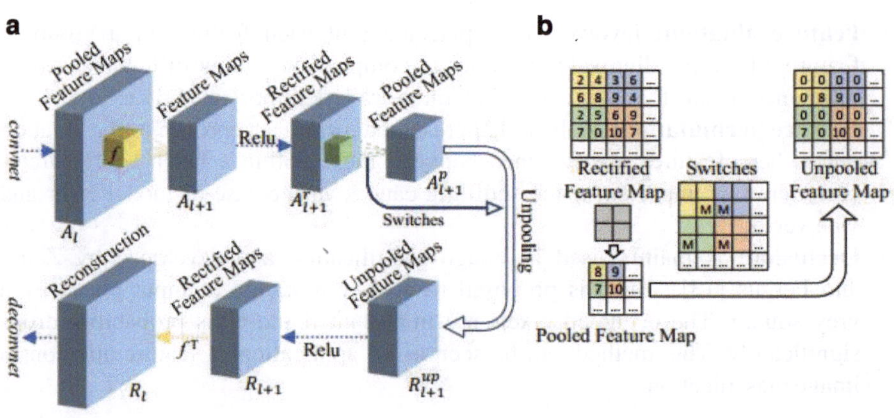

Fig. 16.1 (a) Top: classical operations in a convolutional network (filtering, rectifying, pooling); Bottom: associated deconvolutional operations (filtering, rectifying, unpooling). (b) Illustration of the unpooling operation [14]

for a classification problem to be solved with a convolutional network. The goal is to rank the pixels of I_0 upon their impact on $S_c(I)$. By using the derivative $\frac{\partial S_c}{\partial I}|_{I_0}$, the pixels' importance can be computed. This backpropagation is applicable to any layer (dense layers, for example), whereas the deconvolutional network is only applicable to convolutional layers.

3. **Guided Backpropagation:** is proposed by Springenberg et al. [16], which combines the convolution and backpropagation method with *rectifying* : if at least one of the entry values compared to the top gradient **or** bottom signal data is negative, it will be masked (row 4 of Fig. 16.2 compared to rows 2 and 3). This is the only significant difference from the previous methods. It is called *guided* because it has another guidance from the higher layers compared to classic backpropagation. It erases the backward flow of negative gradients, thus reducing the activation of the higher layer unit we want to visualize.
4. **Class Activation Mapping (CAM)** The authors in [17] proposed to highlight the most discriminative image regions for a chosen class. Based on the fact that convolutional layers retain spatial information and that higher-level

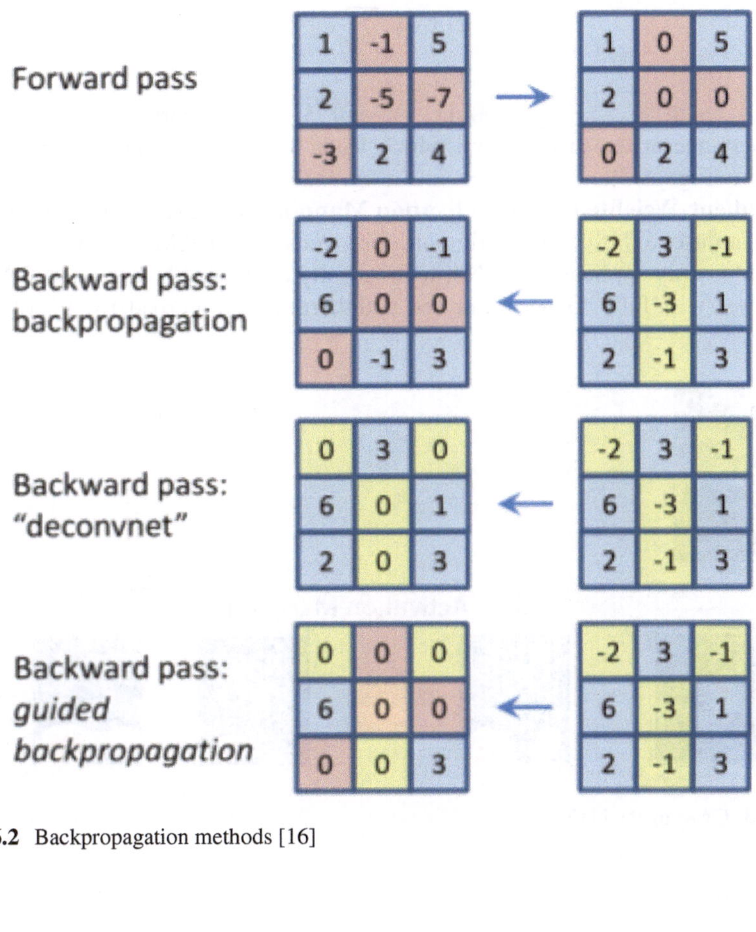

Fig. 16.2 Backpropagation methods [16]

visualizations are represented by the last convolutional layers of CNNs, the best choice for visualization is the last convolutional layer. The neural network includes a succession of convolutional layers, followed finally by a GAP (global average pooling), which will use the features extracted from the last convolutional layer for a fully connected layer, giving the probabilities by class.

For a selected image, we consider $f_k(x, y)$ as the activation unit k, at location (x, y) in the last convolutional layer. The global average pooling operation is represented by $F^k = \sum_{x,y} f_k(x, y)$. For a class c, the probability is calculated as $S_c = \sum_k w_k^c F_k$, where w_k^c is the weight corresponding to class c for unit k. By replacing F_k with S_c, we obtain

$$S_c = \sum_k w_k^c \sum_{x,y} f_k(x, y) = \sum_{x,y} \sum_k w_k^c f_k(x, y). \tag{16.1}$$

M_c represents the class activation map of the class c, as shown in the following equation.

$$M_c(x, y) = \sum_k w_k^c f_k(x, y). \tag{16.2}$$

As a result, $S_c = \sum_{x,y} M_c(x, y)$, and $M_c(x, y)$ represents the activation importance at the pixel (x, y), which leads to affect the class c for the input image (Fig. 16.3).

5. **Gradient-Weighted Class Activation Mapping (Grad-CAM)**: is proposed by Selvaraju et al.[18] representing an improvement of CAM method [17], where CAM is only applicable to CNN without fully connected layers. Grad-CAM can be used with fully connected layers, and therefore for a broader range of CNNs.

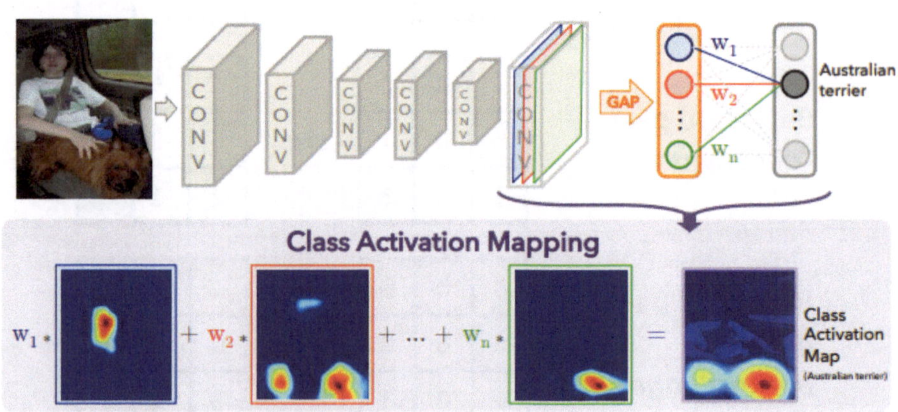

Fig. 16.3 CAM method [17]

Grad-CAM uses the gradient in order to calculate the importance of each feature map from this last convolutional layer for the predicted class.

Other explanation methods exist in the literature, which are also based on the gradient such as "Gradient*input" [19], "Integrated gradient" [20], "SmoothGrad" [21], and Guided Grad-CAM by Selvaraju et al. [18].

16.2.1.3 Relevance-Based Methods

1. **Layer-Wise Relevance Propagation (LRP)**: is a conservative backpropagation technique that uses several purposely designed rules, created by Bach et al. [22]. The conservative property is ensured in this way: the input values that are received by a neuron are redistributed equally to the lower layer, and this is true for any layer (Fig. 16.4). A neuron's weight from the final layer (a class probability for instance), backpropagated to the input layer, will have its weight summed by the neurons of any layer. Several approaches based on LRP are proposed such as LRP-Z (or LRP-0), LRP-ϵ, LRP-$\alpha\beta$, LRP-Flat, and LRP-Preset.
2. **Deep Taylor Decomposition**: it exploits the DNN structure by propagating the explanation from the output to the input layers using a predefined set of rules [24].

16.2.1.4 Proxy Models

Proxy models allow to reduce complexity of deep neural networks (such as ResNet, NasNetLarge, etc.) and other classifiers. A proxy model has a similar behavior to the initial model but is easier to explain.

1. **Linear model: LIME**: is proposed by Ribero et al. [25], which stands for *Local Interpretable Model-agnostic Explanations*. Local means that the provided explanation will be specific to an input image fed to the model, and will not probe the global model behavior. Interpretable specifies that a qualitative understanding between the input and the prediction is needed. This interpretation depends on

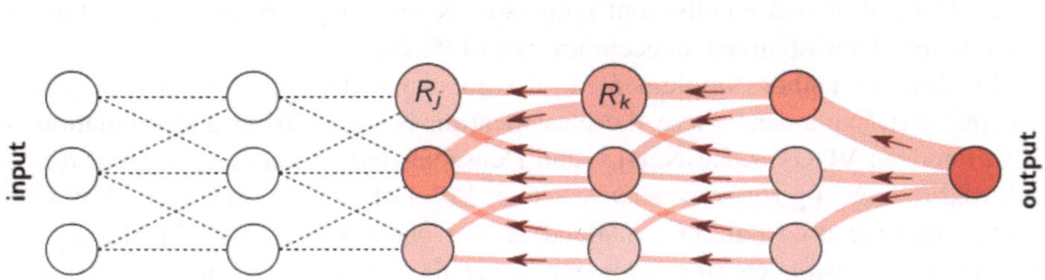

Fig. 16.4 LRP : each neuron redistributes the received values (from higher layer) to the lower one [23]

the audience and the user limitations and therefore should be easy to understand. Finally, model-agnostic relates to the applicability to any classifier that exists or even will be created in the future. Therefore, this technique does not rely on the inner principles of neural networks (layers, units).

2. **Decision Tree**: Decision trees allow to classify an instance, beginning at the root of the tree. On each node, a test is applied to design the convenient branch where a class is assigned by the leaf reached. In the 1990s, research work has been made to decompose shallow neural networks into decision trees, as they are much more interpretable. Now, with the arrival of deep neural networks, new techniques are needed to emerge to generalize to the hidden layers.
3. **DeepRED**: is proposed by [26], which uses a decision tree as a proxy model.

16.2.2 Covid-19 Deep Learning Models

Despite the recent appearance of Covid-19, several studies have been carried out to detect this disease from X-ray and CT-scan images of the chest. Different Deep Learning-based architectures are used for accurate disease detection [27–30]. Other researchers have been interested in proposing explainable architectures to convince doctors about the decision of their models. Among them, we find the work of [31] where the authors proposed a transfer learning approach using the CheXnet model [32]. The obtained DenseNet-121 model was developed and generated using a public database of 13,800 chest radiography images (13,725 patients). The authors proposed an explanation using the Grad-CAM [33] method in order to detect the most relevant areas. Their model achieved an average accuracy of 92.91% using patient-wise k-fold cross-validation. In [34], the authors fine-tuned the SqueezeNet architecture with Bayesian optimization and data augmentation. They generated visual explanations of their model decisions using class activation mapping. The proposed approach was trained and tested on 5949 posteroanterior chest radiography images (2839 patients), and the accuracy of the proposed model reached to 98.3%. In [35], the authors proposed a CNN architecture, called CovXNet, that used depth-wise convolution. In their experiments, the authors implemented different types of CovXNets using different definitions of X-ray images. The Grad-CAM method is used to distinguish inconsistent regions of X-ray images relative to the type of pneumonia. They obtained an accuracy rate of 90.2%.

In [36], the authors implemented an explainable deep neural network, called DeepCOVIDExplainer, where the classification is made using a combination of three models: VGG-19, ResNet-18, and DenseNet-161. Their experimental results allowed to have a positive predictive value (PPV) of 89.61% and a recall of 83%. Notice that the used dataset contained 16,995 chest X-rays. In [37], the authors proposed a transfer learning approach using the VGG-16 architecture, which is completed by the Grad-CAM explanation method. The obtained accuracy is around 98%.

16.3 Covid-19 Detection and Classification

This section is presented in two main parts: Covid-19 detection using X-ray images and Covid-19 detection using CT scans.

16.3.1 Covid-19 Detection Using X-ray Images

Before staring the process of model explanation, we start by their development within four steps: X-ray data collection, data augmentation, transfer learning, and model evaluation.

16.3.1.1 X-ray Data Collection

In this chapter, the used dataset was proposed by [38]. The images were collected from three different sources:

- SIRM Covid-19: images offered by the Italian Society of Medical and Interventional Radiology[39];
- Covid-19 dataset available on GitHub and developed by Cohen et al. [40];
- images obtained from 43 publications.

The final database contains images in PNG (Portable Network Graphics) file format with a size of 1024 × 1024 pixels. To complete the database with viral pneumonia and normal cases, the authors used the images available in the Chest X-ray (pneumonia) image database [41].

16.3.1.2 Data Augmentation

In order to increase our dataset and get a better accuracy, we used a common practice in deep learning, called "data augmentation." This practice has the effect of presenting information in different aspects of the image, which is favorable to the training of the parameters and avoids overfitting. Our augmentation strategy is purely geometric and is applied during training. For each input image, we applied a random combination of operations to provide the network with variations in the information present in the original images at each iteration. The operations used are rotation, zoom, horizontal flip, and rotation. The parameters are random and chosen according to a fixed interval. This process of data augmentation allowed to increase our database volume with a ratio of 30%.

16.3.1.3 Transfer Learning

In order to provide accurate results, we propose to exploit the technique of transfer learning using pre-trained classification models, where the weights are initialized with the ImageNet database.[1] This allows to benefit from previously acquired learning weights for solving another classification problem (Covid-19 images classification). The pre-trained CNN models are composed of multiple layers, which transform the input data (with labels) to a model. For image classification, the input layer is represented by a grid of pixels, while the intermediate analyzes images and pixels for detecting specific features (lines, circles, faces, edges, faces, etc.). The last layer is dedicated to detect the corresponding class. During the learning phase, the initialized weights are updated after each epoch (iteration) in order to classify Covid-19 images (3 classes) instead of ImageNet images (1000 classes). This process allows to accelerate the learning process and increases the accuracy since the models are pre-trained with a huge database. For our Covid-19 detection problem, we applied the transfer learning from CNN classification models: VGG-16, ResNet, Inception, Xception, and DenseNet.

1. **VGG**: is developed by Simonyan and Zisserman [42] and composed of 16 (for VGG-16) or 19 (for VGG-19) convolutional layers, and it contains only 3x3 convolutions, but a lot of filters. At the end of the network, we find two fully connected layers, each containing 4096 nodes, and a softmax function. VGG-16 is one of the most widely used models for the extraction of features from images.
2. **ResNet**: is introduced by Kaiming He et al. [43] and consists of several residual modules where each module represents a layer. It is a new architecture with skip connections applied to each layer of the network before the ReLu activation function, allowing to preserve the gradient. Using this technique, they have been able to form a neural network with 152 layers, but with lower complexity than VGGNet.
3. **Inception**: This architecture uses inception modules and aims to test all kind of convolution configuration to improve its performance by diversifying its attributes. It uses the 1×1 convolution to limit its computational complexity. The first version of Inception was GoogLeNet [44]. The following versions were all named Inception followed by the architecture release (Inception V2, Inception V3, etc.).
4. **Xception**: proposed by François Chollet [45], an extension of Inception's architecture that replaces Inception's standard modules with deeply separable convolutions.
5. **DenseNet**: The name DenseNet refers to Densely Connected Convolutional Networks. It was introduced in 2017 by Huang et al. [46]. Traditional CNNs have connections between each layer and the one that precedes and succeeds it.

[1] IMAGENET. http://www.image-net.org/.

In DenseNet, each layer receives as input all the output characteristics of the previous layers, and this is called a dense block.

16.3.1.4 Model Evaluation

Once the process of learning is completed, we can test the models with the test dataset that is not yet seen by the models. This allows to confirm the accuracy of our models and check the problems of overfitting.

16.3.2 Covid-19 Detection Using CT Scans

The use of CT scans allows to benefit from high-resolution and accurate sectional images or organs (lungs in this case). Within CT scans, doctors can better differentiate between the types of fluids and thus provide an easier diagnosis for Covid-19 detection. Moreover, physicians are also interested by the quantification of the size of Covid-19-related lesions, which is not possible with X-ray images. In this chapter, we employed the database proposed by Zhao et al. [47], which contains 349 CT-scan images from Covid-19, as well as 397 normal images. Actually, we are waiting a new and bigger CT-scan dataset from CHU Ambroise Paré in Mons Belgium.
The classification of Covid-19 using CT scans represents a problem so similar to the one seen in Sect. 16.3.1, where we need to classify images also and the only difference is present in the type of images (CT-scan instead of X-ray images). Thus, we applied the same classification Deep Learning architecture using CT scans.

16.4 Proposed Approach for Models Explanation

This section is devoted to present our approach of Deep Learning explanation based on the related works and our best knowledge. Our explanation approach is based on four steps: problem identification, dataset collection, selection of DL models, and explanation of DL models.

16.4.1 Problem Identification

The explanation approach is always related to the type of application or problem, which is represented by image classification in our case. Before starting the process of explanation, it is so important to take in hand and understand the problem and the required solution. Several questions could be considered: what do we want to solve and why? Is there an interest of explainability? In fact, these questions may be considered before going further. This question is treated in Sect. 16.3 for our Covid-19 detection problem.

16.4.2 Dataset Collection

The problem resolution is highly dependent on the available data that represent the most important element for solving a data science problem. The more you have, the less likely it is to have bias and overfitting problems. Finding sufficient amount of qualitative data representing different situations is always necessary. The visualization of data in various ways is also essential, to understand what is available and the results that will be obtained afterwards. This question is treated in Sects. 16.3.1.1 and 16.3.2 for our Covid-19 detection problem.

16.4.3 Selection of DL Models

The knowledge and identification of appropriate DL models are important before starting explanation. As specified above, our focus is to solve a classification problem related to Covid-19 detection using X-ray and CT-scan images. Thus, we have to identify the best models in terms of accuracy and loss values after dividing data into training, validation, and test sets. The general parameters will be defined, such as learning rate, loss, optimizer, etc., which will be so useful for the explanation. Notice the models architectures and parameters are described in Sects. 16.3.1.3 and 16.3.2.

16.4.4 Explanation of Deep Learning Models

Once the problem is identified and the dataset and DL models are selected, we can start the process of analyzing and explaining neural networks and thus confirm their accuracy. In fact, the use of Explainable Artificial Intelligence methods allows to ensure that the applied process is correct and close to the *Right to Explanation* requested. We propose an explanation based on the six steps: XAI framework's identification and analysis, XAI framework's comparison, XAI method selection, visual comparison of XAI methods against the predicted class, visual comparison of XAI methods against all classes, non-visual evaluation of XAI methods, and models and XAI method selection.

16.4.4.1 XAI Framework's Identification and Analysis

In the literature, one can find several frameworks that use XAI methods that mainly depend on the Deep Learning framework (TensorFlow, Caffe, PyTorch, etc.). In this context, the XAI frameworks of *tf-explain*, *iNNvestigate*, *Skater*,[2] *DeepExplain*,[3] and *Deep Visualization Toolbox*[4] are compatible with TensorFlow. On the other hand, *Captum* is compatible with PyTorch. Since we are working with TensorFlow for DL model development, we propose brief descriptions of tf-explain and iNNvestigate that are compatible with TensorFlow and the most performant in the domain.

1. **tf-explain [48]:** is a Python library well adapted to TensorFlow 2.x. The proposed XAI methods are defined as a class, containing two main functions:
   - *explain*: where we can provide the model, the selected XAI method (defined in Sect. 16.2.1), and its parameters;
   - *save*: allows to save the output of the *explain* function, as well as the path where to save the visualization of the explanation found.

2. **iNNvestigate [49]:** implements several methods of the state of the art with both versions of TensorFlow (1.x and 2.x). Their objective is to simplify the analysis of neural networks.

16.4.4.2 XAI Framework's Comparison and XAI Method Selection

The selected XAI frameworks (iNNvestigate and tf-explain) proposed several methods of explanation as shown in Table 16.1. Notice that the two XAI frameworks provide the implementation of three types of explanation methods: perturbation, gradient, and relevance methods. In order to produce a complete explanation of methods, we start by selecting the XAI methods that are provided by both the libraries: Vanilla Gradient, Gradient * Input, SmoothGrad, and Integrated Gradients. Thereafter, we will apply an analysis of the remaining methods in iNNversitgate framework and proxy models (LIME) provided from *Marco Tulio Correia Ribeiro*.[5] Notice that the last three methods in Table 16.1: PatternNet and PatternAttribution [50] and DeepLift [51], implemented by iNNvestigate, do not provide convenient results for image classification and thus are not selected for this chapter. After this selection, we apply a comparison between the XAI methods in order to identify the most appropriate methods for our classification problem.

[2]Skater. https://github.com/oracle/Skater.

[3]DeepExplain. https://github.com/marcoancona/DeepExplain.

[4]Deep visualization toolbox. https://github.com/yosinski/deep-visualization-toolbox.

[5]https://github.com/marcotcr/lime.

Table 16.1 List of explanation methods implemented by *tf-explain* and *iNNvestigate*

	tf-explain	iNNvestigate
Deconvolution		X
Activations visualization	X	
Vanilla gradient	X	X
Guided backpropagation		X
Grad*Input	X	X
SmoothGrad	X	X
Integrated gradients	X	X
LRP and rules		X
Grad-CAM	X	
Occlusion	X	
DeepTaylor		X
PatternNet		X
PatternAttribution		X
DeepLift		X

16.4.4.3 Visual Comparison of XAI Methods Against the Predicted Class

The results of explanation are dependent on the provided parameters. In this section, we propose to compare visually the results where the idea is to quantify the contribution of input image pixels to the results. First, from the input image, we apply explanation using the class predicted by our model, i.e., the one with the highest probability. We visualize and interpret the results for this class. This approach is useful if the model presents a high score of classification accuracy.

16.4.4.4 Visual Comparison of XAI Methods Against All Classes

In case where models can provide classification results with several candidate classes, it is important to analyze the results for the explanation of other classes, even if the probability is lower. Thus, for each existing class in the produced model, a comparison of the explanations is performed for several methods. This makes it possible to answer questions such as: "Why class A rather than class B?"

16.4.4.5 Non-visual Evaluation of XAI Methods

In the literature, the major methods of neural networks explanation provide a visual inspection of the result, which might not be sufficient in several situations mainly where the input images present high resolutions or where the target classes are present with very small sizes such as presented in a medical context. Therefore, we propose to offer a non-visual evaluation, inspired from the research of Samek et al. [52], which supposes that perturbing important regions will have the most impact on the classification score. Taking into account that the saliency maps produce a decreasing ranking of the pixels related to their importance for the class score, a deletion of the most important pixels is made per step. This process is called *most relevant first*, abbreviated as MoRF. After each information removal, the effect and classification scores are calculated. The evolution of the class score for different methods at each step (at each deleted pixel) is performed using this approach. This allows to evaluate the quality of the produced method.

16.4.4.6 Model and XAI Method Selection

The last step consists of comparing the DL classification models (related to our problem) taking into account both accuracy and explainability. The idea is to determine the best compromise between the most complete explanation and the accuracy. Based on this analysis, we can select the appropriate model and explanation method.

16.5 Experimental Results

Experimentations are presented within three subsections where the first one describes the related results (accuracy and loss) for both X-ray and CT-scan Covid-19 detection models. The second subsection is devoted to present the results of explaining the X-ray Covid-19 detection models, while the third subsection illustrates the results of explaining CT-scan Covid-19 detection models. Notice that the dataset is splitted as follows: 70% for training, 15% for validation, and 15% for test.

16.5.1 Covid-19 Classification Using X-ray Images

Table 16.2 presents the obtained values of loss and accuracy of our DL models (Sect. 16.3.1) for the detection of Covid-19 in X-ray images. As shown in the table, the models present a high accuracy ranging from 93% to more than 97%.

Table 16.2 Results of different models using X-ray images

Model	Acc.	Loss
VGG-16	0,9311	0,2239
VGG-19	0,9361	0,1649
InceptionResNetV2	0,9741	0,1873
Inception v3	0,9568	0,2137
Xception	0,9435	0,1369
DenseNet	0,9601	0,1388
ResNet50	0,9686	0,1435

16.5.2 *Covid-19 Classification Using CT Scans*

According to our model of Covid-19 detection using CT-scan images, the best result was obtained by applying a transfer learning from the VGG-16 architecture (where the weights are initiated using the ImageNet database). The obtained test accuracy is about 90% for classification, which can be considered as a good result in a medical context, but we need to validate this accuracy using our explanation approach (Sect. 16.4). In fact, the validation of these models needs a deep evaluation of several questions:

- Among the literature, which explanation methods can explain and interpret these models?
- How can we evaluate the accuracy of the selected explanation methods?
- Which models provide the best ratio accuracy/explainability?

These three questions are treated in the next two subsections.

16.5.3 *Explainable Covid-19 Classification Using X-ray*

The explanation of our X-ray Covid-19 classification models is applied with our approach proposed in Sect. 16.4. Several steps are followed:

16.5.3.1 Visual Comparison of XAI Methods Against the Predicted Class

The first results are carried out on the DenseNet-121 model using a Covid-19 image. With the deconvolution method (Fig. 16.5c), the result is too noisy to define areas of interest. The occlusion method (Fig. 16.5e) produces, in this case, inconsistent results with respect to the patch size parameter. Small variations in size produce large variations in results for any chosen size. The result obtained is therefore unreliable : https://www.youtube.com/watch?v=wzYAUFu0IYQ.

The gradient methods (Fig. 16.5f–i) give very similar results, which do not inform of the positive and negative contributions among the highlighted pixels. With the Guided Backpropagation (Fig. 16.5d), the interest is mainly focused on two areas: top left where we find letters ("upina") and top right. This letter detection is also observable for the Grad-CAM method (Fig. 16.5j), LIME (Fig. 16.5p), and DeepTaylor (Fig. 16.5o) where the explanation proves to be much more intense on these letters than in the rest of the image. It is also a part of the detection done for LRP-rules, especially via LRP-PresetAFlat (Fig. 16.5m), which only detects the letters in question. All this means that the main element contributing to the positive prediction of Covid-19 is the detection of the letters present in the top-left corner of the image.

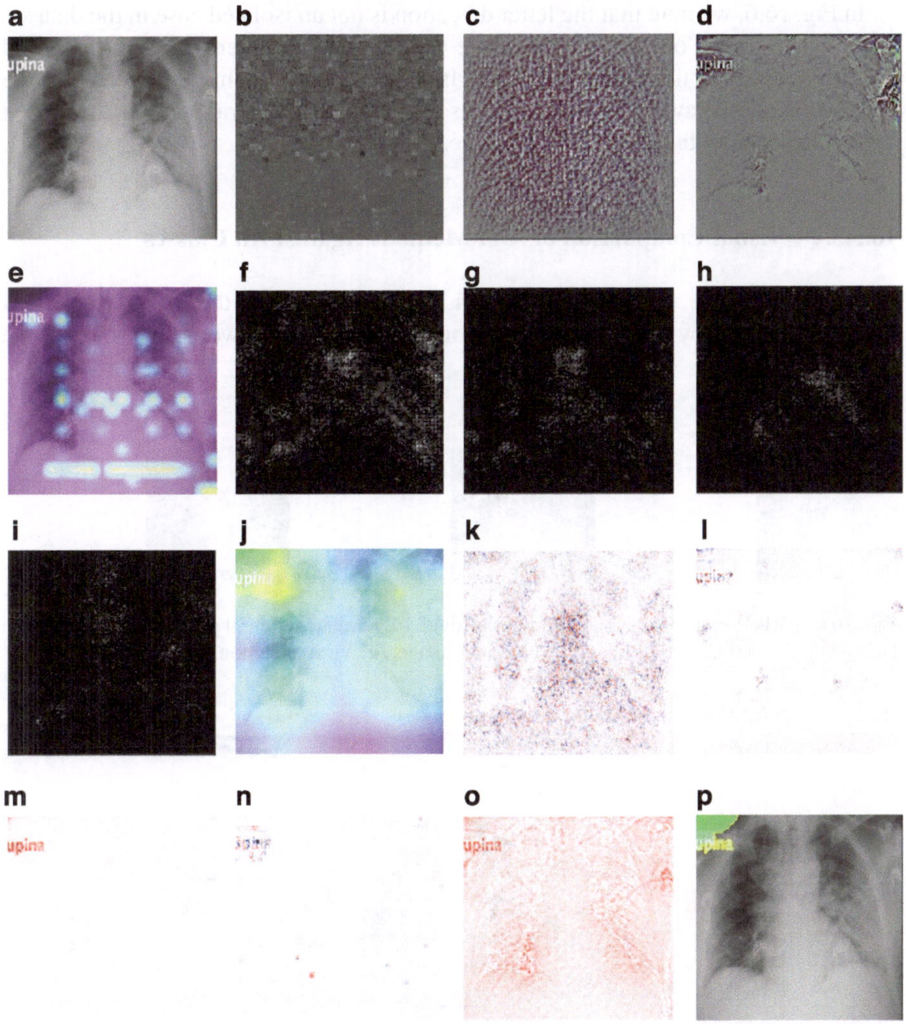

Fig. 16.5 DenseNet-121 explanation with each method for a Covid-19 image. (**a**) Input. (**b**) Visualization. (**c**) Deconvolution. (**d**) Guided. (**e**) Occlusion. (**f**) Gradient. (**g**) Grad*Input. (**h**) SmoothGrad. (**i**) Integrated. (**j**) Grad-CAM. (**k**) Z-rule. (**l**) ϵ-rule. (**m**) PresetAFlat. (**n**) PresetBFlat. (**o**) DeepTaylor. (**p**) LIME

In Fig. 16.6, we note that the letter detection is not an isolated case in the dataset. The model focuses on parts of the image where there are letters (L,R), or it should logically focus on the lungs to distinguish the class of an image. Therefore, the conclusion to be drawn is that the patterns detected by the neural network are biased by the presence of the letters in the image.

16.5.3.2 Visual Comparison of XAI Methods Against All Classes

In Fig. 16.7 (image without letters in this case), we observe that the normal class is explained only by negative contributions by LRP, and by weights too low to be

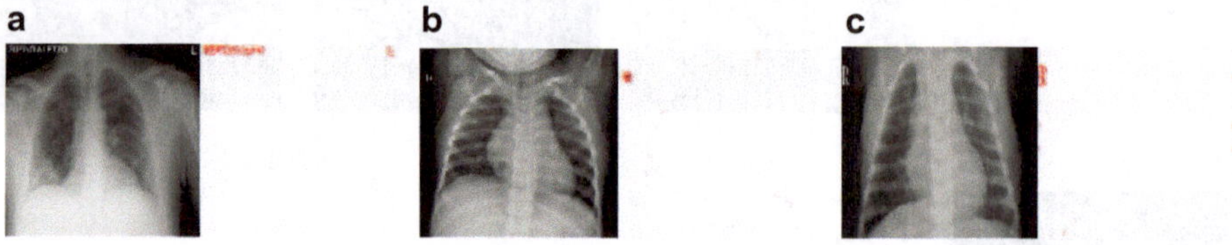

Fig. 16.6 LRP-PresetAFlat explanation for a Covid-19, normal, and viral pneumonia images with DenseNet-121. (**a**) Covid-19 image. (**b**) Normal image. (**c**) Viral pneumonia image

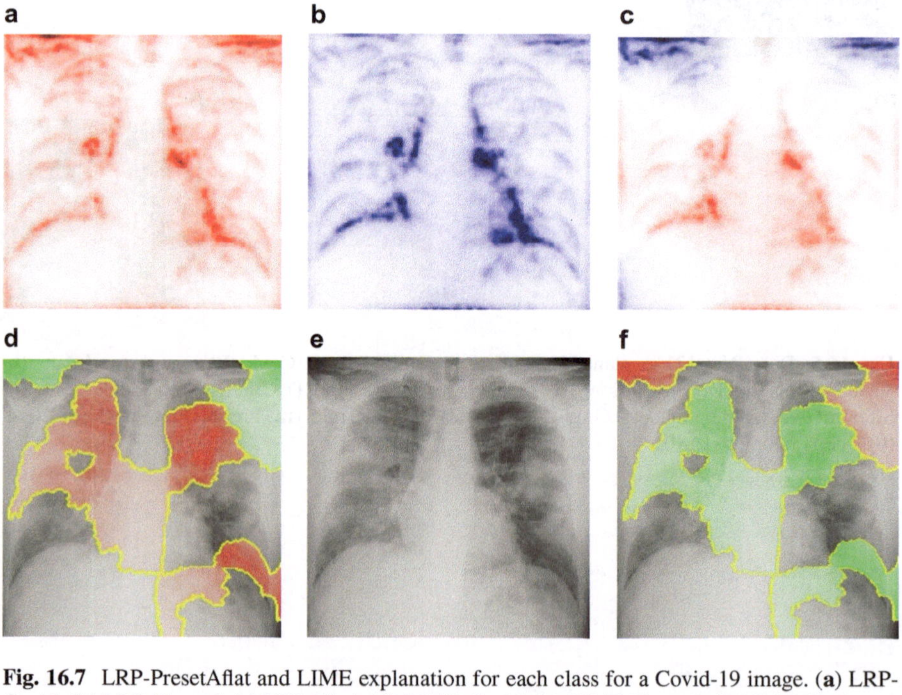

Fig. 16.7 LRP-PresetAflat and LIME explanation for each class for a Covid-19 image. (**a**) LRP-Covid. (**b**) LRP-Normal. (**c**) LRP-Viral. (**d**) LIME-Covid. (**e**) LIME-Normal. (**f**) LIME-Viral

represented by the threshold defined with LIME (0.003), which is in agreement with the associated probability of 0.01%. Then, whether LRP or LIME is used, the viral pneumonia class offers the same perspective, predicting elements negatively at the level of the shoulder blades, and positively inside the lungs for a final probability of 2.2%. For the class predicted (Covid-19) with 97.7%, the scapulae are a strong element of prediction whether it is with LIME where they are the main positive weights, or with LRP where it is a more intense part of the prediction. This should not be the case and is another possible bias in the model.

16.5.3.3 Non-visual Evaluation of XAI Methods

In Fig. 16.8, the value by which the pixels are replaced is black (the minimum value). LRP-rules, Guided Backpropagation, Input*Gradient, and Integrated Gradients get a high score. Notice that some methods not yet integrated in iNNvestigate are not tested, such as LIME and Grad-CAM that gave promising visual results, in line with the other methods (Fig. 16.9).

16.5.3.4 Model and XAI Method Selection

Following this detected bias, we applied our analysis on all available models in order to compare and confirm results. In this context, the VGG-16 model, while clearly using letters for detection, seems to use other information in the images as seen in Fig. 16.10. We note multiple red areas that are not related to the letters at all. These red areas are generally related to the lungs, suggesting a better model than conventionally expected. For the normal class, it is not only the letters that are considered. The attention is also focused on the top of the picture, at the head and shoulder level. By looking at the data (Fig. 16.11), two elements can be noticed : the

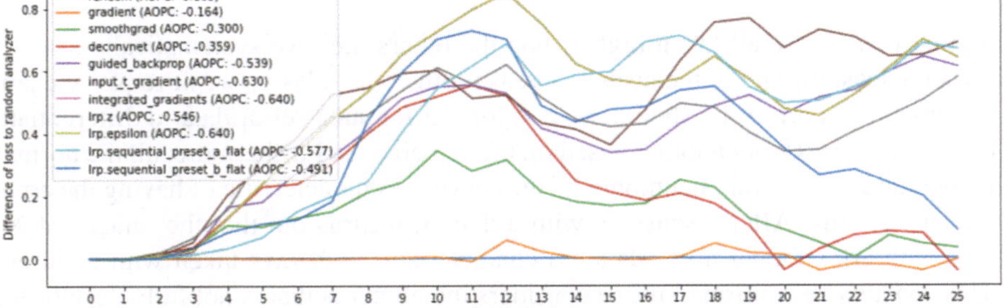

Fig. 16.8 The loss difference between different iNNvestigate methods compared to a random analyzer at each perturbation step, using the VGG-16 model applied to the Covid-19 dataset

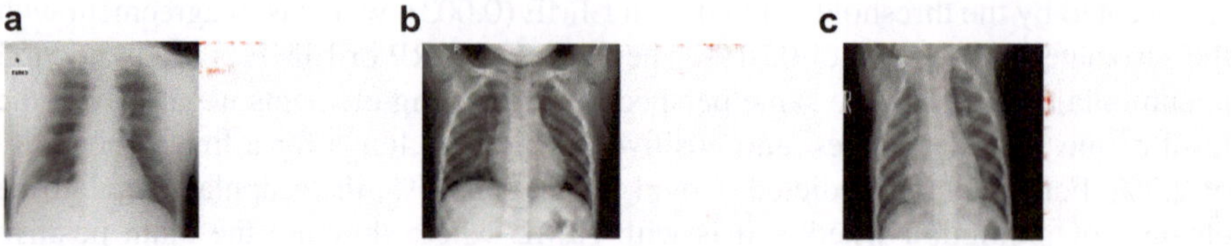

Fig. 16.9 LRP-PresetAFlat explanation for a Covid-19, normal, and viral pneumonia images with ResNet50. (**a**) Covid-19 image. (**b**) Normal image. (**c**) Viral pneumonia image

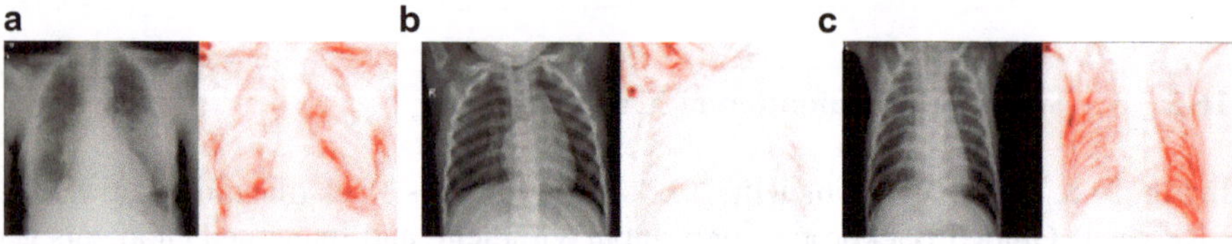

Fig. 16.10 LRP-PresetAFlat explanation for a Covid-19, normal, and viral pneumonia images with VGG-16. (**a**) Covid-19 image. (**b**) Normal image. (**c**) Viral pneumonia image

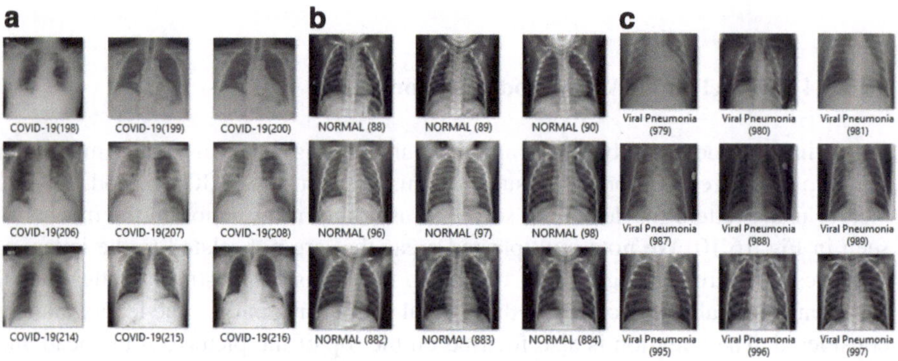

Fig. 16.11 Comparison between images from Covid-19, normal, and viral pneumonia classes. (**a**) Covid-19 images. (**b**) Normal images. (**c**) Viral pneumonia images

normal images are all taken higher than the others, i.e., we systematically see the jaw or at least the end of the neck, whereas for the other classes we never see the jaw or sometimes part of the shoulders. It is logical for such set of data to differentiate one normal class from another based on those elements. Furthermore, all the normal images and some viral pneumonia images have the characteristic of having the arms facing upwards. After discussion with a doctor, it turns out that the images of X-rays with arms facing upwards are a characteristic of X-rays taken with children. This can also be confirmed if one considers the humerus that is not fully developed.

16.5.3.5 Global Analysis

The methods of explicability have allowed to get an important observation: the identification of bias. Thanks to XAI, the defects of the dataset could be detected: for the normal class, arms mostly turned upwards, X-ray image taken higher than the other classes (showing the shoulder blades and the bottom of the head), and images only of children. Apart from that, for all classes, we find letters in the pictures for which the models give importance, when they should not. Therefore, we cannot rely on the models obtained. Among these, the explainability methods allowed to select the "best" model according to the plausibility of the explanations obtained (VGG-16 provides more plausible explanations, with interest not only in the letters but also in the lungs). Without the explicability methods, anyone would have stopped at the test score obtained by the model(s) and would have selected the highest precision, which proves that this is a very bad practice.

16.5.4 Explainable Covid-19 Classification Using CT-Scan Images

In this part, only the methods giving the most interesting results are presented. In case of Covid-19 detection using CT-scan images (Fig. 16.12), the Integrated Gradients method has a majority of pixels outside the lungs, which is supposed to be the area of interest. In addition to this, LRP-PresetAFlat and LIME show the greatest interest in the upper-right corner of the image, totally outside of what the CT-scan detects. This again represents a bias that should not exist, and the model is unreliable (Fig. 16.13).

As a result of all these biases detected with X-ray as well as CT-scan images, classification alone is most probably not sufficient to correctly detect Covid-19 in the images with the available datasets. A new approach is brought to give to the neural network only the areas that are of interest: the lungs segmentation.

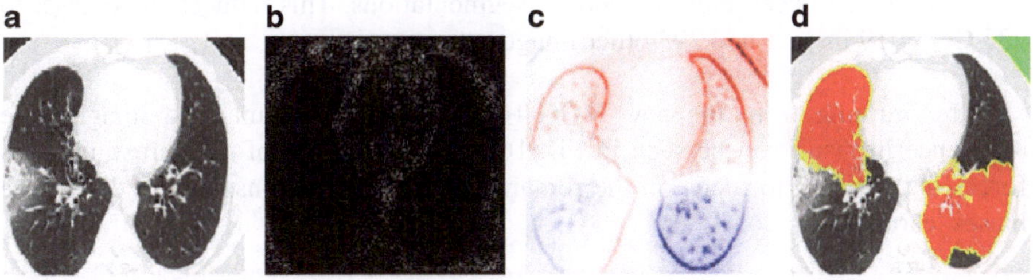

Fig. 16.12 Unsegmented Covid-19 CT scan explained for a VGG-16 model. (**a**) Unsegmented Covid-19 image. (**b**) Integrated gradients. (**c**) LRP PresetAFlat. (**d**) LIME proxy model

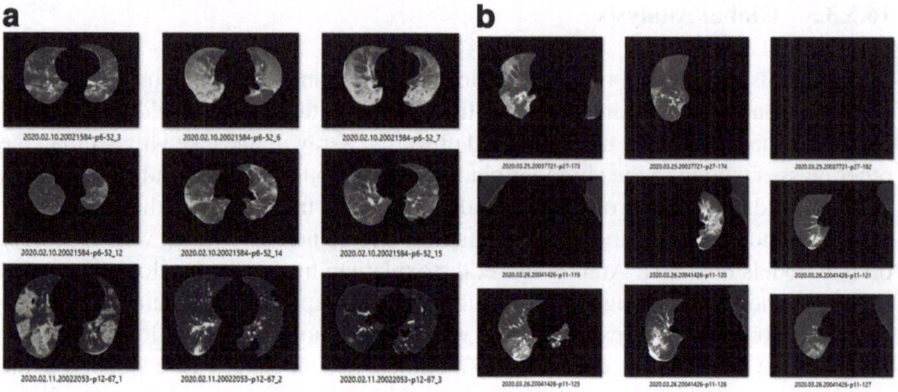

Fig. 16.13 Visualization of good and bad results sorted from lungs segmentation. (**a**) Successful segmentation. (**b**) Failed segmentation

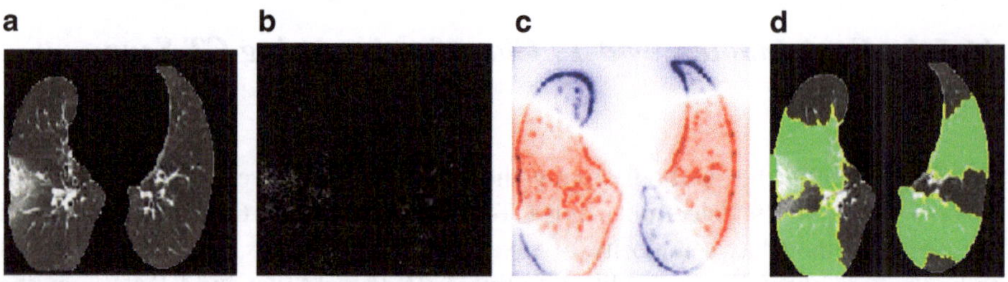

Fig. 16.14 Segmented Covid-19 CT scan explained for a VGG-16 model. (**a**) Segmented Covid-19 image. (**b**) Integrated gradients. (**c**) LRP PresetAFlat. (**d**) LIME proxy model

16.5.4.1 Preprocessing Segmentation

To focus the interest of the network on the lungs, the other areas of the image must be removed. To do this, the lung segmentation model R231-CovidWeb (U-Net) from Hofmanninger et al. [53] is used on all images in the dataset. The results are sorted in order to keep only the correct segmentations. This reduces the dataset to 233 Covid-19 images and 293 other images.

After training from the new VGG-16 model on the remaining images, the difference in result can be seen in Fig. 16.14. The removal of uninteresting areas forces the network to focus on the remaining area, which consequently limits the biases learned.

16.6 Conclusion

This book chapter addressed the problem of Covid-19 diagnosis with the use of chest X-ray and CT-scan images. In order to confirm the ability of our models to differentiate Covid-19 X-ray and CT-scan images from both healthy persons and pneumonia patients, we performed a study on different DL models for the classification of Covid-19 images. For this aim, two public databases were employed, one for X-ray images and the other for CT-scan images representing three classes (normal, Covid-19, viral pneumonia). The obtained results showed that the transfer learning of the models applied to the used datasets offers good performances. Moreover, we performed a large explainability analysis to interpret and visualize how our models work. Experimental results showed the interest of our explanation approach to detect the most interpretable DL model, to measure the positive and negative contributions of input parameters in the decision of DL models, and to detect data biases. The provided explanations were evaluated by doctors and physicians who confirmed the efficiency of our results. As a future work, we plan to extend our dataset in order to train new accurate models and reduce bias data, thanks to DL explanation. We also plan to deploy our solution on cloud platforms [54, 55] in order to increase the availability of our explainable models.

References

1. S.A. Mahmoudi, P. Manneback, Multi-CPU/multi-GPU based framework for multimedia processing, in *Computer Science and Its Applications*, ed. by A. Amine, L. Bellatreche, Z. Elberrichi, E.J. Neuhold, R. Wrembel (Springer International Publishing, Cham, 2015), pp. 54–65
2. S.A. Mahmoudi, P. Manneback, Multi-GPU based event detection and localization using high definition videos, in *2014 International Conference on Multimedia Computing and Systems (ICMCS)* (2014), pp. 81–86
3. P.d.C. Possa, S.A. Mahmoudi, N. Harb, C. Valderrama, A new self-adapting architecture for feature detection, in *22nd International Conference on Field Programmable Logic and Applications (FPL)* (2012), pp. 643–646
4. M.A. Larhmam, S.A. Mahmoudi, M. Benjelloun, S. Mahmoudi, P. Manneback, A portable multi-CPU/multi-GPU based vertebra localization in sagittal MR images, in *Image Analysis and Recognition*, ed. by A. Campilho, M. Kamel (Springer International Publishing, Cham, 2014), pp. 209–218
5. S.A. Mahmoudi, M. Ammar, G.L. Joris, A. Abbou, Real time GPU-based segmentation and tracking of the left ventricle on 2D echocardiography, in *Bioinformatics and Biomedical Engineering*, ed. by F. Ortuño, I. Rojas (Springer International Publishing, Cham, 2016), pp. 602–614
6. A. Krizhevsky, I. Sutskever, G.E. Hinton, ImageNet classification with deep convolutional neural networks, in *Advances in Neural Information Processing Systems*, ed. by F. Pereira, C.J.C. Burges, L. Bottou, K.Q. Weinberger, vol. 25 (Curran Associates, Red Hook, 2012), pp. 1097–1105. http://papers.nips.cc/paper/4824-imagenet-classification-with-deep-convolutional-neural-networks.pdf

7. S. Mahmoudi, M.A. Belarbi, G. Belalem, Towards a smart selection of resources in the cloud for low-energy multimedia processing, Concurr. Comput. Pract. Exper. **30**, e4372 (2018)
8. S.A. Mahmoudi, E. Ozkan, P. Manneback, S. Tosun, *Taking Advantage of Heterogeneous Platforms in Image and Video Processing*, ch. 22 (Wiley, Hoboken, 2014), pp. 429–449
9. S.A. Mahmoudi, M.A. Belarbi, S. Mahmoudi, G. Belalem, P. Manneback, Multimedia processing using deep learning technologies, high-performance computing cloud resources, and big data volumes. Concurr. Comput. Pract. Exp. **32**, e5699 (2020)
10. L.H. Gilpin, D. Bau, B.Z. Yuan, A. Bajwa, M. Specter, L. Kagal, Explaining explanations: An overview of interpretability of machine learning, in *2018 IEEE 5th International Conference on Data Science and Advanced Analytics (DSAA)* (IEEE, Piscataway, 2018), pp. 80–89
11. F. Doshi-Velez, B. Kim, Towards a rigorous science of interpretable machine learning (2017). Preprint arXiv:1702.08608
12. C. Molnar, *Interpretable Machine Learning* (2019), https://christophm.github.io/interpretable-ml-book/.
13. M.D. Zeiler, R. Fergus, Visualizing and understanding convolutional networks, in *European Conference on Computer Vision* (Springer, Berlin, 2014), pp. 818–833
14. Z. Qin, F. Yu, C. Liu, X. Chen, How convolutional neural network see the world:a survey of convolutional neural network visualization methods (2018). Preprint arXiv:1804.11191
15. K. Simonyan, A. Vedaldi, A. Zisserman, Deep inside convolutional networks: Visualising image classification models and saliency maps (2013). Preprint arXiv:1312.6034
16. J.T. Springenberg, A. Dosovitskiy, T. Brox, M. Riedmiller, Striving for simplicity: The all convolutional net (2014). Preprint arXiv:1412.6806
17. B. Zhou, A. Khosla, A. Lapedriza, A. Oliva, A. Torralba, Learning deep features for discriminative localization, in *Proceedings of the IEEE Conference on Computer Vision and Pattern Recognition* (2016), pp. 2921–2929
18. R.R. Selvaraju, M. Cogswell, A. Das, R. Vedantam, D. Parikh, D. Batra, Grad-CAM: Visual explanations from deep networks via gradient-based localization, in *Proceedings of the IEEE International Conference on Computer Vision* (2017), pp. 618–626
19. P.-J. Kindermans, K. Schütt, K.-R. Müller, S. Dähne, Investigating the influence of noise and distractors on the interpretation of neural networks (2016). Preprint arXiv:1611.07270
20. M. Sundararajan, A. Taly, Q. Yan, Axiomatic attribution for deep networks, in *Proceedings of the 34th International Conference on Machine Learning-Volume 70*, JMLR.org (2017), pp. 3319–3328.
21. D. Smilkov, N. Thorat, B. Kim, F. Viégas, M. Wattenberg, SmoothGrad: Removing noise by adding noise (2017).Preprint arXiv:1706.03825
22. S. Bach, A. Binder, G. Montavon, F. Klauschen, K.-R. Müller, W. Samek, On pixel-wise explanations for non-linear classifier decisions by layer-wise relevance propagation. PloS one **10**(7), e0130140 (2015)
23. G. Montavon, A. Binder, S. Lapuschkin, W. Samek, K.-R. Müller, Layer-wise relevance propagation: an overview, in *Explainable AI: Interpreting, Explaining and Visualizing Deep Learning* (Springer, Berlin, 2019), pp. 193–209
24. G. Montavon, S. Lapuschkin, A. Binder, W. Samek, K.-R. Müller, Explaining nonlinear classification decisions with DeepTaylor decomposition. Pattern Recogn. **65**, 211–222 (2017)
25. M.T. Ribeiro, S. Singh, C. Guestrin, "Why should I trust you?" explaining the predictions of any classifier, in *Proceedings of the 22nd ACM SIGKDD International Conference on Knowledge Discovery and Data Mining* (2016), pp. 1135–1144
26. J.R. Zilke, E.L. Mencía, F. Janssen, DeepRED–rule extraction from deep neural networks, in *International Conference on Discovery Science* (Springer, Berlin, 2016), pp. 457–473
27. X. Xu, X. Jiang, C. Ma, P. Du, X. Li, S. Lv, L. Yu, Q. Ni, Y. Chen, J. Su, G. Lang, Y. Li, H. Zhao, J. Liu, K. Xu, L. Ruan, J. Sheng, Y. Qiu, W. Wu, T. Liang, L. Li, A deep learning system to screen novel coronavirus disease 2019 pneumonia, *Engineering***6**, 1122–1129 (2020). http://www.sciencedirect.com/science/article/pii/S2095809920301636
28. M. Rahimzadeh, A. Attar, A modified deep convolutional neural network for detecting Covid-19 and pneumonia from chest X-ray images based on the concatenation of Xception and

ResNet50v2. Inf. Med. Unlocked **19**, 100360 (2020). http://www.sciencedirect.com/science/article/pii/S2352914820302537
29. N. Narayan Das, N. Kumar, M. Kaur, V. Kumar, D. Singh, Automated deep transfer learning-based approach for detection of Covid-19 infection in chest X-rays. *IRBM* (2020). http://www.sciencedirect.com/science/article/pii/S1959031820301172
30. Y. Pathak, P. Shukla, A. Tiwari, S. Stalin, S. Singh, P. Shukla, Deep transfer learning based classification model for Covid-19 disease. *IRBM* (2020). http://www.sciencedirect.com/science/article/pii/S1959031820300993
31. L. Sarker, M. Islam, T. Hannan, Z. Ahmed, Covid-DenseNet: A deep learning architecture to detect Covid-19 from chest radiology images. Preprints (2020). https://www.preprints.org/manuscript/202005.0151/v1
32. P. Rajpurkar, J. Irvin, K. Zhu, B. Yang, H. Mehta, T. Duan, D. Ding, A. Bagul, C. Langlotz, K. Shpanskaya, M.P. Lungren, A.Y. Ng, CheXNet: Radiologist-level pneumonia detection on chest X-rays with deep learning. (2017).
33. R.R. Selvaraju, M. Cogswell, A. Das, R. Vedantam, D. Parikh, D. Batra, Grad-CAM: Visual explanations from deep networks via gradient-based localization, in *Proceedings of the IEEE International Conference on Computer Vision (ICCV)* (2017)
34. F. Ucar, D. Korkmaz, COVIDiagnosis-net: Deep Bayes-SqueezeNet based diagnosis of the coronavirus disease 2019 (Covid-19) from X-ray images. Med. Hypotheses **140**, 109761 (2020). http://www.sciencedirect.com/science/article/pii/S0306987720307702
35. T. Mahmud, M.A. Rahman, S.A. Fattah, CovXNet: A multi-dilation convolutional neural network for automatic Covid-19 and other pneumonia detection from chest X-ray images with transferable multi-receptive feature optimization. Comput. Biol. Med. **122**, 103869 (2020). http://www.sciencedirect.com/science/article/pii/S0010482520302250
36. M.R. Karim, T. Dohmen, D. Rebholz-Schuhmann, S. Decker, M. Cochez, O. Beyan, Deep-CovidExplainer: Explainable Covid-19 diagnosis based on chest X-ray images (2020)
37. L. Brunese, F. Mercaldo, A. Reginelli, A. Santone, Explainable deep learning for pulmonary disease and coronavirus Covid-19 detection from X-rays. Comput. Methods Programs Biomed. **196**, 105608 (2020). http://www.sciencedirect.com/science/article/pii/S0169260720314413
38. M.E.H. Chowdhury, T. Rahman, A. Khandakar, R. Mazhar, M.A. Kadir, Z.B. Mahbub, K.R. Islam, M.S. Khan, A. Iqbal, N. Al-Emadi, M.B.I. Reaz, T.I. Islam, Can AI help in screening viral and Covid-19 pneumonia? IEEE Access **8**, 132665–132676 (2020)
39. S.I. di Radiologia Medica e Interventistica, Covid-19 database: Casistica radiologica italiana (2020)
40. J.P. Cohen, P. Morrison, L. Dao, Covid-19 image data collection 2020.
41. D.S.K. et al., Identifying medical diagnoses and treatable diseases by image-based deep learning. Cell **172**, 1122–1131 (2020). https://www.cell.com/cell/fulltext/S0092-8674(18)30154-5
42. K. Simonyan, A. Zisserman, Very deep convolutional networks for large-scale image recognition (2014). Preprint arXiv:1409.1556
43. K. He, X. Zhang, S. Ren, J. Sun, Deep residual learning for image recognition, in *Proceedings of the IEEE Conference on Computer Vision and Pattern Recognition* (2016), pp. 770–778
44. C. Szegedy, W. Liu, Y. Jia, P. Sermanet, S. Reed, D. Anguelov, D. Erhan, V. Vanhoucke, A. Rabinovich, Going deeper with convolutions, in *Proceedings of the IEEE Conference on Computer Vision and Pattern Recognition* (2015), pp. 1–9
45. F. Chollet, Xception: Deep learning with depthwise separable convolutions (2016). arxiv:1610.02357. http://arxiv.org/abs/1610.02357
46. G. Huang, Z. Liu, L. Van Der Maaten, K.Q. Weinberger, Densely connected convolutional networks, in *Proceedings of the IEEE Conference on Computer Vision and Pattern Recognition* (2017), pp. 4700–4708
47. J. Zhao, Y. Zhang, X. He, P. Xie, COVID-CT-Dataset: a CT scan dataset about Covid-19 (2020). Preprint arXiv:2003.13865
48. tf-explain, https://tf-explain.readthedocs.io/en/latest/. Accessed 28 May 2020
49. M. Alber, S. Lapuschkin, P. Seegerer, M. Hägele, K.T. Schütt, G. Montavon, W. Samek, K.-R. Müller, S. Dähne, P.-J. Kindermans, Investigate neural networks. J. Mach. Learn. Res. **20**(93), 1–8 (2019)

50. P.-J. Kindermans, K.T. Schütt, M. Alber, K.-R. Müller, D. Erhan, B. Kim, S. Dähne, Learning how to explain neural networks: PatternNet and PatternAttribution (2017). Preprint arXiv:1705.05598
51. A. Shrikumar, P. Greenside, A. Kundaje, Learning important features through propagating activation differences, in *Proceedings of the 34th International Conference on Machine Learning-Volume 70*. JMLR.org (2017), pp. 3145–3153
52. W. Samek, A. Binder, G. Montavon, S. Lapuschkin, K.-R. Müller, Evaluating the visualization of what a deep neural network has learned. IEEE Trans. Neural Netw. Learn. Syst. **28**(11), 2660–2673 (2016)
53. J. Hofmanninger, F. Prayer, J. Pan, S. Rohrich, H. Prosch, G. Langs, Automatic lung segmentation in routine imaging is a data diversity problem, not a methodology problem (2020).Preprint arXiv:2001.11767
54. S.A. Mahmoudi, M.E. Adoui, M.A. Belarbi, M.A. Larhmam, F. Lecron, Cloud-based platform for computer vision applications, in *Proceedings of the 2017 International Conference on Smart Digital Environment*, ser. ICSDE '17 (Association for Computing Machinery, New York, 2017), pp. 195–200. https://doi.org/10.1145/3128128.3128158
55. S.A. Mahmoudi, et al., Real time web-based toolbox for computer vision. J. Sci. Technol. Arts **10**(2), 3–13 (2018)

Chapter 17
Innovative Solutions to the Clinical Challenges of COVID-19

S. M. Kadri, Samir Mattoo, Ailbhe H. Brady, and Marija Petkovic

17.1 Introduction

This paper will address the clinical challenges of COVID-19 through the lens of informatics, detailing examples of how these challenges have been tackled.

COVID-19 emerged from Wuhan, China, in late 2019. Coronaviruses represent a large family of viruses that cause infective disorders ranging from a mild cold to severe disease. Since the epidemic was initially noted in China, COVID-19 spread rapidly throughout the globe. Initially marked as a 'Public Health Emergency of International Concern' by WHO, it was later declared a pandemic on the March 11, 2020. To our knowledge, there have been more than 6.6 million confirmed cases on the worldwide.

On February 21, 2020, six special envoys on COVID-19 were appointed to provide strategic and high-level political advocacy and engagement in different parts of the world [1].

The main goal of the special envoys on COVID-19 is to apply WHO recommendations on COVID-19 preparedness. Additionally, it is necessary to monitor COVID-19 hotspots and provide further strategic plans and reports to the corresponding government bodies [2].

S. M. Kadri (✉)
Disease Control, Directorate of Health Services, Kashmir, UT of Jammu and Kashmir, India

S. Mattoo
Directorate of Health Services, Kashmir, UT of Jammu and Kashmir, India

A. H. Brady
National Health Service, Manchester, United Kingdom

M. Petkovic
University of Medicine, Belgrade, Serbia

L. Garg et al. (eds.), *Healthcare Informatics for Fighting COVID-19 and Future Epidemics*, EAI/Springer Innovations in Communication and Computing,
https://doi.org/10.1007/978-3-030-72752-9_17

To improve strategic healthcare measures, prevention and monitoring in this pandemic, it is of utmost importance to enhance government readiness and actions both within healthcare and wider society- ultimately aiming to minimize risk and adverse outcomes.

As of July 20, 2020, there have been the following PPE had been delivered to 128 countries: 646,464 goggles, 1.8 million gowns, 5.5 million face shields, 10.2 million respirators and 41.1 million medical masks.

To improve laboratory capacity, 14,000 oxygen concentrators were allocated to more than 120 countries. In the diagnostic area, approximately 6 million polymerase chain reaction (PCR) tests and 5.2 million sample collection kits have been delivered [3].

Of global importance was collaboration of the covid-19 special envoys with more than 50 digital companies and social media platforms to combat misinformation and promote science-based health messages globally such as Facebook, Google, WhatsApp, Viber, Youtube, Tinder and Governments.

17.2 SARS-CoV-2 Characteristics

SARS-CoV-2 is an enveloped virus consisting of the spike (S) protein, membrane protein (M) and envelope protein (E). It is single-stranded, positive 26–32 kb RNA betacoronavirus belonging to the subfamily Coronavirinaea (*Nidovirales coronaviridae*). Coronaviruses are zoonotic, which implies that they are transmitted between animals and humans.

SARS-CoV-2 genome has 88% similarity with the bat-SL-CoVYC45 and bat-SL-CoVZXC21 sequences. It was 96.2% identical to another bat CoVRaTG13. It was also demonstrated that the protein-coding genes of coronavirus have 79.5% and 51% sequence similarity to SARS-CoV and MERS-CoV. It has been concluded that SARS-CoV-2 virus has the angiotensin-converting enzyme 2 (ACE2) receptor [4] (Fig. 17.1).

The initial symptoms are upper and lower respiratory tract symptoms, fever, cough and breathing difficulties. There are pneumonia, severe acute respiratory symptoms, renal insufficiency and lethal outcome in the more advanced cases. More serious cases have manifested as pneumonia, acute respiratory distress syndrome (ARDS), venous thromboembolism (VTE) renal insufficiency and death.

Nations have been striving to 'flatten the curve', to reduce the burden on healthcare systems and reduce the number of deaths. Globally we have had to get to grip with diagnosing, treating and navigating this novel coronavirus in a time-critical manner.

COVID-19 has negatively affected economies worldwide, as well as overwhelming healthcare systems and hugely impacting on day-to-day life. According to A. Kalil, it is of great importance to conduct controlled trials of treatment in the emerging pandemic.

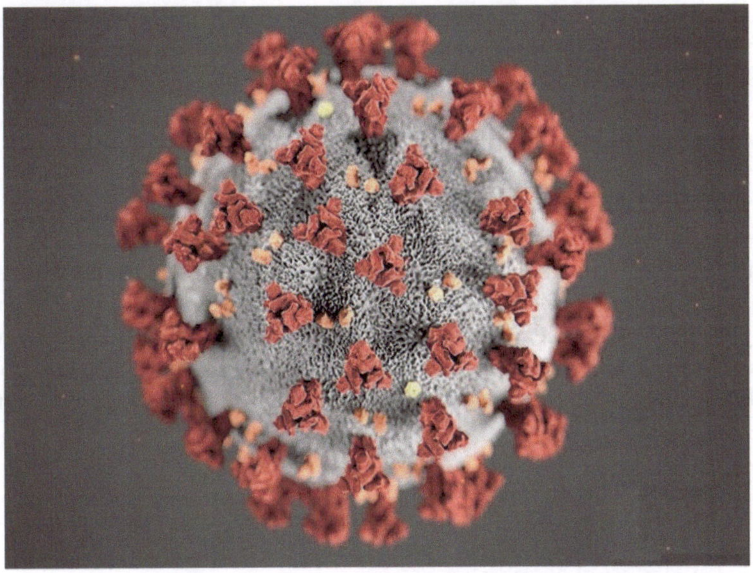

Fig. 17.1 SARS-CoV-2 virus

At time of writing, trials are being conducted with outcomes eagerly awaited. Up to this date, the variety of combined drug treatment has experimented. But in the case of no proven clinical trials, there is no documented medical benefit.

A research study concluded that the covid-19 virus may be viable for approximately 72 h, particularly on plastic and stainless steel, and furthermore up to 4 h on copper and 24 h on the cardboard [5].

17.3 Clinical Evaluation

The initial symptoms include fever, breathing difficulties- including shortness of breath, tachypnoea and cough- and gastrointestinal symptoms. Additionally, there is confusion, chest pain, vomiting, nausea, sneezing, nasal congestion, increased sputum production, anosmia and dyspepsia [6].

The positive laboratory values are cytokine elevation, sepsis, anaemia, increased lactate dehydrogenase, aspartate aminotransferase, alanine transaminase, C-reactive protein (CRP), creatine kinase, erythrocyte sedimentation rate, elevated white blood cell, D-dimer, procalcitonin, urea and creatinine. In certain individuals, there is decreased haemoglobin, lymphocyte and eosinophil number and albumin.

The most common radiological changes are a ground-glass opacity in the parenchyma of the lung [7].

In the case of the emerging pandemics, such as COVID-19, there is no vaccine available at the moment. Consequently, the vaccine may be developed in several years.

17.4 Methods

Informed by a retrospective review of the body of COVID-19 literature, first-hand clinical experience and overreaching public and global health principles, we propose the key clinical challenges faced in the fight against COVID-19. These will be explored, with current and potential informatics solutions elaborated upon. We will study healthcare systems and how information has been transformed within these during the pandemic.

17.5 Results

We have identified a number of clinical challenges faced in the wake of COVID-19. These challenges vary between countries, however without doubt there is considerable commonality. The key challenges identified were testing and laboratory capacity; understanding presentations of COVID-19; rapid formulation of treatment guidelines and dissemination of these; contact tracing; use of technology for communication; human resources; personal protective equipment supplies; information sharing within the scientific community; running clinical trials; finding a vaccine; increasing hospital capacity; ensuring appropriate use of healthcare facilities; secondary impacts, e.g. delayed presentation; misinformation; use of infographics; training of healthcare professionals; performing aerosol-generating procedures; and quarantining clinical areas.

17.6 Transmission of COVID-19

The new strain of coronavirus is transmitted via direct pathway (droplet, human-to-human transmission) and indirect contact (contaminated objects, airborne contagion, tracheal intubation, noninvasive ventilation, tracheotomy, cardiopulmonary resuscitation, manual ventilation, bronchoscopy, etc.). It is possible to transmit COVID-19 from an asymptomatic individual without any radiological findings [8].

In the case of the faecal-oral transmission, there is a significant correlation, according to WHO-China report [9].

17.7 Epidemiology of COVID-19

Currently, in Brazil, there are more than 87,000 lethal outcomes and 2.42 million new cases as of July 26, 2020.

In the majority of countries worldwide, there has been a rapid development of the intensive care units in the emergency setting, especially field hospitals and vehicle transport.

MIRAGRODEP'S projections have evaluated the impact on per capita gross national income (GNI). GNI is a model predicting the influence of COVID-19 on malnutrition and mortality. According to those investigations, there has been a prediction of an increase in wasting to child mortality on 1.26 million children (177 Demographic and Health Surveys—DHS) in the period of 1990–2018 [10].

It has been noted that lockdown measures in accordance with severe mobility and food disruption have been experienced in most LMICs. In those cases, there is a 7–9% decrease in GNI per capita reactive to pre-COVID-19 projections. There has been a decrease in GNI per capita in correlation with a significant increase in child wasting.

Consequently, there is an expectation that COVID-19 pandemic leads to a higher risk of various malnutrition. COVID-19 pandemic has a great impact on the food system crisis, malnutrition and both maternal and child malnutrition [10].

A key challenge in any type of pandemic is maintaining balance in the effectiveness of clinical care and conducting thorough clinical research. According to a legal international obligation by the Nuremberg Code of 1947, provided by the International Conference on Harmonization, it is necessary to provide the main elements such as to protect the rights, safety and welfare of humans participating in the research.

17.8 Diagnosis

Before any hospital discharge, it is necessary to have the data on two consecutive RT-PCR negative results in the 24 h interval. Additionally, it is necessary to confirm the complete resolution of the acute exudative respiratory lesions on computed tomography (CT) imaging and the decrease of temperature in 72 h [11].

The therapeutic approach is supportive, not curative. For example, in China, strict preventive measures and isolation resulted in a significant decrease in new cases. Afterwards, the infection spread to Europe, especially Italy and Spain [12].

17.9 Preventive Measures

In the case of COVID-19, there are several recommended measures such as washing hands often with the application of alcohol-based hand rub or using soap and water. Furthermore, it is advised to maintain social distancing at least 1 m (3 ft). Nevertheless, it is advised to avoid touching eyes, nose and region of the lips. In the epidemiological chain, there is a known infection transmission pathway. A most common route of transmission is by hands. Thus, hands may transfer the virus to the eyes, nose or mouth, entering the respiratory and gastrointestinal system.

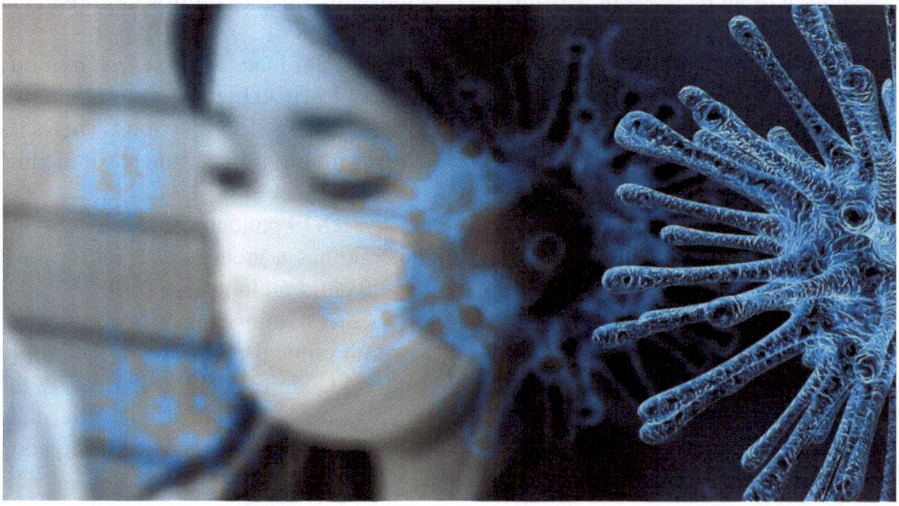

In case of respiratory hygiene, it is necessary to regularly cover the mouth and nose and dispose the used tissue.

Thus, it is necessary to perform self-quarantine. To improve the healthcare system, it is necessary to follow the national and local authorities on the current pandemic guidelines.

In case you reach a healthcare provider promptly, there is advice for the healthcare facility. Such an act will protect and prevent the spread of viruses and other possible infective diseases [2].

The basic preventive actions in the hospital settings are infection prevention and control (IPC) strategies to manage COVID-19 transmissions such as an appropriate triage, source control, performing standard precautions and additional preventive measures.

Administrative control aims to provide guidelines for infection prevention and control (IPC measures). The following are recommended: an adequate infrastructure, transparent IPC policies, increased laboratory testing capacities, a timely mannered triage as well as professional healthcare education. The most important action in these types of pandemics is to reduce the transmission and the contamination of surfaces and other objects [13].

17.10 WHO COVID-19 Report

The WHO supported the fundings and trials for vaccines that were presented at the Global Vaccine Summit. Health Cluster partners continually enhance the implementation of the Global Humanitarian Response Plan for COVID-19 in 29 countries experiencing a humanitarian crisis, affecting 63 million people. The major activities include an increased community awareness of COVID-19 signs and symptoms, related risk factors, the importance of seeking early treatment and protection measures, including isolation and quarantine. Furthermore, it is necessary to support community-based surveillance and early screening and establish treatment centres and train health workers in COVID-19 case management protocols.

GOARN partners are providing support in epidemiology, surveillance, laboratory, infection prevention and control (IPC), case control, risk estimation and community actions and coordination [14].

UNICEF, IFRC, OCHA and US Centers for Disease Control and Prevention collaborate closely with WHO supporting all current strategies.

As of June 7, 2020, the Emergency Medical Teams (EMT) network has deployed 23 international EMTs to the most affected areas mainly in Europe and Africa. Furthermore, 43 national teams, in the process of international classification, have been mobilized to support the national health system. More than 500 national teams have used the EMT methodology to respond to the COVID-19 crisis.

17.11 Current Clinical Challenges

In a retrospective, single-centre study from January to January 20, 2020 in Wuhan, China, 99 individuals diagnosed with coronavirus were admitted. The epidemiological, demographic, clinical, laboratory and prognostic information were obtained and followed until January 25, 2020. In the diagnostic approach, throat swab specimens were collected from the upper pulmonary pathway [15].

The most common symptoms were shortness of respiratory ventilation, muscle weakness, headache, respiratory difficulties and diarrhoea. In 17% of cases, ARDS has been present, in 8% acute respiratory injury, in 3% acute renal injury, in 4% septic shock and in 1% ventilator-associated pneumonia [16].

In the laboratory values, leucocytes were lower in 9% of patients and elevated in 24%. In 38% of cases, neutrophils were significantly increased. In the majority of patients, lymphocytes and haemoglobin were elevated. Additionally, platelets were decreased, and liver function was impaired (elevated AST and ALT). In regard to the heart function, there was increased creatine kinase and lactate dehydrogenase.

In 75% of cases, bilateral pneumonia has been confirmed by radiologic examination (multiple mottling and ground-glass opacities).

The confirmed case has been isolated and treated by antiviral medications for 3–14 days such as oseltamivir (75 mg two times/day orally), ganciclovir (0–25 g two times per day, intravenously) and lopinavir and ritonavir tablets (500 mg two times per day, orally). Additionally, antibiotic treatment has been included for the most common pathogens.

In 13 patients, noninvasive ventilator mechanical ventilation has been necessary for 4–22 days. Assisted ventilation has been applied in 4 patients for 3–20 days (inhaled oxygen concentration was 35–100%), and the positive end expiratory pressure was 6–12 cm H_2O.

In the prediction of mortality in case of viral pneumonia, MuLBSTA score has been applied [17].

Overall, nine patients died, of whom eight had lymphopenia, seven had bilateral pneumonia, five were older than 60 years old, three had hypertension, and one patient was a smoker.

17.12 Ongoing Clinical Trials

The use of convalescent plasma from recovered patients in individuals with COVID-19 has been investigated (Roback et al.). In the Shenzhen Hospital (China), the combination of convalescent plasma and antiviral drugs such as lopinavir/ritonavir and interferon leads to their enhanced recovery in the period of 1 week. In those patients, there has been significant improvement in Sequential Organ Failure Assessment scores.

To be up to date with the current COVID-19 pandemic, 200 vaccine trials are trending (The Lancet). The two early phases of COVID-19 vaccine trial conclusion included an adenoviral vector with the humoral response to the SARS-CoV-2 receptor-binding domain on 28th day and T-cell response. Noted adverse effects are fever, fatigue and local injection pain [18].

Andrew Polland et al. have reached phase 1/2 randomised trial of one injection of chimpanzee adenovirus-vectored COVID-19 vaccine in the group of 1077 healthy individuals in 28 days [18]. The neutralizing antibodies have been produced in more than 90% of participants.

In the study of Weil Chen et al. in phase 2 randomised trial, a non-replicating adenovirus-vectored COVID-19 vaccine was tested against placebo (508 healthy individuals).

The reported seroconversion was detected in more than 96% of individuals, while neutralizing antibodies were present in 85%.

It may be concluded that both trials used adenovirus vectors to generate COVID-19 vaccine in the pandemic peak. Such type of vaccine showed a great ability to enhance humoral, cellular and innate immune mechanisms. Further results from these ongoing studies are expected.

There is a worldwide initiative to provide effective preventive actions to decrease the mortality rate. The most prominent act is the strict healthcare measures that may affect the quality of life in the future in all human spheres. Healthcare organizations have outlined the directives and specific measures in COVID-19 treatment and prevention.

Simultaneously, there is a tremendous scientific focus on developing the thesis such as the etiopathogenesis, route of transmission, clinical challenges, novel diagnostic approach and possible therapeutic modalities. It is yet no clear the virus-host connection in the midst of the pandemic.

Currently, proposed treatment strategies are supportive but not curative. Up to date, strict isolation measures held in China have led to a significant decline in the morbidity and mortality from COVID-19 [19].

Consequently, the pandemic spread to Europe, especially Italy and Spain. Those healthcare governments acted promptly and have managed to localize the pandemic peak. As of June 20, 2020, there have been 2,282,000 cases detected in the United States. Out of that number, 121,000 have been lethal. In Brazil, the estimated number of new cases is 1,000,000 and approximately 50,000 lethal outcomes.

Notably, the number of new cases and mortality rate in COVID-19 pandemic is statistically lower than in the SARS and MERS. The only difference is that SARS-CoV-2 virus is larger with higher mortality rates. In the setting of chronic comorbidities, there is an estimated risk that 1/5 patients are at an increased risk for a severe form of COVID-19.

In the COVID-19 ring-based prevention trial, there have been conducted 854 interventional trials registered. The most commonly applied treatment has been lopinavir-ritonavir treatment in one randomized, controlled trial (RCT) [20].

In the midst of a global health emergency, we have identified and addressed many clinical challenges. We have adapted rapidly out of necessity. Lessons have been learned, and future challenges will arise. We must reflect on our progress and failings thus far, to ensure maximum learning. Recommendations for future pandemics are open information sharing, easily accessible knowledge hubs, a continuous commitment to analyse and learn from our actions and the pursuit of innovative solutions utilising informatics.

17.13 Global Strategic Objectives

Up to March 2020, there have been 79,424 confirmed cases, including 2626 associated lethal outcomes. In China, there are 77,262 confirmed cases, and out of that number, there are 2595 deaths. Outside China, there are 2162 confirmed cases and 17 deaths from 33 countries. In Iran, there are 61 confirmed cases with 12 deaths. There is one case reported in Iraq in Najaf (one religious student travelling back from Iran and four from the same family in Kirkuk with the recent travel history to Iran).

To obtain control of the pandemic crisis, the following are recommended:

- Reduce the human-to-human transmission.
- Identify, isolate and monitor for patients.
- To point out the main clinical severity, route of transmission and infection, treatment modalities, diagnostic approach and vaccines.
- To elaborate on the main risk and event data to avoid misinformation.
- To identify and reduce transmission from the animal source.

17.14 Results

17.14.1 Testing and Laboratory Capacity

The recommended COVID-19 testing is by molecular diagnosis by real-time RT-PCR. RdRp gene assay is performed on oral swabs [21].

According to the communicable disease protocols and communication strategy, the operational framework is based on federal, state and local pandemic plans. The additional plans are staff management, workforce management, innate management, visitor management, government processes and corresponding guidelines (COVID-19 PPE guidelines for health and custodial staff, COVID-19 environmental cleaning guidelines for rooms and non-emergency transport, "Help Stop the Spread of COVID-19" posters and pamphlet in inmate and visitor areas).

17.14.2 Understanding Presentations of COVID-19

The pandemic mitigation strategy is to delay the outbreak peak, to reduce peak burden on services and corresponding systems and to diminish overall cases and health impacts [22].

17.14.3 Contact Tracing [33]

The main healthcare staff responsibilities are to (1) identify patients at risk, use COVID-19 screening form, (2) to isolate as to place a surgical mask on the inmate, (3) to inform the corresponding healthcare services, (4) to monitor inmates for symptoms of respiratory compromise and deterioration.

17.14.4 Use of Technology for Communication

In the era of digital technologies, the COVID-19 pandemic uses various next-generation telecommunication networks, big data analytics, artificial intelligence, etc. The aforementioned computer technology is necessary to understand and enhance the pandemic crisis, such as COVID-19 [23].

The most accurate global COVID-19 pandemic monitor may be found on https://www.worldometers.info/coronavirus/. The following social media is incorporated in the COVID-19 news and education: WhatsApp, Facebook, Twitter, SenseTime, Sunell and e-virtual learning platforms. In China, there is a platform that may identify individuals with an elevated body temperature: https://apnews.com/PR%20Newswire/354aae0738073bc95331ee72a458cb50 [24].

17.14.5 Human Resources

In the workplace setting, it is crucial to have robust business continuity plans, with frequent review of service delivery mechanisms. The aim is to minimize disease transmission amongst the workforce, so as to ensure that adequate levels of staffing are maintained. In order to accommodate those who are required to shield, role substitution needs be addressed- are there other members of staff who could take up their duties? Staff illness will require flexible working within teams. Throughout it is crucial to ensure workforce wellbeing and resilience- this can be achieved by interventions at the local level- counseling etc. Additionally, workforce unions have an important role to plan in advocating for their members. A healthy workforce is necessary to delivery good patient care.

17.14.6 Personal Protective Equipment Supplies

PPE includes gloves, medical and/or surgical face masks, eyeglasses, face shield, gowns and specific procedures-filtering facepiece respirators. In the case of COVID-19 pandemic, the main goal is to protect the frontline healthcare staff and coworkers. The suggested strategies are to include minimizing the need for PPE in healthcare. Also, it is necessary to provide rational and appropriate use of PPE [25].

Currently, there is a lack of PPE supplies globally despite the efforts of the manufacturing companies. According to WHO, there are last-resort temporary measures such as PPE extended use, reprocessing followed by reuse and including alternative items.

17.14.7 Information Sharing Within the Scientific Community

In the sphere of scientific data exchange, WHO has the main role to ensure global pandemic awareness and data presentation. The aim is to provide the best evidence-based guidance and operational support for all individuals [25].

17.14.8 Increasing Hospital Capacity

There are four current strategies posited by WHO for increasing hospital capacity.

1. Staff, to ensure a sufficient 345 number of healthcare and social workers.
2. Space, to focus on making adequate space in hospitals and other institutions that provide healthcare.
3. Supplies, to guarantee an adequate number of supplies and equipment for the patient and healthcare professionals' safety.
4. Systems, to coordinate action to respond to the surge in demand for services.

17.14.9 Secondary Impacts, E.g. Delayed Presentation

In the COVID-19 pandemic, the indirect impacts are seen through the effect of fear on the population or as a consequence of the measures necessary to monitor the pandemic [26]. Worldwide it has been noted that patients have delayed seeking medical attention when they most certainly need to. Fear of attending hospitals with a significant number of COVID 19 patients has been a major contributer to this change in health-seeking behavior. Delayed presentations impact adversely on patient outcomes.

17.14.10 Training of Healthcare Professionals

Healthcare professionals have had to adapt rapidly to this new disease. In order to determine best practice, clinical trials have been running. Healthcare professionals have had to manage critically unwell patients- trialling novel treatment strategies whilst developing their infection control skills. Due to limited resources and overwhelming demand, treatment has had to be rationalized- for instance drug shortages and ventilators. Doctors have been learning more and more about the disease's trajectory, learning when it is necessary to intubate and ventilate Vs when a patient would be better managed with CPAP. The healthcare professionals' training is to identify, regulate and provide the medical care for patients in the case of the coronavirus pandemic. The basic topics are symptoms and sign in patients with

COVID-19 and an adequate stabilization of patients. There is a swell need for intubation and ventilator management [27].

17.14.11 Performing Aerosol-Generating Procedures

The aerosol-generating procedures (AGPs) generate a higher concentration of infective respiratory aerosols in comparison with coughing, sneezing, speech or breathing. The procedures mentioned earlier are open suctioning of airway secretions, sputum production, cardiopulmonary resuscitation (CPR), endotracheal intubation, extubation and intussusception noninvasive positive pressure ventilation (NIPPV, BIPAP, CPAP), bronchoscopy and manual ventilation.

17.14.12 Quarantining Clinical Areas

The proposed quarantine measures are in the form of the restrictions of activities or the separation of the infected individuals in a proper way to monitor the objective symptomatology or detect emerging cases. WHO recommends that the patients with laboratory-confirmed COVID-19 be in quarantine for 14 days since the last time they were exposed to the patient [28]. In the hospital setting, cohorts of COVID 19 patients have been assigned to specific wards, so as to allow for 'clean' areas within hospitals. In Intensive Care Units this has resulted in moving patients around and opening new areas, so as to allow for both COVID 19 and non COVID 19 patients to be accommodated. This takes considerable planning, communication and manpower amongst multiple specialties.

17.15 Conclusion

The coronavirus disease 2019 (COVID-19) pandemic is due to severe acute respiratory syndrome coronavirus 2 (SARS-CoV-2) which emerged in the Wuhan, China, in 2019, causing significant burden in numerous healthcare systems worldwide.

Currently, there is an increase in viral disease worldwide. The first unexplained respiratory infection in Wuhan was been noted on December 31, 2019 by the WHO.

The high contagious potential of these viruses is a serious public health risk.

In regard to that attribute, WHO states that the CoV epidemic had its peak on February 28, 2020. By March, the number of COVID 19 cases worldwide had tripled. There have been more than 118,000 cases in 114 countries and over 4000 deaths [29].

There has been a conclusion that the rigorous measures such as the lockdown may save more than three million individuals in Europe.

References

1. S. Perlman, J. Netland, Coronaviruses post-SARS: Update on replication and pathogenesis. Nat. Rev. Microbiol. **7**(6), 439–450 (2009)
2. M. Lotfi et al., COVID-19: Transmission, prevention, and potential therapeutic opportunities. Clin. Chim. Acta **508**, 254–266 (2020)
3. Cochrane COVID-19 study register, https://covid-19.cochrane.org/. Last updated 28 Apr 2020. Accessed 28 Apr 2020
4. R. Lu, X. Zhao, J. Li, P. Niu, B. Yang, H. Wu, W. Wang, H. Song, B. Huang, N. Zhu, et al., Genomic characterisation and epidemiology of 2019 novel coronavirus: Implications for virus origins and receptor binding. Lancet **395**, 565–574 (2020)
5. N. van Doremalen et al., Aerosol and surface stability of SARS-CoV-2 as compared with SARS-CoV-1. N. Engl. J. Med. **382**, 1564–1567 (2020)
6. N. Chen, M. Zhou, X. Dong, J. Qu, F. Gong, Y. Han, Epidemiological and clinical characteristics of 99 cases of 2019 novel coronavirus pneumonia in Wuhan, China: A descriptive study. Lancet **395**(10223), 507–513 (2020)
7. A.R. Sahin, A. Erdogan, P.M. Agaoglu, Y. Dineri, A.Y. Cakirci, M.E. Senel, 2019 Novel coronavirus (COVID-19) outbreak: A review of the current literature. EJMO **4**(1), 1–7 (2020)
8. C. Rothe, M. Schunk, P. Sothmann, G. Bretzel, G. Froeschl, C. Wallrauch, Transmission of 2019-nCoV infection from an asymptomatic contact in Germany. N. Engl. J. Med. **382**(10), 970–971 (2020)
9. K. McIntosh, M.S. Hirsch, A. Bloom, Coronavirus disease 2019 (COVID-19), in *UpToDate*, ed. by M. S. Hirsch, A. Bloom, Accessed 5 Mar 2020
10. D. Headey, Impacts of COVID-19 on childhood malnutrition and nutrition-related mortality. Lancet **396**(10250), 519–521 (2020)
11. F. Pan, T. Ye, P. Sun, S. Gui, B. Liang, L. Li, et al., Time course of lung changes on chest CT during recovery from 2019 novel coronavirus (COVID-19) pneumonia. Radiology **295**(3), 715–721 (2020)
12. N. Chen et al., Epidemiological and clinical characteristics of 99 cases of 2019 novel coronavirus pneumonia in Wuhan, China: A descriptive study. Lancet **395**(10223), 507–513 (2020)
13. World Health Organization, WHO Director-General's opening remarks at the media briefing on COVID-19 - 11 Mar 2020, https://www.who.int/dg/speeches/detail/who-director-general-s-opening-remarks-at-the-media-briefing-on-covid-19%2D%2D-11-march-2020
14. https://www.cdc.gov/coronavirus/2019-ncov/global-covid-19/pre-deployment-processes-COVID-19-considerations.html. Accessed 20 Jan 2021
15. M.D. Fei Zhou, Clinical course and risk factors for mortality of adult inpatients with COVID-19 in Wuhan, China: A retrospective cohort study. Lancet **395**(10229), 1054–1062 (2020)
16. F. Jiang, Review of the clinical characteristics of coronavirus disease 2019 (COVID-19). J. Gen. Intern. Med. **35**(5), 1545–1549 (2020)
17. L. Guo, Clinical features predicting mortality risk in patients with viral pneumonia: The MuLBSTA score. Front. Microbiol **10**, 2752 (2019)
18. P.M. Folegatti et al., Safety and immunogenicity of the ChAdOx1 nCoV-19 vaccine against SARS-CoV-2: A preliminary report of a phase 1/2, single-blind, randomised controlled trial. Lancet **396**(10249), 467–478 (2020)
19. M.D. Fujun Peng, Management and treatment of COVID-19: The Chinese experience. Can. J. Cardiol. **36**(6), 915–930 (2020)
20. D. Tan, *COVID-19 Ring-Based Prevention Trial with Lopinavir/Ritonavir (CORIPREV-LR)* (St. Michael's Hospital, Toronto)
21. S. Mahendiratta, Molecular diagnosis of COVID-19 in the different biologic matrix, their diagnostic validity and clinical relevance: A systematic review. Life Sci. **258**, 118207 (2020)

22. N. Madhav, B. Oppenheim, M. Gallivan, P. Mulembakani, E. Rubin, N. Wolfe, Chapter 17: Pandemics: Risks, impacts, and mitigation, in *Disease Control Priorities: Improving Health and Reducing Poverty*, 3rd edn., (The World Bank Group, Washington)
23. A. Kumar, A review of modern technologies for tackling COVID-19 pandemic. Diabet. Metab. Syndr. **14**(4), 569–573 (2020)
24. D.S.W. Ting, Digital technology and COVID-19. Nat. Med. **26**, 1–3 (2020)
25. M. Saiful Islam et al., Current knowledge of COVID-19 and infection prevention and control strategies in healthcare settings: A global analysis. Infect. Control Hosp. Epidemiol. **15**, 1–11 (2020)
26. C. Maringe et al., The impact of the COVID-19 pandemic on cancer deaths due to delays in diagnosis in England, UK: A national, population-based, modelling study. Lancet **21**(8), 1023–1034 (2020)
27. https://www.who.int/docs/default-source/coronaviruse/clinical-management-of-novel-cov.pd. Accessed 20 Jan 2021
28. S.M. Lemon et al., *Ethical and Legal Considerations in Mitigating Pandemic Disease: Workshop Summary* (Institute of Medicine (US) Forum on Microbial Threats, National Academies Press, Washington, DC, 2007)
29. I. Rudan, A cascade of causes that led to the COVID-19 tragedy in Italy and other European Union countries. J. Glob. Health **10**(1), 010335 (2020)
30. A. Clark, M. Jit, C. Warren-Gash, B. Guthrie, H.H.X. Wang, S.W. Mercer, C. Sanderson, M. McKee, C. Troeger, K.L. Ong, F. Checchi, P. Perel, S. Joseph, H.P. Gibbs, A. Banerjee, R.M. Eggo, Centre for the Mathematical Modelling of Infectious Diseases COVID-19 Working Group, Global, regional, and national estimates of the population at increased risk of severe COVID-19 due to underlying health conditions in 2020: a modelling study. Lancet Glob. Health (2020)

Chapter 18
Being Resilient to Deal with Attrition of Nurses in Private COVID-19 Hospitals: Critical Analysis with Respect to the Crisis in Kolkata, India

Soumik Gangopadhyay and Amitava Ukil

18.1 Introduction

The entire world is experiencing the biggest catastrophe of this century in the form of COVID-19 pandemic [47]. From salience to the resonance of the corona attack, countries are competing in a number of affected patients of COVID-19. Countless count in several crisscross attacks, a sharp rise in mortality of COVID-19 has compelled the world community to face a new health challenge [44]. This wildfire epidemic of COVID-19, which originated from China, has made its roaring presence with a myriad count among Indians. The first case of corona victimisation was detected on 30 January 2020 in India. According to The Hindu, 17 March 2020, West Bengal marked its presence in the list of victimisation on 15 March 2020 in Kolkata, the oldest metro of India. Incidentally, urban India has also witnessed a dramatic paradigm shift in the dominance of mortality burden from non-communicable to infectious diseases. High infectivity rate, zero preventive option, silent attack, unwarranted therapeutic option and inestimable death have left no option other than 'lockdown' before the human being. Social distancing has a profound potentiality to break the contagious infection chain of COVID-19. According to WHO, it is an attempt to arrest the intensity of community infection and scale up tertiary care preparation. Adhering with WHO guidelines, the lockdown was imposed at every nook and corner of India on 24 March 2020 and unlock started from 8 June 2020. India has registered approximately 10 lakh cases

S. Gangopadhyay (✉)
Business Administration Institute of Engineering and Management, Kolkata, India
e-mail: soumik.gangopadhyay@iemcal.com

A. Ukil
Department of Business Administration, Eminent College of Management & Technology, Kolkata, India

L. Garg et al. (eds.), *Healthcare Informatics for Fighting COVID-19 and Future Epidemics*, EAI/Springer Innovations in Communication and Computing,
https://doi.org/10.1007/978-3-030-72752-9_18

of the disease even after ensuring social distancing through nationwide 'lockdown' of residents for approximately 74 days. Mondal [1] observed that even with a less than average Global Health Security score (GHS-2019), i.e. 46.5, India has given an encouraging fight against corona attack as compared to many developed nations. Indian research in the treatment of corona attack with hydroxychloroquine and self-reliant initiatives for vaccine development to prevent the disease has justified its dedication to protect health of the world community.

Sound tertiary care facilities and adequate emergency healthcare infrastructure are the fundamental options before the COVID-19 victims to combat the escalating trend in corona victimisation [48]. But, Anand and Fan [2] report indicates the proportional shortage in a number of hospital beds, doctors and nurses in pre covid-19 era of West Bengal regarding population compared to WHO standards. Per capita expenditure on health is near the average for Indian states at US$3.50 per head (42). Moreover, 44.7% of West Bengal residents do not use government health facilities compared to the Indian national average of 55.1% [43]. Poor access to medical care, too long waiting time and poor quality of care are the three major causes of non-usage of state government health facilities among the non-users (4th round of National Family Health Survey, 2015–2016). Evidenced-based analytical research of Rana and Mishra [3] has revealed that poor motivation level of clinical staff, improper coordination, poor work culture, the overcrowded and outdated infrastructure of government clinical establishments blended with the accompanying stench of an unhealthy environment backed by nepotism and a delayed response in treatment give goose bumps to the residents of West Bengal. Further, COVID-19 pandemic has imposed a new burden of healthcare/welfare expenses on the world community [4]. In essence, even the improved emotional responses to COVID-19, combined with the latest medical technology currently available and accessible in public tertiary care, have failed to combat this deadly trend effectively. Therefore, private hospitals seem to have a pivotal role in treating and/or moderation of patients' individual psyche [5]. In this decade of conscious consumerism, private COVID-19 hospitals are becoming relatively reliable searching for customised care. Prospective patients will prioritise the hospitals for COVID-19 treatment based on these establishments' available clinical skills rather than opportunistic occupancy [40].

Further, Kolkata is the highest corona affected zone in West Bengal with highest death toll [6]. So, uncontrolled escalation in several victims has created a mismatch between the current provision of available occupancy and expected skilled care demand [35]. These are becoming an inevitable deciding factor of choosing private hospitals for COVID-19 treatment, promoting positive word of mouth. Incidentally, COVID-19 caregivers are becoming victims that are variably interrupting the smooth care process of COVID-19 victims [7] and adding value to the existing shortage of population vs doctor/nurse ratio.

18.1.1 Problems Behind the Problem

Healthcare is a labour-intensive industry that depends on specific skills. Underprepared, quasi-prepared health systems of several countries are fighting to save their residents' life on the face of COVID-19 pandemic. Sundararaman [8] has stated that inadequate public healthcare facility, improper health surveillance system and an insufficient workforce in dealing such a menace are the obstacles in effectively dealing with such a disease outbreak in India.

So, the Indian community has been compelled to pause and ponder on this current, burgeoning health crisis. Several researchers like Singh [9] have spotted the damaging effects of COVID-19 on the national economy and its impact on the negative economic outcome [44]. According to the Government of West Bengal Health Department, around 6500 nurses work in private hospitals in Kolkata and its suburbs. Almost, 80% of them (more than 5000) hail from outside West Bengal. Kolkata's private hospitals have faced a fresh crisis of nurses in recent times when 500 nurses have resigned in May 2020 from major hospitals [36], including R.N. Tagore International Institute of Cardiac Sciences, BelleVue and Fortis, Medica, IRIS Multispeciality Hospital, Apollo Gleneagles Hospitals Limited, AMRI Hospitals, Fortis Healthcare Limited, Charnock Hospital and BelleVue Hospital [10]. Atri [11] has mentioned that approximately 500 nurses have gone back to their home states, including 318, 43, 32 and 2, respectively, from Manipur, Tripura, Orissa and Jharkhand. Based on the exit interview of Manipur bound nurses, The Week, May (2020) have cited work station related dissatisfiers such as agitated mental health and/depression incubated from poor pay protective gear, extended working hours, zero extra payment for overtime at a private hospital, lack of adequate leave, more accountability and work pressure, job insecurity, shortage of personal protection equipment (PPE) etc [41]. Apart from the existing problem, few revealed other discouraging reasons: personal safety and security, poor access to food during quarantine, ill-treated by the landlord and uncomfortable accommodation. The Organization of Manipuris in Kolkata (MIK) has expressed several issues like social ostracism, racism, social discrimination, social stigma and mental distress. They sincerely voiced for justice, well-deserved respect and legitimate recognition of their invaluable contributions to humanity's services during this crisis period. Shortage of nursing staff is a perennial problem in Bengal because there are not many training colleges. The majority of trained nurses are occupied with government hospital job because of more salaries and other facilities. Mondal [1] reported that a nurse in the government hospital gets around INR25,000 at the entry level, whereas private hospitals offer between INR16,000 and INR18,000.

On the contrary, concerning hospital authorities have also questioned the professional commitment of the concerned nurses on the face of emergency medical care and blamed this whimsical decision as an act of violation of code of ethical and moral conduct. Moreover, administrators have expressed their serious concerns regarding the state's healthcare system, apprehending a significant nursing care crisis. Interestingly, Andel et al. [12] has proved that cost of poor quality or error in healthcare is very high. Current low occupancy across all hospitals may not affect the operational affairs in the short run, but long-term crisis is guaranteed. Fallible decisions are inevitable in most organisations, as the impact on safety is indirect and invisible. In the wake of the current epidemic, necessary care for COVID-19 patients will be compromised during these difficult times due to short supply of caregivers. This may even give birth to an unhealthy competition of employees poaching among competing hospitals (Table 18.1).

Eighty percent of adverse events in medicine are caused by human error. Human error is the dominant cause of injury and death in hospitals [13]. This will add negative value to potentiate the contemporary fear psychosis among the COVID-19 fighters.

18.2 Survey of Literature

Domenico et al. [14] have observed that equity in access to palliative care is a legitimate right of COVID-19 patients and clinical staff have a crucial role to play in it. But, American Hospital Association [15] has proved that decreased staff satisfaction results in 52% of workforce shortage. Stirling and Harmston [16] proved the irrefutable importance of hospital staff. They play a special role as a communicator and carry out routine procedures in treating such infectious diseases. Research of Lai et al. [17] evidenced, nurses and other frontline health professionals have shown maximum mental setback in the fight against the coronavirus. Moreover, Zhang et al. [18] mentioned that the importance of both the caregivers and care receivers' mental health has to be ensured. But, Zhenyu et al. [19] specified that duty-bound dedicated healthcare professionals become physically and mentally stressed due to the perceived threat of being a victim of COVID-19. Chen et al. [20, 21] derived the reasons of such are poor access to recommended personal protective equipment, the probability to be an asymptomatic carrier to their family or a victim, inadequate or late access to testing if they develop COVID-19 symptoms and the concomitant fear of propagating infection at work, the uncertainty of support from an employer for self and family protection, isolation from home, improper support for personal and family needs as work hours increase, uncertainty with respect to professional competency in a new environment with the constrained facility, lack of access to up-to-date information and poor communication. Further, Stirling et al. [22] mentioned that with a perceived probability of self-victimisation in caring MERS-CoV patients, nurses become depressed. Zhenyu et al. [19] have termed this as 'vicarious traumatisation'. Adams and Walls [23] heard the remorse sound of homesick, overloaded, overstressed, isolated caregivers seeking relief from these life-risk assignments. The disturbed souls demand 'hear me', 'protect me', 'prepare me', 'support me' and 'care for me' [24].

Nurses were in a conundrum. In the battle against corona, these warriors fight between role and obligation. Obligation backed by a perceived threat of physical existence due to the increased probability of infection became a priority. Perceived

Table 18.1 Information on Covid-19 treatment facilities and nurse attrition of private hospitals of Kolkata

Sl. No.	Name of the private hospital	No of isolation beds for COVID-19 patients	No of ventilators	No. of nurses left
1	AMRI Hospital, Dhakuria	7	25	72
2	AMRI Hospital, Mukundapur	5	23	
3	AMRI Hospital, Salt Lake	10	25	
4	Apollo Gleneagles Hospitals	13	63	10
5	BelleVue Clinic	8	30	37
6	Bhagirathi Neotia Hospital, Kolkata	1	2	11
7	Calcutta Heart Clinic, Salt Lake	6	8	00
8	Charnock Hospital	23	19	41
9	CMRI	12	65	00
10	Columbia Asia Hospital, Salt Lake	4	7	00
11	Desun Hospital	5	28	76
12	Divine Nursing Home	7	4	00
13	EEDF Medicare Centre (Sri Aurobindo Seva Kendra)	5	2	52
14	Fortis Hospital Ltd.	8	42	16
15	Genesis Hospital	4	3	NA
16	ILS Dumdum	5	2	NA
17	ILS Hospital, Salt Lake	3	4	NA
18	Institute of Neurosciences	2	28	NA
19	Medica Superspecialty Hospital	10	45	93
20	Narayana Superspeciality Hospital	1	25	NA
21	Nightingale Hospital	2	1	NA
22	North City Hospital	6	2	NA
23	Peerless Hospital	8	24	37
24	R.N. Tagore International Institute of Cardiac Science	5	60	10
25	Ruby General Hospital	2	14	6
26	Woodlands Multispeciality Hospital	2	22	NA
27	IRIS Hospital	NA	NA	11
	Total	158	571	472

Source: Covid19_Pvt_Hospitals_Kol_Isolation_22_March_20.pdf.; Eisamay, News18, 16th May '20 [37]
NA not available

dissatisfaction has shifted from job satisfaction-related aspects, i.e. workload or poor remuneration to an aspect of self-existence. Hence, the problems potentiate further, and job-related reason becomes the escape route. Wu et al. [25] have shown that detecting signs of emotional stress, identifying cause and treatment and promoting health and happiness protocols must be designed to handle such psychological, occupational hazards effectively. Blake et al. [26] stressed on a prototype-based design validation to check the acceptability, usability, demand, implementation, practicability, adaptation and integration before execution.

18.2.1 Role of Automation in Healthcare

The intervention of technology in disease detection, prevention, mitigation and monitoring has immense potential to combat highly infectious diseases like COIVD-19. Contactless Bluetooth-driven devices are now uniformly used in many clinical premises to measure body temperature and blood pressure to combat COVID-19. Thus, semi-skilled jobs can be performed by non-clinical staff to reduce the workload of nurses to engage them more in specialised clinical work. Installation of robot at the interface between patients and doctors has opened the scope of large-scale intervention. Recently, Spot, a robot dog of Boston Dynamics, has been used to assess patients of US hospitals. The Hindu, April (2020), reported that even in India, 'Maitri', a mobile-operated robot, effectively serves Vijayawada-based hospital to monitor and serve the COVID-19 patients [45]. KARMI-Bot, a robot, was deployed to assist patients at COVID-19 isolation wards of Ernakulam Government Medical College of Kerala to reduce the risk of infection of doctors and other health workers. Jaipur-based Sawai Man Singh Hospital has also started using robots in isolation wards to deliver food and other items among COVID-19 patients [46]. Such operational changes reduce 10% chance of exposure per round of visits by a robot compared to a clinical staff [27].

Artificial intelligence (AI) is the new oil in the emerging field of health that functions at the intersection of medical informatics, public health and business, referring to health services and information delivered or enhanced through the internet and related technologies. With the application of artificial intelligence (AI), risk of transmission of contagious viruses can be minimised. Stanczyk [28] observed that such alternative initiatives are very efficient and effective in the automatic diagnosis of diseases, research and development of a vaccine and disinfection of remote or inaccessible areas of hospitals as it has successfully fulfilled expected objectives in recent past. Machine learning has been applied even to analyse the pattern of infection and death of victims from big data. Keith [29] has mentioned regarding the usage of BlueDot, a Canadian AI initiative that has alerted the entire world on the first outbreak of corona at its epicentre in China. So, a proactive technology-based preparedness turns a hospital ready to combat unforeseen future challenges.

e-Health can provide extra revenue earning for hospitals by providing health service to home-quarantined patients [30]. Telemedicine for patients with other diseases can be given additional support. m-Health apps such as 'Aarogya Setu' have been designed to trace and track possible carriers of contagious diseases that can offload the pressure on critical COVID-19 care. Such algorithm-based contact tracing apps are widely being used in China, Singapore, Hong Kong, South Korea, Italy, Israel and so on, which has helped detect cross-infection risk through real-time inter-sectoral integration. These apps can even exchange updated health information with the patients, doctors booking, brand promotion, etc. Prior to such implementations, a need-based survey is a necessity to justify the relevance, effectiveness and feasibility. Some of the affected private hospitals of Kolkata have already started e-health and m-health services for the COVID-19 patients [39]. The offer includes a remote monitoring package that contains a digital thermometer, pulse oximeter, doctor's telephonic advice/video conferencing and routine visit at home for mild symptomatic home-quarantined patients at minimum cost. Moreover, the distant monitoring system helps solve the bed crisis for the COVID-19 patients as doctors can access the patient's report, uploaded in a hospital app. Atri [11] has confirmed that patients with other diseases also get the benefits of doctor's booking, doctor's consultation and updated information through this system.

So, it is not reliable to depend on human healthcare as it is unsafe and insecure, which can be replaced by machine for non-skilled work.

18.3 Proposed Model

Radical acceptance of change is an antidote to uncertainty. Resilience can be brought with thought, behaviour and action-oriented changes. Innovention is partial innovation. it is a fusion of invention and innovation. Several approaches deriving robots or applying AI are complying such term. A blend of proactive (information, integration) and reactive (innovention) approach may help them adapt to such situations.

18.3.1 Information

Time is the essence of quality care which is crucial in treating COVID-19. Motivation cannot be mass-produced, but complacency in dealing with caregiver's working station-related problems may pile up issues to germinate crises. Moreover, a proactive real-time information collection can uncover a hidden problem derived due to underreporting. So, the information should be collected at legitimate intervals from different sources regarding the dissatisfaction of clinical employees which can be collected for better surveillance. Continuous monitoring of workforce requirement must be based on triage rather than on statute. Even the workload can be monitored to create a better work-life balance of caregivers of paramount importance [38]. Primary data-based research of Ackerson and Stiles [31] has proved training as an effective tool to retain nurses that reduces organisational expenses. However, attention to nurses' requirements, affection for them and legitimate appreciation for good work are key to retaining nurses.

18.3.2 *Integration*

The future breakdown is unpredictable that may occur at a more critical time, leading to higher losses. Also, the strong focus on keeping the process going to reduce interruptions is a self-defeating endeavour as future problems will cause more interruptions and loss of time. So, collaboration with nursing colleges with the help of a mutually beneficial contract can ensure nurses' uninterrupted flow. These nurses can use hospitals for the inheritance of knowledge. Liaisons with other workforce supply chains such as external recruiting agencies can bring long-term relief.

18.3.3 *Innovention*

This term is a fusion of act of invention and innovation. Virtual, augmented reality and robotics will consolidate business more resilient for the future. A Czechoslovakia-based hospital has installed auto-updating basic information of patients. Bluetooth-driven stethoscope is also an example. The recent work of Baru [32] emanated that China, the epicentre of the COVID-19 epidemic, plans to incorporate telemedicine and public-private sector partnerships to face a similar inevitable epidemic in the future. Workforce to machine power can help to cope up with the changing needs of the situation. IoT-based automated contact tracing [33] and remote patient monitoring [34] have also demonstrated their effectiveness during COVID-19 pandemic.

18.4 Conclusion

As the disease progresses, healthcare system capacity and response need to be enhanced. A comprehensive emergency plan concentrated on collective approach may help to attain short-term crisis. Real-time public display of several available and occupied beds, doctors, nurses, ventilators and so on at hospital premises updated at reasonable intervals can clarify the victims. Moreover, other paramedical staff or locals can be trained for nominal healthcare activities to provide saline and oxygen support and check blood pressure or temperature to help with the short-term crisis.

But, it can be complementary, not substitute. Further, flexibility and adaptability training will prepare the nurses better to cope up with a new system for change management. Mental mapping of the nurses is a prerequisite to infuse emotional resilience. This can be a strategy to establish behavioural competence among caregivers. The identical health crisis is sure to arrive in future, and dependency on human capital may not be guaranteed. Machines are more commit-mental than a human being as it doesn't have an emotion that makes them comparatively reliable. In such a scenario, dependency on technology-based system and devices shall be a more reliable, cost-effective and outstanding progressive step for hospitals. So, a quest for technology-based innovation, being agile with updated information and integrating with healthcare stakeholders, can turn these hospitals to be resilient. Thus a hospital can create a game-changing strategy to sustain a competitive environment with a perfect caregiver balance.

References

1. S. Mondal, Nurse exodus leaves private hospitals in crisis in Calcutta, The Telegraph Online, 8 Mar 2019, https://www.telegraphindia.com/west-bengal/nurse-exodus-leaves-private-hospitals-in-crisis-in-calcutta/cid/1686413
2. S. Anand, V. Fan, *The Health Workforce in India*, Human Resources for Health Observer Series, vol 16 (World Health Organization, Geneva, 2016) http://www.who.int/hrh/resources/16058health_workforce_India.pdf?ua=1
3. K.P. Rana, P.B. Mishra, Ailing health status in West Bengal critical analysis. J. Law Policy Glob. **2**, 1–6 (2012)
4. WHO announces COVID-19 outbreak a pandemic, 12 Mar 2020, https://www.euro.who.int/en/health-topics/health-emergencies/coronavirus-covid-19/news/news/2020/3/who-announces-covid-19-outbreak-a-pandemic
5. S. Gangopadhyay, Noncommunicable diseases, a potential danger of Indian health disparity: Wait until dark, in *Special Issue of The Indian Economic Journal on Inequality and Human Development in Proceedings of the 98th Annual Conference of Indian Economic Association on Growth, in association with Centre for Economic & Social Studies, Hyderabad and IPE, Hyderabad*, (2015), pp. 212–221
6. Nurses leave for home, Kolkata private hospitals stare at crisis, Sumati Yengkhom | TN N, The Times of India, 16 May 2020, https://timesofindia.indiatimes.com/city/kolkata/nurses-leave-for-home-kol-pvt-hospitals-stare-at-crisis/articleshow/75768370.cms
7. Senior Bengal health official detected with corona dies Outlook, The News Scroll, 26 Apr 2020., https://www.outlookindia.com/newsscroll/senior-bengal-health-official-detected-with-corona-dies/1815104
8. T. Sundararaman, Health systems preparedness for COVID-19 pandemic. Indian J. Public Health **64**(6), 91–93 (2020)
9. S.S. Singh, Coronavirus | Kolkata reports first case. Kolkata, 18 Mar 2020, https://www.thehindu.com/news/national/other-states/coronavirus-west-bengal-reports-first-case/article31093265.ece
10. 'Maitri' robot to serve COVID-19 patients in Vijayawada, The New Indian Express, 25 May 2020, https://www.newindianexpress.com/cities/vijayawada/2020/may/25/maitri-robot-to-serve-covid-19-patients-in-vijayawada-2147602.html
11. M. Atri, 'No pay, heckling': 300 nurses leave Kolkata hospitals, go back to Manipur, The Indian express, Atri Mitra | Kolkata, 20 May 2020., https://indianexpress.com/article/india/no-pay-heckling-300-nurses-leave-kolkata-hospitals-go-back-to-manipur-cornavirus-6418278/

12. C. Andel, L.S. Davidow, M. Hollander, A.D. Moreno, The economics of health care quality and medical errors. J. Health Care Finance **39**(1), 39–50 (2012)
13. Institute of Medicine (US) Committee on Quality of Health Care in America, in *To Err is Human: Building a Safer Health System*, Errors in Health Care: A Leading Cause of Death and Injury, ed. by L. T. Kohn, J. M. Corrigan, M. S. Donaldson, vol. 2, (National Academies Press, Washington, DC, 2000) https://www.ncbi.nlm.nih.gov/books/NBK225187/
14. G.B. Domenico, G. Claudia, O. Monika, J. Ralf, COVID-19: Decision making and palliative care. Swiss Med. Wkly. **150**, w20233 (2020). https://doi.org/10.4414/smw.2020.20233
15. American Hospital Association, The state of America's Hospitals—Taking the Pulse (2006), http://www.ahapolicyforum.org/ahapolicyforum/reports/
16. B. Stirling, J. Harmston, Readying nurses for clinical practice: Protecting students during an outbreak of Middle Eastern-Coronavirus in Saudi Arabia. Int. J. Educ. Pract. **5**, 34 (2015)
17. J. Lai, M. Simeng, W. Ying, C. Zhongxiang, H. Jianbo, W. Ning, W. Jiang, Factors associated with mental health outcomes among health care workers exposed to coronavirus disease 2019. JAMA **3**(3) (2020). https://doi.org/10.1001/jamanetworkopen.2020.3976
18. S. Zhang, L. Jing, A.J. Asghar, N. Khaled, Y. Ali, L. Jizhen, S. Shuhua, At the height of the storm: Healthcare Staff's health conditions and job satisfaction and their associated predictors during the epidemic peak of COVID-19. Brain Behav. Immun. (2020). https://doi.org/10.1016/j.bbi.2020.05.010
19. L. Zhenyu, J. Ge, M. Yang, J. Feng, M. Qiao, R. Jiang, J. Bi, G. Zhan, X. Xu, L. Wang, Q. Zhou, C. Zhou, Y. Pan, S. Liu, H. Zhang, J. Yang, B. Zhu, Y. Hu, K. Hashimoto, Y. Jia, H. Wang, R. Wang, C. Liu, C. Yang, Vicarious traumatization traumatisation in the general public, members, and non-members of medical teams aiding in COVID-19 control. Brain Behav. Immun. (2020). https://doi.org/10.1016/j.bbi.2020.03.007
20. Chen, K.Y., Yang, C.M., & Lien, C.H. (2013). Burnout, job satisfaction, and medical malpractice among physicians. Int. J. Med. Sci., 10(11),1471–1478
21. Chen, Q., Liang, M & Li, Y. (2020). Mental health care for medical staff in China during the COVID-19 outbreak. Lancet Psychiatry, 7(4), e15-e16
22. B. Stirling, J. Hatcher, J. Harmston, Communicating the changing role of a nurse in an epidemic: The example of the MERS-CoV outbreak in Saudi Arabia. J Healthc. Commun. **2**(3) (2017). https://doi.org/10.4172/2472-1654.100070
23. J.G. Adams, R.M. Walls, Supporting the health care workforce during the COVID-19 global epidemic. JAMA **323**(15), 1439–1440 (2020). https://doi.org/10.1001/jama.2020.3972
24. T. Shanafelt, J. Ripp, M. Trockel, Understanding and addressing sources of anxiety among health care professionals during the COVID-19 pandemic. JAMA (2020). https://doi.org/10.1001/jama.2020.5893
25. E. Wu, S.R. Peter, L.W. Gold, Mitigating the psychological effects of COVID-19 on health care workers. CMAJ **192**, E459–E460 (2020). https://doi.org/10.1503/cmaj.200519
26. H. Blake, F. Bermingham, G. Johnson, A. Tabner, Mitigating the psychological impact of COVID-19 on healthcare workers: A digital learning package. Int. J. Environ. Res. Public Health **17**(2997), 2–15 (2020). https://doi.org/10.3390/ijerph17092997
27. S. Baneerjee, SMS Hospital brings in robots to serve COVID-19 patients, 26 Mar 2020, http://health.economictimes.indiatimes.com/news/industry/sms-hospitals-brings-in-robots-to-serve-covid-19-patients/74827822
28. B. Stanczyk, AI in the times of corona: Robots can reduce human contact, transmission of Covid-19. Healthworld.com, The Economic Times, 9 May 2020
29. D. Keith, How artificial intelligence is helping prevent the spread of the covid-19 pandemic, https://www.bbvaopenmind.com/en/technology/artificial-intelligence/how-ai-is-helping-prevent-the-spread-of-the-covid-19-pandemic/
30. I. Hernández-García, T. Giménez-Júlvez, Assessment of health information about COVID-19 prevention on the internet: Infodemiological study. JMIR Public Health Surveill. **6**(2), e18717 (2020). https://doi.org/10.2196/18717

31. K. Ackerson, A.K. Stiles, Value of nurse residency programs in retaining new graduate nurses and their potential effect on the nursing shortage. J. Cont. Educ. Nurs. **49**(6), 282–288 (2018). https://doi.org/10.3928/00220124-20180517-09
32. R.V. Baru, Health systems preparedness during COVID-19 pandemic: China and India. IJPH **64**(6), 96–98 (2020) http://www.ijph.in/text.asp?2020/64/6/96/285619
33. L. Garg, E. Chukwu, N. Nasser, C. Chakraborty, G. Garg, Anonymity preserving IoT-based covid-19 and other infectious disease contact tracing model. IEEE Access **8**, 159402–159414 (2020)
34. M. Jayalakshmi, L. Garg, K. Maharajan, K. Srinivasan, K. Jayakumar, A.K. Bashir, K. Ramesh, Fuzzy logic-based health monitoring system for COVID'19 patients. Comput. Mater. Continua (2022)
35. T. Chatterjee, Migrant nurses leaving Bengal for safety; private hospitals face manpower shortage, Hindustan Times, Kolkata, 16 May 2020, https://www.hindustantimes.com/kolkata/migrant-nurses-leaving-bengal-for-safety-private-hospitals-face-manpower-shortage/story-htJzRdHYup8IP713ZOObAM.html
36. Eisamay, News18, 16 May 2020, https://eisamay.indiatimes.com/west-bengal-news/kolkata-news/west-bengal-cm-mamata-banerjee-says-about-alternative-way-to-fight-against-nurses-crisis-in-bengal/articleshow/75805199.cms
37. Covid-19_Pvt_Hospitals_Kol_Isolation_22_March_20.pdf, http://wbhealth.gov.in/uploaded_files/corona/Covid-19_Pvt_Hospitals_Kol_Isolation_22_March_20.pdf.i
38. Q. Liu, D. Luo, E.J. Haase, Q. Guo, Q.X. Wang, S. Liu, L. Xia, Z. Liu, J. Yang, X.B. Yang, The experiences of healthcare providers during the covid-19 crisis in China: A qualitative study. Lancet Glob. Health **8**(6), e790–e798 (2020). https://doi.org/10.1016/S2214-109X(20)30204-7
39. M. Prithvijit, Private hospitals in Kolkata offer mild patients home-monitoring packages, Times of India, Kolkata dt, 16 Jun 2020., https://timesofindia.indiatimes.com/city/kolkata/pvt-hosps-offer-mild-patients-home-monitoring-packages/articleshow/76395594.cms
40. B.S. Neogi, G.S. Preetha, Assessing health systems' responsiveness in tackling COVID-19 pandemic. Indian J. Public Health **64**(6), 211–216 (2020) http://www.ijph.in
41. PTI report on 'Contrary to pvt hospital body's claim in WB Manipuri nurses say lack of safety reason to quit job', The Week, 18 May 2020, https://www.theweek.in/wire-updates/national/2020/05/18/cal23-mn-nurses-bengal.html
42. PWC report, https://www.pwc.in/assets/pdfs/publications/2018/reimagining-the-possible-in-the-indian-healthcare-ecosystem-with-emerging-technologies.pdf
43. https://www.iiste.org/Journals/index.php/JLPG/article/download/1212/1133
44. K.M. Singh, Y. Neog, Contagion effect of COVID-19 outbreak: Another recipe for disaster on Indian economy. J. Public Affairs **20**, e2171 (2020). https://doi.org/10.1002/pa.2171
45. https://health.economictimes.indiatimes.com/news/health-it/ai-in-the-times-of-corona-robots-can-reduce-human-contact-transmission-of-covid-19/75646859d-1
46. Kerala government hospital deploys robot to serve COVID-19 patients, The Hindu, 25 Apr 2020, https://www.thehindu.com/news/national/kerala/kerala-government-hospital-deploys-robot-to-serve-covid-19-patients/article31432663.ece
47. WHO Director-General's opening remarks at the media briefing on COVID-19, 11 Mar 2020, https://www.who.int/dg/speeches/detail/who-director-general-s-opening-remarks-at-the-media-briefing-on-covid-19%2D%2D-11-march-2020
48. West Bengal sees 2,000+ new cases in a day for first time, The Times of India, 19 Jul 2020, https://timesofindia.indiatimes.com/city/kolkata/west-bengal-sees-2000-new-cases-in-a-day-for-first-time-toll-at-a-high-of-27/articleshow/77045371.cms

Chapter 19
Healthcare Technology for Reducing the Risk and the Spread of COVID-19 Pandemic and Other Epidemics

Suchandra Dutta, Dhrubasish Sarkar, Premananda Jana, and Dipak K. Kole

19.1 Introduction

In today's time when the entire world has been fighting with COVID-19, it is essential to track the disease's spread in a trajectory to curb down the spread rate and the growth rate as much as possible. COVID-19 possesses an infectious spread where the disease spreads through droplets of infected individuals and a substantial format without any precautions. Due to the absence of any medication, it is crucial to curb down the disease's spread. Cough and cold, acute fever, headache, nausea, and loss of taste are some of the very common symptoms of the disease, similar to the very primary influenza virus. Modern healthcare technology helps in the control of such diseases which may cause future epidemics.

Modern healthcare technologies can make an easy epidemic method and reply in unique and difficult to obtain sequentially. A few countries had already incorporated modern technology into federal government-coordinated contingency and prevention methods, along with monitoring, checking, contact tracing, and tight quarantine that might be correlated with the initial weakening of one's prevalence graphs. As a result, healthcare technology will assist in making the task of treating the corona virus disease easier.

S. Dutta · D. Sarkar (✉)
Amity Institute of Information Technology, Amity University, Kolkata, West Bengal, India

P. Jana
Netaji Subhas Open University, Kalyani, West Bengal, India

D. K. Kole
Department of CSE, Jalpaiguri Government Engineering College, Jalpaiguri, West Bengal, India
e-mail: dipak.kole@cse.jgec.ac.in

L. Garg et al. (eds.), *Healthcare Informatics for Fighting COVID-19 and Future Epidemics*, EAI/Springer Innovations in Communication and Computing,
https://doi.org/10.1007/978-3-030-72752-9_19

19.2 Discussion on the Spread of COVID-19 and Other Epidemics

At first, we spoke about what a coronavirus is. Over the course of nearly two decades, researchers and scientists have been mapping the source of the deadly infectious disease across China's highest peaks and even most elusive canyons and grottos. Researchers ended up discovering these in the 'Shitou' canyon bats. This disease at issue had been a coronavirus which triggered a series, Severe Acute Respiratory Syndrome (SARS) outbreak in 2003. A coronavirus is a collection of viruses coated in small clusters of protein that appear in Latin as a crown or 'corona'.

Hundreds of known coronaviruses occur globally; seven of these can affect human beings and cause disease. The seventh, which produces COVID-19, has functionalities; it grows fast but can severely affect the lung. Droplets that hold the virus spill out after infected individual coughs. Once the droplets touch the patient's nose or mouth, the virus will affect a new individual. Coronavirus better communicates in enclosed areas, where individuals are close to one another.

Cold atmosphere persists in its sensitive casing from keeping soaking, making it possible for the virus to survive longer among servers, even when ultraviolet exposure to sunlight can harm it. This temperature difference is much more critical for the accepted virus since none is immune from new viruses, which have many other prospective servers. It needs not even an optimum environment to stretch.

In the human body, sharp protein rise is embedded in the infected cells and fuses with them, allowing the virus to infiltrate gene-encoding machines to reproduce its genes. Coronavirus places its genes on ribonucleic acid (RNA).

All viruses consist of either RNA viruses or DNA viruses; coronavirus tends to be narrower, cum lesser genes, which means that to attendees are infected as well as replicated rapidly in these attendees. Generally, coronavirus does not have a rereading method, whereas DNA viruses do.

The dynamic model of COVID-19 was modified by selecting the objective functions of $f_1(y)$ and $f_2(y)$ based on proof and collected with the help of data obtained over a prolonged time from various regions among the country. One might, too, determine time reliance on parameters β and n to have a much more accurate estimation of y [1].

The dynamic model can be arithmetically amended by considering the incredible variety of catastrophe organisational schemes in different areas of just such a big country. This model's fundamental presumption is that the client is instantly put in total secrecy if an indicative issue is identified. That's far from how this happens in the real world in several instances [1].

Droplet transmission through one or more droplets generated one infected person Coughs to a neighbouring person. Contact transfers infection through when a person touches the infected surface and then the nose or eyes and mouth.

The transmission of aerosols in one respecter droplet contains the virus mixture into the air and then into the health. COVID-19 is stable for up to 24 h on cartons, 23 days on plastics and stainless steel, and up to 3 h on aerosols, including fog, dust, and smog. Thus it is possible to get afflicted by touching contaminated objects or through the air. The implantation timeframe is the time between infection and onset of symptoms for illness. COVID-19 incubation forecasts ranged from 2 to 14 days but are widely expected to be around (median) 5 days.

There is too much controversy in the latent period between infection and infectiousness. It has become short that persons with COVID-19 may be infectious ever since they show symptoms and display a latent period shorter than the incubation period. A patient is sick in one place and confirmed to be ill in another, according to an imported case.

Local transmission throughout a traveller infects others. If there is a regionally and expanded group, such supported care for the patients and the same family is easily identified. Prevalent interpretation, along all, if there is no consistent cause of infection, contagiousness can be measured using:

$$\text{Measured by } R_0 = \text{REPRODUCTION NUMBER}$$

This is several mean cases that an infected person will cause throughout their infectious timespan, so, if $R_0 = 3$.

The infected person will infect an average of three other people who get afflicted. There are two important types are in R_0, these are as follows:

(a) The basic reproduction number: It identifies the highest potential of the pathogen to infect humans. Essentially, will it happen if an infectious person enters a group with several prior immunities?
(b) The effective reproduction number: It represents the group of people's situation vulnerability based on whether people have immunity from vaccination or previous exposure. The efficacy does not decrease in the duration of an outbreak.

Both basic and effective reproduction numbers rely on environmental factors (e.g. climate) and demography (e.g. population and group statistics, i.e. age, education, religion, race, gender, and socioeconomic status) additament to telepathy and contagiousness.

The achievement of public health interventions is to bring R_0 down to less than 1, causing the disease to die over time.

High R_0 estimates mean there is much greater potential for spread of COVID-19 than for the flu.

Will see how much more there is.

Consider the following example: let's say the flu $R_0 = 1.5$ and COVID-19 $R_0 = 3$.

After three cycles of infection 11 people had the flu and 40 people were infected through COVID-19 but after the ten cycles of infection, flu becomes 171 people for the flu and over 88,573 people for COVID-19 (Fig. 19.1) [2].

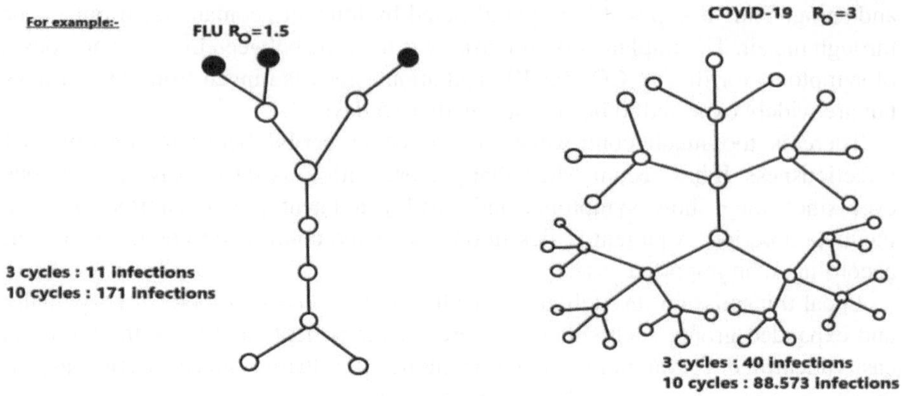

Fig. 19.1 Chain of flu and COVID-19

19.3 Overview of Healthcare Technologies

So what is healthcare technology? Mobile healthcare technology refers to all IT (information technology) tools or technologies built to improve healthcare centres and organisational performance, offer comprehensive data via therapy and treatment, and improve the consistency of medication provided. The number of patient waiting is decreasing; for such involvement of AI and data analytics is unavoidable, hospitals are functioning that efficiently. The involvement of ultra-precise devices for robotics is unquestionable for operations and more dishonest raptors in other procedures; even clinical procedures like recovery levels are being reduced.

The paper asserts that perhaps the WWW (World Wide Web) is a site. The appropriate basis for the use of work process techniques in the healthcare industry. Massive techniques (e.g. mobile information technology, JavaScript, Java applets, Java servlets, and Dynamic HTML) are used to supply the flow of workout over the World Wide Web. Trying to apply this one to mobile computing, the design code proposals for web-based WFMS are then explored.

Some of the researchers conclude that even a healthcare-based 'workflow management system' (WFMS), utilising 'object-orientated' (OO) technology, must be transmitted and diverse and also that the World Wide Web (WWW) is an appropriate basis for the use of workflow systems [3].

Private technology is leading to a new era of healthcare. It is radically changing where and how medical decisions are taken, and diagnosis is created through a confluence of wearable health monitoring techniques. Telemedicine, home diagnosis, and even a pop-up retail setting are examples of healthcare technologies.

Electronic health records, or EHRs, track almost any aspect of one's health, from visits to doctors to major surgery. With the growing acceptance of EHRs, healthcare practitioners need to maintain and secure this information. There are even more software and healthcare in history today than every other time, which increases the need for expertise and advanced technologies for people.

Healthcare professionals have begun to recognise the significance of mobile treatment of patients. In 2014, 2.3 billion dollars was lifted for healthcare technology start-ups, and between 2011 and 2014, 1.9 billion dollars was brought up for data management companies.

By 2018, 70% of healthcare providers are advised to spend in mobile health devices with approximately 1.5 trillion dollars in differential healthcare control technologies and the android app, an increasing craze in distant health care services.

'House Calls Plus'—It has permitted more quick and efficient medication for patients and their homes to reduce overall resources needed to sustain and enhance care quality.

'Pilot Programs'—It is displaying outstanding outcomes, although one program in the US decreasing hospital admissions registers by 18% for its pediatric patients to use monitoring systems and interaction and admittance also dumped by 31% of all expenses to the test center by 7% and lowered alternative to care facility-run health programs is driving patients to wearable and Some customised machines can obtain a wide range of readings that can be compared to several targets and determine to choose whether or not continue to health care providers.

Alternatively, some patients could choose to communicate health social media networks to share the information from computerised readings, consult a doctor throughout question and answer meetings, and sometimes pursue psychological support. Patients could also use a mobile app to identify the similarity between symptoms and medication interactions.

Poor clinical habits enable choices over how to enhance patient clinically. For further in-depth research, patients may opt to use home kits for customised genomics programs, plasma, and other biomarkers monitoring environmental research and even maintaining a healthcare model. To those who want to contact the healthcare specialists and the number of choices reached to diverts the person far from the hospital pharmacy stores in traditional town centres. Hospitals in rural areas will accept patients, evaluate their records, and determine to either proceed with additional treatment by a doctor; on-call physicians are also widely available to answer questions. Or include medical guidance to clients wherever thru video calling, cellphone emails.

'Telemedicine'—Telemedicine has developed rapidly with up to 80% of hospitals and up to 60% of medical doctors in the USA presently offering these facilities. Telehealth systems have seen a yearly increase of around 30% in recent years. The associated risks with developing customised healthcare technologies believe that technologies will assume the doctor's position.

One hundred forty-two million healthcare and medical applications are estimated to be installed, and approximately 65% of customer healthcare purchases are to be made via smartphones. No fewer clinics and healthcare practitioners are anticipated to have been at the root of all treatment decisions, particularly in specific situations and a revised view of healthcare industries' function in the global supply chain.

Industry 4.0 provides a standardised answer for a variety of applications. Producing and some other public industries. It includes various products and digital data innovations to collect, transfer, store, analyse, and monitor data systems. New technologies include a creative approach to technology. Appropriate separation of an infectious person to reduce the risk of death, accelerate drug production, diagnosis, and treatment. By applying these devices, people have to work from their home; people are finding out a new office environment, work schedules, virtual offices, video conferences, and substantial formal communication processes [2].

19.3.1 Advantages as Well as Usefulness of Healthcare Technologies

Due to radiation treatment and even chemotherapy, technology has been implemented in the healthcare industry to render care for people as easy as possible and improve the industry's efficiency. The different areas where healthcare technology is used that's are basically

1. Management or administrative health care centres as well as hospitals.
2. Use for surgeries.
3. Also, use in the drug development process.
4. Use for self-health care as well as fitness.
5. Treatment and prevention of errors.
6. Also, help to combat depression as well as mental health.

Also, healthcare technologies are progressively being embraced for fighting against the COVID-19 pandemic.

19.4 Primary Healthcare Through Online (Telemedicine): Home-Confined Medical Treatment

Day by day, the hospitals become overcrowded by the coronavirus-affected patient, so in that case or in that situation, if we use telemedicine for the first stage care, we can reduce overcrowded situations in the hospitals and also able to decrease the spread of the virus.

Telemedicine includes providing digital healthcare services using computerised video and auditory methodologies, mainly through real-life relationships between the patient and the provider's healthcare insurer. If anyone catches the coronavirus disease, they don't immediately hurry up to see a doctor.

Telemedicine visit life cycles [4]:

- Planning
- Record

- Measuring with visual acuity
- Intraocular pressure
- Accessary testing
- Experiment
- Intervening
- Preparation as well as working out

It isn't the best approach. It doesn't appear to be caused by supporting the country or emergency individuals with problems they contact the doctor rather than an urgent care facility. Such day doctors can also decide whether somebody is ill with the coronavirus and yet if they need to be checked.

Fast acceptance of telemedicine access panel to also coherence for the patient's care whilst also restricting unneeded care exposed to infectious diseases, like COVID-19. One such kit offers the required guidance for providers, and a patient knows how to fully execute the telehealth program and cooperate through both the bill payment documentary evidence and criteria for coding. Since this is a mainly unknown territory with most procedures, this approach typically must ease integrating a telemedicine scheme [5].

Telemedicine is a choice for those patients who feel sick, and you should have risk going to the hospital and putting your health at future risk or other situation, which has been a disease outbreak explosion. Sufferers may ask physicians about their symptoms or are checked for certain illnesses from the sitting at home; it decreases excessive medication, enabling doctors to concentrate on emergency conditions needing immediate medical care.

The thought that is compulsory for telemedicine technologies must be considered as like

- Various channels include free ones.
- Doctors require both a camera and a microphone.
- Patients require a video camera, computer, as well as a mic or mobile phone.
- Both need excellent accessibility, better communication, and efficient networking such as Wi-Fi or 4G or 5G network.

We all know that the population in India is how much high. So if the spread of the virus is increasing day by day, then the situation will not be in our hands. In this situation, telemedicine will improve the Indian current healthcare system to meet the requirement of this imminent global catastrophe.

India has no healthcare practitioner's shortage, but that could lead to a disastrous situation when the doctors should be quarantined themselves. Sustaining sick patients out of health centres is an important aspect of coronavirus treatment.

Virtual meetings could curb down on unnecessary consultation. More attention is required in such a potential disease setting maintaining healthcare professionals.

There may also be a must for involving patients to recommend accessible and valuable alternatives. There is no time to hesitate. It's indeed conclusive to use every feasible device to prevent feelings of isolation, stress, anxiety, and flutter that may deteriorate the physical effects. It is hoped that the COVID-19 epidemic could

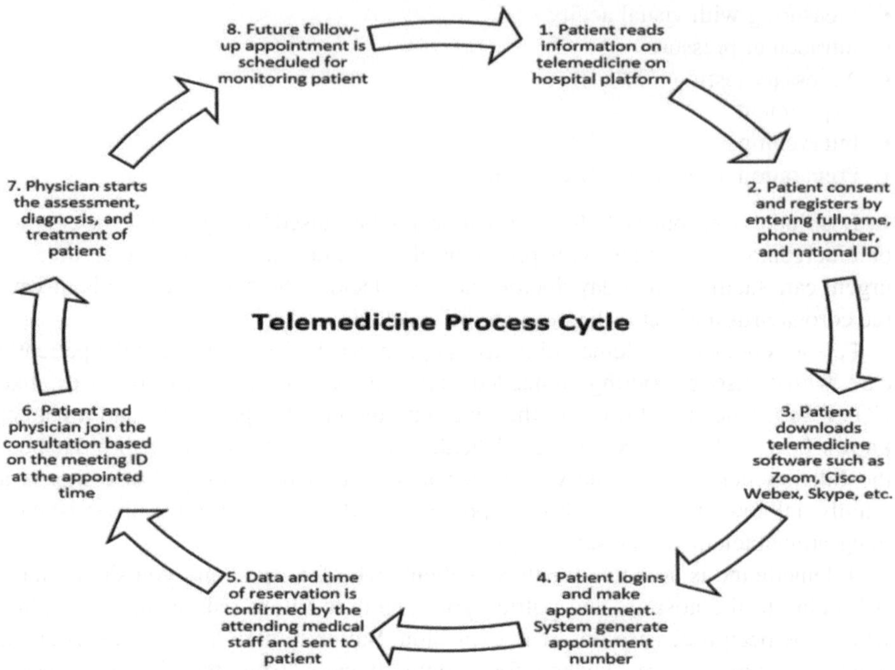

Fig. 19.2 Telemedicine process cycle [14]

even profit from current technologies and help resolve patient data requirements and continued social contact throughout quarantine [6].

The telemedicine processing cycle is shown in the Fig. 19.2.

19.5 Artificial Intelligence to Combat Against the COVID-19

All AI and machine learning are specifically relevant for coronavirus assessment and control and responding. Suppose we can begin mining that data with current artificial intelligence technology. In that case, researchers can receive significant messages of things, occurring in peoples that would have been essential from the viewpoint of responding. Such data alone could be extremely useful for WHO, including public health departments such as the CDC when they just seek to catch a grip about how this epidemic is progressing.

And there's an entire lot of data that we'll get by extracting such unorthodox resources, namely, Twitter data, Facebook data, internet forums and chat rooms, and Google search query data. A wide variety of how people communicate with the internet.

19.5.1 AI Temperature Checking System

Hospitals are fitted with a temperature control alert machine. People in India and over the world are slowly returning to work. AI temperature testing is named in public areas like banks, subways, commercial buildings, and other gathering places.

The world's first intelligent AR temperature measuring glasses were also put into use during the COVID-19 outbreak. The device can scan the people's body temperature in real-time and show it to the weather by way of thermal imaging up to 100 people can be screened within 2 min.

19.5.2 Conducting Follow-Up Visits

Utilising large information, speech detection, and concrete comprehension technologies, AI could help all individuals at risk of disease. Such technologies can make 10,000 phone calls daily while taking a rest.

Jobs can't be achieved with staff and artificial intelligence; they can obtain information with demarcated details for their investigations within only 2 h.

19.5.3 Online Diagnosis

Unless it becomes completely essential, it only needs to stay away from the hospital throughout viral outbreaks. And what if illness hits?—Artificial intelligence could even give a helping hand throughout the shape of online doctors. It takes only 1 min from the independent inquiry stage to try age and trying to connect the patient with a suitable doctor. It also can offer regular medication consultants and health development.

19.5.4 AI Helped to Identify Coronavirus Genetic Sequence in Just a Few Days

Even during SARS (Severe Acute Respiratory Syndrome), epidemics took months to recognise the virus's genetic material. Artificial intelligence plays an essential role. The scientist initially collected BAL (Broncho Alveolar lavage) fluid samples of patients, separated the DNA and RNA pattern of the genetic material by comparing them. Artificial intelligence's advantage is its capacity to identify behaviours despite a massive amount of data.

The coronavirus genetic testing is involved in searching for a thread in a haystack searching for genotype with unique features in a large genetic pool. This follows a subset of current artificial intelligence, a fever-stick target machine.

Paired with micro genomic computation and a virus library, this artificial intelligence technology could also be used to monitor virus mutation. Let's imagine it as an efficient search engine; this search algorithm can shorten month-long genetic sequencing to weeks or even just a few days to identify a virus.

Artificial intelligence does not just assist scientists but can also support the patient by increasing the quality of treatment. China also introduced a genomics program, which can run on multiple virus gene correlations and generate a comprehensive report under 60 s. Such a methodology has been put into use in China and shared with the world for free.

19.5.5 Detection with the Diagnosis of AI

Throughout this case, people will have to diagnose if an individual has COVID-19 both in the internal and external state. The passive or incubation stage can stretch among 2 and 3 days and therefore can quickly be unidentified. Infrared cameras have been used to identify fever symptoms, but the machine won't tell the patients whether it's just the ordinary flu or coronavirus. Some researchers are also using a deep-learning model for detecting the coronavirus on high resolution computed tomography, also known as CT scan. Also, some techniques use saliva to help identify the type of infectious disease instantly. Along with the corona experiment move, there have become more prevalent across the world. Let's take a glance at all of these methods of diagnosis. Thus, the swab test includes obtaining samples from patients, swabbing for their saliva, and monitoring for specific samples. The types of molecules that occur in the genetic information of the new coronavirus. Also, the use of the process called Nucleic Acid Detection.

Nucleic Acid Test—The whole method was helped identify the specific nucleic acid pattern and, therefore, identify and select a certain species for a subspecies of the organism. Sometimes a virus or bacteria which behave as a pathogen in the tissue, blood, or urine. Throughout this case, researchers have used it to detect COVID-19.

Since these designs are affordable, readily available, and reasonably accurate, experiment kits could be in store with an increasing number of coronary artery situations. Artificial intelligence and state treatment plan could significantly reduce the burden of the doctor, that's are basically

- Fast treatment
- Easily separation or isolation
- Decrease the spread of the virus

Artificial intelligence aid treatment has reduced the reading time by 65%. Therefore, it has enormous potential to enhance the doctor's effective diagnosis and recovery stress in training and soothe the already overstressed and tired doctors infer vision and 'Alibaba' are both using CT scan imaging for the corona treatment plan.

It also aids in the monitoring of infected people's conditions [7]. This can considerably improve the reliability of diagnosis and decision-making by implementing effective methodologies. AI is also beneficial for treating infected COVID-19 patients and careful oversight of one's wellness. This could monitor the recession of COVID-19 on a range of venues such as medical, biochemical, and pharmacological systems. It is quite beneficial to facilitate research into this virus by collecting and analysing information.

19.6 Using Mobile Apps to Tracing COVID-19 Patients

Considering that the novel coronavirus afflicts an infinite amount of individuals, traditional detection methodologies are not enough to classify others with the viral infection and restrict spread. And for this reason, governments worldwide have needed to resort to such a task using modern technologies.

By monitoring mobile consumers, agencies may determine who's where and then warn anyone who may have been in the vicinity of anyone with COVID-19. In just 13 days, 'Aarogya Setu', India's contact-tracing app, has been downloaded by over 50 million users. By mid-May, Apple and Google decide to publish the first edition of their contact-tracing program.

Covid-19 had already attacked over 600,000 people and caused a deep recession. Governments would like to get people into work. A crucial part of it is the contact tracking technology that enables officials to trace down the virus and alert residents who might be affected to stay at home or even get checked.

As the worldwide battle against the COVID-19 epidemic persists, almost the entire world is strapping its aspirations of reducing lockdowns so that persons who could have been infected with the virus can be easily detected. However, these 'contact tracing' is usually an arduous, slow process focused on speeches and special agent work throughout-person.

Enter the mobile phone: a new type of software seeks to speed up the process of trying to follow the steps of an individual to identify someone who may have been affected by the coronavirus and potentially alert certain persons as quickly as possible.

These applications are continued to demonstrate their usefulness. The simulation indicates those who may effectively slow virus expand, and just if they are used by so much of the population.

Researchers have no illusions that perhaps the contact-tracing application creators and similar technologies are very well-intentioned. Yet until they are generally implemented, we encourage these technologies' designers to step up and consider the shortcomings of such systems. These can consider as a limitation of these technologies.

Contact tracing can become an essential element of an outbreak solution, especially if disease susceptibility is small. These measures are most successful where testing is easy and readily accessible, and where diseases are reasonably rare disorders that are uncommon in America at present.

Optimally, physical contact tracing by qualified professionals can help classify test applicants and quarantine to prevent coronavirus spread.

Furthermore, contact tracing applications can't guarantee that walking out is safe only since no disease has been identified in the area. Essentially, contact tracing is a global health initiative, not personal health interference. It can minimise disease spread throughout the population, but it doesn't provide direct security to any patient.

The list of some mobile app is shown in Fig. 19.3 [7].

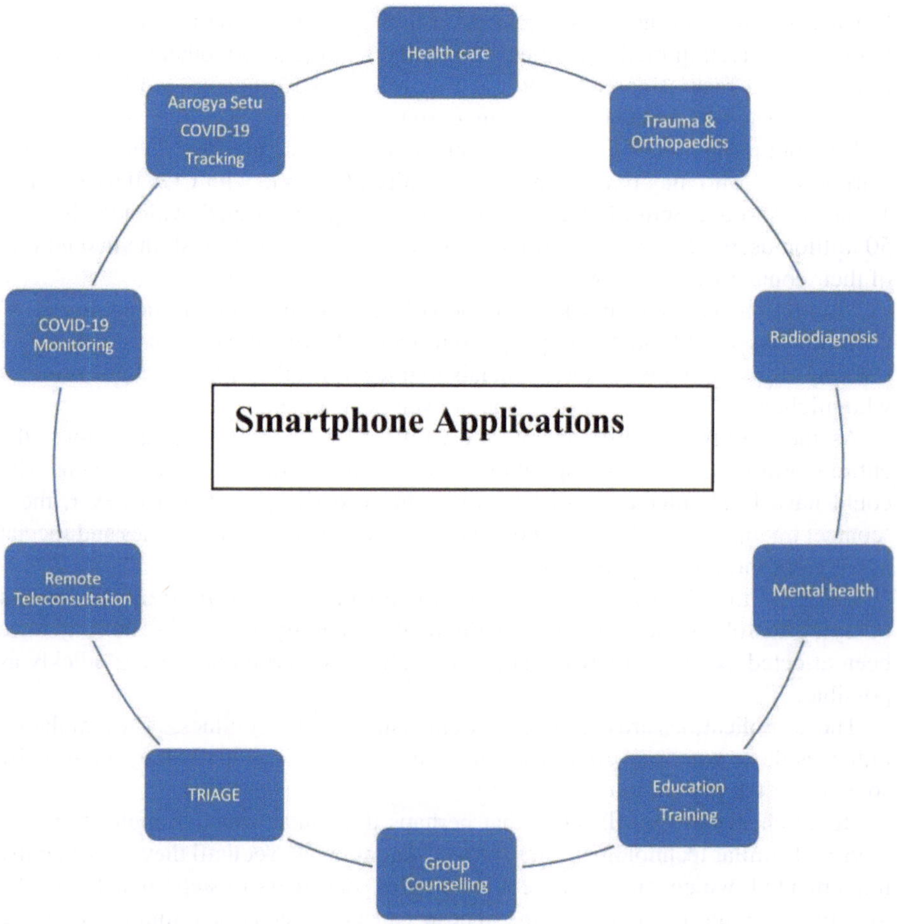

Fig. 19.3 Mobile apps for healthcare as well as COVID-19

19.7 Sampling Genes to Identify Probable Vaccinations

Throughout the ethnicity to improve a coronavirus disease vaccination (Covid-19), thousands of worldwide scientists use multiple forums for developing vaccines concurrently, including platforms based on Deoxyribonucleic acid (DNA) as well as Ribonucleic acid (RNA) leading the charge due to one's speed possibility.

RNA and DNA are genetic material pieces. In recent January China synthesised and released the genome of the Severe Acute Respiratory Syndrome Coronavirus 2 (Sars-CoV-2), the disease that causes COVID-2019. Several other countries also synthesised the virus then, India is also included.

Such genetic samples are being utilised to evolve the active virus and research its nature, as to how it reaches individual cells and triggers the disease, which is crucial to the production of medicines and vaccines for combat disease.

Research upon the COVID-2019 vaccination started shortly since the first gene excerpt became accessible, as well as the Moderna's m-Ribonucleic acid (RNA)-based Sars-CoV-2 patients entering a phase-1 trial (to check for security as well as an injection in helpers with good health) at the middle of the march. A no-replicative vector-based vaccine also obtained governmental permission to launch phase 1 studies in China, although nucleic-acid vaccine permits phase one trials launched in April.

Vaccine production is a costly proposition with large failure rates, with researchers adopting a sequential number of actions that require extensive analysis of data and fabrication-process controls.

According to a new paper in the New England Journal of Medicine (NEJM), rapidly building a vaccine holds a more significant investment risk. It necessitates a fast start and several stages implemented in tandem before verifying a positive result. For example, phase 1 clinical experiments could be allowed to continue in tandem with testing on animals of systems that have been evaluated in people.

19.8 Using Nanotechnology for Combat Against COVID-19

One of the scientists specialising in producing nano-scale medicines and disease management technologies is a contingent of researchers who contribute innovations and expertise to the COVID-19 infection management and control centres.

The nanomaterial concept says that scientists would be that the inside COVID-19 virus is a size close to its nanomaterial size. Material is incredibly small at that scale, approximately ten thousand times less than the thickness of a singular branch of hair.

The worldwide consortium has built a nanotechnology method to stop propagating viruses that can be used to combat COVID-19.

Nanotechnology provides new opportunities to establish practical and efficient identification, reliable protective devices, and more successful medical technologies. Nanosensors now demonstrate improved capacity to detect bacteria or viruses at quite small quantities, and alert doctors well before signs have arisen or on clients with really low infection rates.

Scientists have begun exploring the feasibility of utilising nanoparticles to manage microbial and viral diseases for decades now. For example, Gold nanoparticles are designed to bind to viruses such as Ebola or influenza, and nanoparticles could instead demolish the virus's framework through warming particles with some electromagnetic wavelengths. Often nanoparticles can be utilised for drug delivery.

In light of such developments in growth, we believe that nanotechnology might help prevent the Covid-19 epidemic. While the coronavirus epidemic threatens to interrupt company processes globally, the health care sector needs to identify an efficient solution rather quickly. More researchers are exploring technological innovations, even nanotechnology.

NANO-SENSORS WHICH ARE USE FOR IDENTIFICATION OF THE DISEASE: Nanotechnology can help build approaches that can help in COVID-19 prevention, treatment, and care. Nanotechnology will offer new opportunities for creating inexpensive and efficient mechanisms of identification, secure appliances for public safety, and more successful medical applications.

Nanosensors are now available on the market, with a broad and diverse usage environment. The application is already developed for the identification of viruses and bacteria. Researchers are now attempting to change and adapt current processes and procedures to build Nano and bio-sensors to assist in coronavirus identification.

By the help of Nano-technology some areas which help to fight against coronavirus these are given below

- Rapid point of care treatment
- Surveillance
- Monitoring
- Therapeutics
- Vaccine development (Fig. 19.4) [8].

19.9 Use of Robotic Technologies to Bail Out Against COVID-19

The novel coronavirus recession had already expanded interests of the public in robotic technologies and artificial intelligence, used as an efficacious means of fighting the epidemic.

In hospitals, robots could be implemented besides dechlorination, food, and medical supplies service, surveillance of vital signs, thus considerably reducing the risk of contamination of all staff.

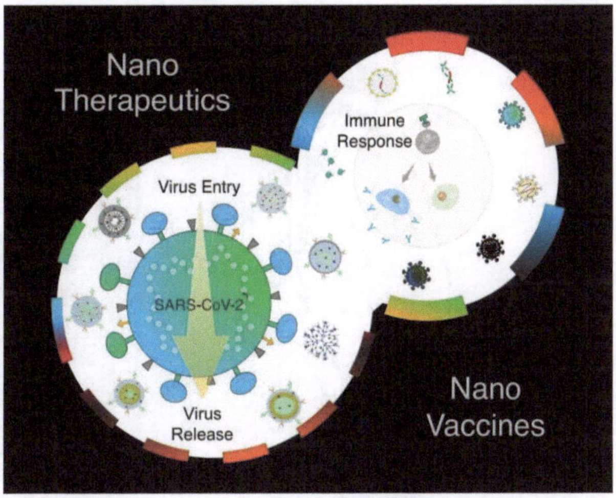

Fig. 19.4 Nanotechnology [8]

Robots that can sanitise the hospitals independently: Independent sanitisation robots can clean up infected zones independently, even without medical personnel's interference.

The robot is designed Ultraviolet light and a standalone robotic platform.

Robots distribute prescription drugs, medical tests, meals, and hospital logistic support in particular. **Robotics can distribute meals and bring items such as drugs and tests along in hospitals and other health care centres by using robotics technology**.

Robots are helping doctors to stay away from coronavirus and keep safe. Robots are helping to boost up the coronavirus tests. Because of the extremely contagious nature of coronavirus, robots will provide contact-free possible solutions. Robots are a game-changer in disease outbreaks from the decontamination of hospitals and public areas to healthcare services.

A cylindrical robot turns into a medical room to enable healthcare staff to take temperatures digitally and evaluate blood pressure and respiration rate from patients attached to the ventilator.

Research organisations and start-ups are developing new robots, such as enabling health care staff to keep taking blood samples vaguely and conduct oral swabs and tissue samples. Such new designs are doubtful to make a significant difference right now. Even so, robots under advancement can make a significant difference in disaster risks if the trend for an investigation into robotics keeps going. For smarter or even worse, robots are replacing many humans in their works, experts say, and the coronavirus epidemic accelerates the process.

Figure 19.5 [9] gives the idea of the robotic technology and also show how it can help to maintain the social distancing.

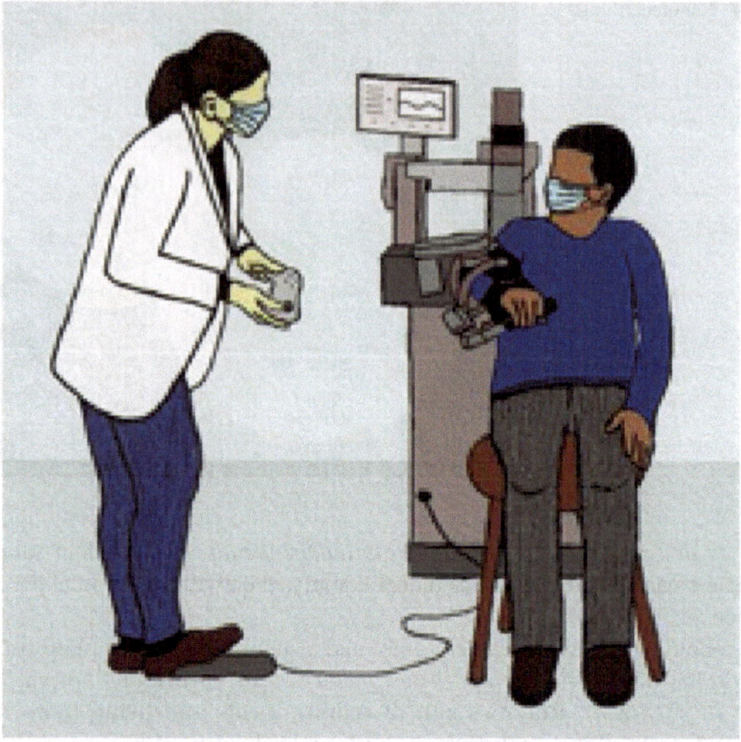

Fig. 19.5 Use of robotic technology [9]

19.10 Three-Dimensional (3-D) Printing Technology Which Could Help Sustains the Pressure of Government as Well as Health Care Centers

Because as COVID-19 pandemic is depleting essential medical equipment world-wide, 3D printer suppliers and 3D printer designers, are adapting manufacturing technologies to create such crucial products and tools.

Experts of the worldwide 3D printing group donate sufficient time and money to create such life-saving materials in huge competition and absurdly short availability.

The 3-D printing technology used Protective glasses: By using the 3-D printing technology, 3-D printer designers are making 3-D printers for the mass-production of protective glasses for healthcare staff. By 3-D Printing Technology, the virus's spreading can be reduced, so coronavirus's death rate also decreases.

Many developers of 3D printing technology manufacture nasal swabs (which is mandatory for the people's corona test for every day) and oxygen valves (which has also a crucial role in ventilator patients in ventilation) using 3D printing. That has a vital role in detection and diagnosis for the coronavirus.

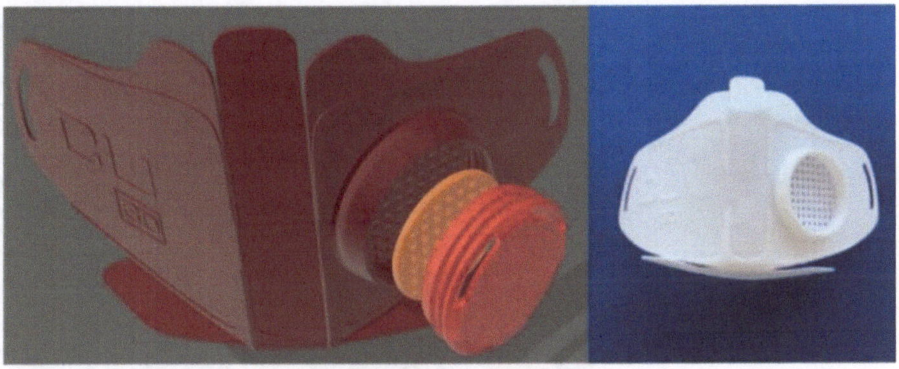

Fig. 19.6 Creating mask with the help of 3-D printing technology

Way across to design reflective face masks (shown at Fig. 19.6 [10]) for healthcare professionals and first responders.

Some countries have used 3D printers and laser cutters round the clock to produce masks for local hospitals.

3-D printing also helps make ventilator splitter, allowing a single ventilator to support multiple patients during times of acute equipment shortages.

This is helpful for the treatment of coronavirus affected people all over the world.

3D printing has already played a vital role in combating the COVID-19 epidemic and keeping people safe. Ideally, more producers and distributors will pursue such trends and change their manufacturing plants to produce equipment that will save lives.

The 3D-printing company developed **a hands-free door** opener and an oxygen-mask adapter to take COVID-19 patients off ventilators. As per scientists, coronavirus is susceptible to living on materials for prolonged amounts of time, and door handles pose a high risk of infection, causing people to contact them regularly. At an executive discussion at Materialize, the organisation set up plans to help protect workers and guests, and this is where the concept for a door opener came into being.

One of the famous companies has built the 3D printed door opener (shown at Fig. 19.7) [10] to connect it to existing door controls without making holes or removing the handle. It contains a paddle-shaped extension that enables people to enter and close doors by using their arms rather than their hands since most doors can't stay open for health reasons.

If the coronavirus, nowadays an epidemic, hits the world, we foresee countries enforcing travel bans, social distancing initiatives, contact tracing [11], remote monitoring [12], and remote working [13]. Also, the more advanced countries are seeing COVID-19 overloading and fatiguing their healthcare networks.

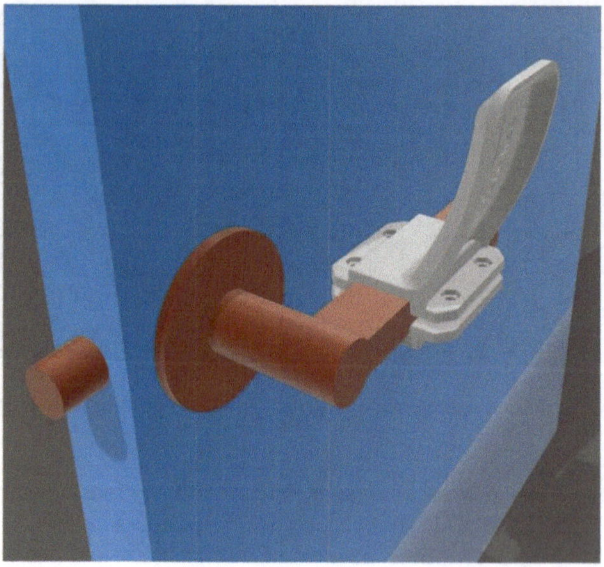

Fig. 19.7 Use of 3-D printing

19.11 Conclusion

Many modern technologies have emerged in the battle against COVID-19 and have also been accepted in different aspects of disease prevention, health care, and people's daily lives and work. New technologies alone cannot substitute or compensate for all other public government policies, but it has a progressively vital role to play in the reaction to evacuation situations. Covid-19, the very first significant epidemic of the twenty-first century.

This offers an essential chance for policymakers and regulatory agencies to represent legislative validity, moral validity. Evolving tenability and efficiency of HealthCare Technology under time constraints. The correct stunning equilibrium would be important to ensure people's trust in evidence-based treatments in human health.

Finally, healthcare organisations worldwide are going to switch with the above-mentioned evolving technologies to enable ease of their tasks, either through helping speed up diagnosis or encouraging physicians to monitor patients who have also been locked up vaguely.

References

1. S. Roy, K.R. Bhattacharya, Spread of COVID-19 in India: A mathematical model. J. Sci. Technol. **05**(03), 41–47 (2020)

2. M. Javaid, A. Haleem, R. Vaishya, S. Bahl, R. Suman, A. Vaish, Industry 4.0 Technologies and Their Applications in Fighting COVID-19 Pandemic (2020). https://doi.org/10.1016/j.dsx.2020.04.032
3. A. Dwivedi, R.K. Bali, A.E. James, R.N.G. Naguib, Workflow Management Systems: The Healthcare Technology of the Future? (2020). https://research.tue.nl/en/studentthesis/a-comparison-of-workflow-management-systems-and-clinical-decision-support-systems-in-supporting-clinical-processes(59e4681b-256e-407a-b81d-84393e9cf112).html
4. S.M. Saleem, L.R. Pasquale, P.A. Sidoti, J.C. Tsai, Virtual Ophthalmology: Telemedicine in a COVID-19 Era, **216**, 237–242 (2020). https://doi.org/10.1016/j.ajo.2020.04.029
5. W.R. Smith, A.J. Atala, R.P. Terlecki, E.E. Kelly, C.A. Matthews, Implementation Guide for Rapid Integration of an Outpatient Telemedicine Program During the COVID-19 Pandemic (2020). https://doi.org/10.1016/j.jamcollsurg.2020.04.030
6. N. Pappot, G.A. Taarnhoj, H. Pappot, Telemedicine and e-Health Solutions for COVID-19: Patients' Perspective (2020). https://doi.org/10.1089/tmj.2020.0099
7. K. Iyengar, G.K. Upadhyaya, R. Vaishya, V. Jain, COVID-19 and applications of smartphone technology in the current pandemic (2020). https://doi.org/10.1016/j.dsx.2020.05.033
8. G. Chauhan, M.J. Madou, S. Kalra, V. Chopra, D. Ghosh, S.O. Martinez Chapa, Nanotechnology for COVID-19: Therapeutics and Vaccine Research (2020). https://doi.org/10.1021/acsnano.0c04006
9. M. Tavakoli, J. Carriere, A. Torabi, Robotics, Smart Wearable Technologies and Autonomous Intelligent Systems for Healthcare During the COVID-19 Pandemic: An Analysis of the State of the Art and Future Vision (2020). https://doi.org/10.1002/aisy.202000071
10. R. Tino, R. Moore, S. Antoline, P. Ravi, N. Wake, C.N. Ionita, J.M. Morris, S.J. Decker, A. Sheikh, F.J. Rybicki, L.L. Chepelev, COVID-19 and the role of 3D printing in medicine (2020). https://doi.org/10.1186/s41205-020-00064-7
11. L. Garg, E. Chukwu, N. Nidal, C. Chakraborty, G. Garg, Anonymity preserving IoT-based COVID-19 and other infectious disease contact tracing model. IEEE Access **8**, 159402–159414 (2020). https://doi.org/10.1109/ACCESS.2020.3020513
12. M. Jayalakshmi, L. Garg, K. Maharajan, K. Srinivasan, K. Jayakumar, A.K. Bashir, K. Ramesh, Fuzzy logic-based health monitoring system for COVID'19 patients. Comput. Mater. Continua (2020). https://www.techscience.com/cmc/v67n2/41372
13. A.K. Bhardwaj, L. Garg, A. Garg, Y. Gajpal, E-Learning during COVID-19 outbreak: Cloud computing adoption in Indian Public Universities. Comput. Mater. Continua **66**(3), 2471–2492 (2022). https://doi.org/10.32604/cmc.2021.014099
14. B. Anthony Jr, Use of Telemedicine and Virtual Care for Remote Treatment in Response to COVID-19 Pandemic (2020). https://doi.org/10.1007/s10916-020-01596-5

Chapter 20
Real-Time Alert System for Delivery Operators Through Artificial Intelligence in Last-Mile Delivery

Vinod Kumar Shukla, Leena Wanganoo, and Nibhrita Tiwari

20.1 Introduction

During the pandemic time, which started in January 2020 in most of the world, lockdown and social distancing norms have become the "new normal". Pharmaceuticals and healthcare products have seen an unprecedented rise through an online distribution channel. However, earlier the sector struggled due to stringent regulatory issues. With the sudden need and transformation in customer buying behaviour, the revenue turnover is estimated to rise from its initial value of USD 33.71 billion in 2018 to approximately USD 101.69 billion by 2026 registering a CAGR of 14.80% in the forecast period of 2019–2026 [1].

Though the sector's future growth will depend upon governmental regulation, the factor that influences the success of the e-pharma is a robust end-to-end integrated last-mile operation. Specifically, activities like handling, storage, packaging and transportation within the city till the customer's doorstep pose a new set of challenges to the logistics. Last mile is a key difference to sustain in the competitive ecosystem. It has become imperative for the retailer to satisfy the customer demand of "anytime, anywhere" delivery. The digital platform facilitates the order process,

V. K. Shukla (✉)
Department of Engineering and Architecture, Amity University, Dubai, UAE
e-mail: vshukla@amityuniversity.ae

L. Wanganoo
Department of Management and Commerce, Amity University, Dubai, UAE
e-mail: lwanganoo@amityuniversity.ae

N. Tiwari
Radicon Institute of Radiology, Dubai, UAE

L. Garg et al. (eds.), *Healthcare Informatics for Fighting COVID-19 and Future Epidemics*, EAI/Springer Innovations in Communication and Computing,
https://doi.org/10.1007/978-3-030-72752-9_20

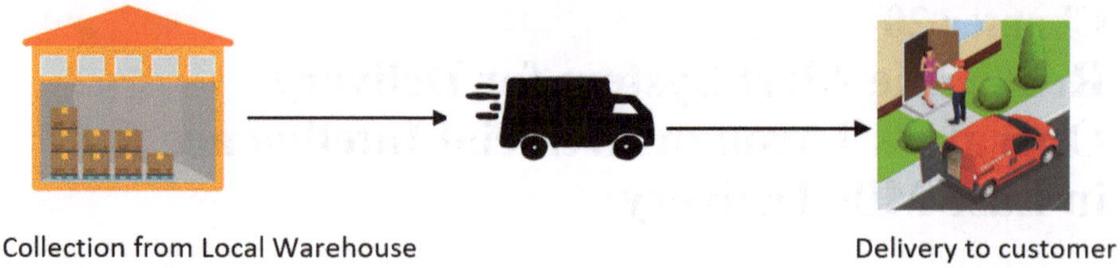

Fig. 20.1 Activities in last-mile delivery

but last mile still lags the integration and collaboration to enhance real-time visibility for operational excellence.

Last-Mile Delivery With the growing demand of e-pharmacy now, the pharma drugs, the last-mile journey starts from the distributor's warehouse to customer doorstep. The "last-mile" delivery is defined as the last step of the supply chain. Strategically, it is a key driver to customer loyalty, though it is the most expensive and time-consuming part of the logistics process. The focal point of this stage of last-mile delivery is the agility and responsiveness. Hence, the prime responsibility lies with the logistics provider to plan an effective operation to deliver [2].

In the "last mile", the logistics provider performs collection/distribution/ communication to the end customer under urban conditions. The process has higher complexities due to constraints of fulfilment, higher cost and increased operational complexities [3]. Hence, last-mile delivery is costly and increases the municipal level due to its operational inefficiency [4] (Fig. 20.1).

For a sustainable competitive advantage, the companies need to implement a robust last-first strategy. The collaborative and integrated supply chain will enhance customer experiences, accelerate the speed, minimise costs, and ensure transparency in the delivery channel.

For a valid e-pharmacy success in the marketplace, the service quality of delivery is paramount because it is one of the primary decision-making criteria for the customers. One of the conjoint analyses conducted by Mckinsey & Company [5] concluded that the customer is willing to pay approximately 25% additional cost for the same day or instant delivery (Fig. 20.2).

Though the customer is willing to pay an additional for the same-day delivery, "last-mile" delivery is one of the most expensive operations and a significant bottleneck of e-logistics. Its cost around 30% of total e-logistics cost. The higher cost of service is because the operational cost is higher than what consumers are willing to pay for the delivery [6]. Hence, it is the least efficient stage [7] in the supply chain. Also, fragmented and uncoordinated, the supply chain usually engages different logistics service providers and carriers for the cities' delivery [8]. The widespread transport mode adopted in the last-mile delivery is road [7], which faces a dual challenge: satisfying the customer demands and meeting environmental requirements [9].

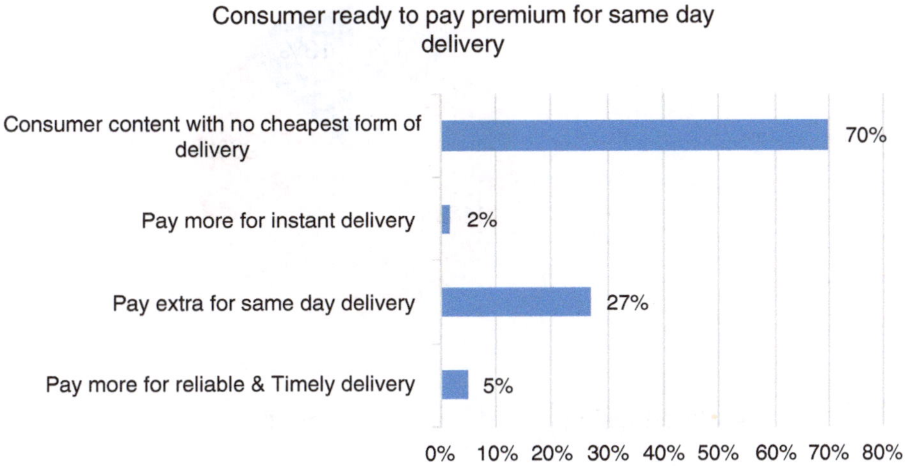

Fig. 20.2 Customer expectation from last-mile delivery. (Source: Mckinsey & Company)

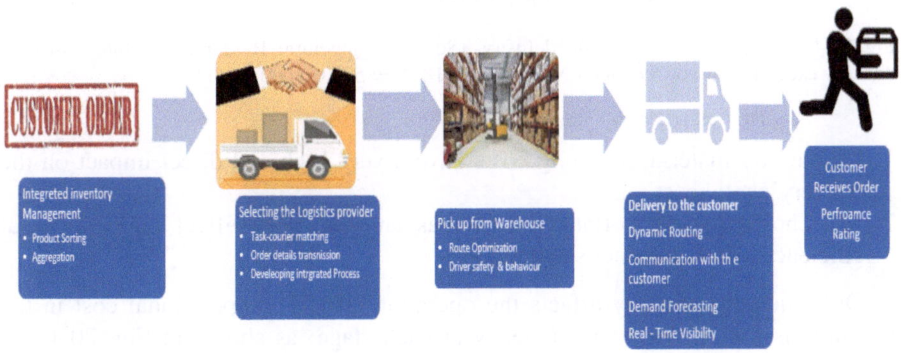

Fig. 20.3 Task performed at each stage of the last-mile delivery process

Following are the elements the customer expects from the last mile delivery:

1. Fast delivery
2. Precise order picking
3. Security and insurance
4. Specialisation
5. Convenience
6. The precision of the product deliveries

To meet the customer expectation following task (Fig. 20.3) needs to perform seamlessly in the supply chain.

Following are the significant challenges in the last-mile delivery for B2C e-pharma:

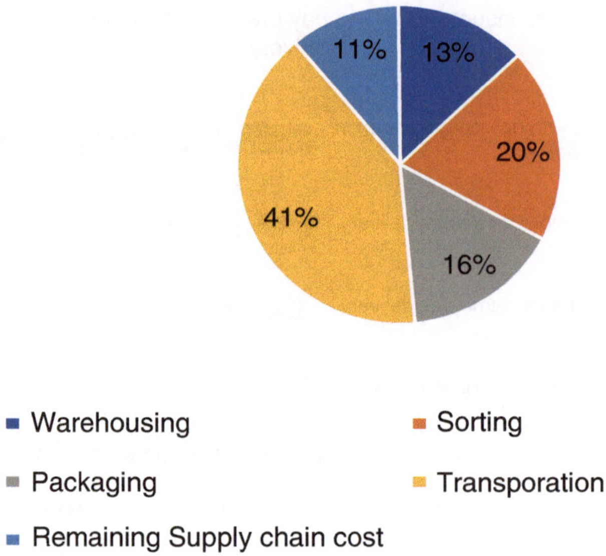

Fig. 20.4 Key drivers in last-mile delivery. (Source: Capgemini Research Institute, last-mile delivery executive survey, October–November 2018, $N = 500$ executives [11])

1. Labour and material handling costs have a very high and direct impact on the delivery's total cost.
2. The choice of transportation mode has an immediate effect on operational efficiencies and customer satisfaction.

Order quantity directly affects the operation [10]. The operational cost in the last mile is higher due to inefficiency at each stage; as shown in Fig. 20.4, the transportation cost is the most significant driver accounting for approximately 47% of the total cost per the report published by Capgemini.

Challenges in Last-Mile Delivery Specifically, for the pharma supply, "last-mile delivery" is a big last leap, with high service quality expectation facing several challenges:

- Truck capacity constraints
- Shortage of specialised drivers
- Non-refrigerated pharma supplies
- Cold-chain pharma products
- Lower visibility in logistics
- Variations in temperature
- Traffic constraints
- Special storage requirements
- Difficulty in fulfilling the sudden rise of on-demand deliveries
- Emergency security measures

- Pharma goods that require refrigeration
- Distribution safety guidelines for various geographies

Specifically, in e-pharma transportation, the major challenge is the specialised delivery operator who understands the transport requirements and specific storage well. There is also a shortage of experienced delivery staff in the pharma industry. There are increased demand and the value of experienced and specialised drivers. Secondly, they can manage the implications that arise during the delivery process, with the increased volume of e-pharmacy and leading to a higher number of freight vehicles to local streets. There has been limited investigation behind the causes of traffic accidents in urban areas related to increased online delivery [12].

Previous research is focused on the emission, operational cost, and customer satisfaction; however, limited attention is paid to how long-distance driving impacts driver behaviour and directly impacts road safety. Hence, whether the logistics provider or the retailer, last-mile visibility of the driver behaviour in the last-mile delivery is essential; the considerable cost involved in the logistics driver safety and behaviour pattern can be measured and monitored through technology. Technology is the only option for pharma companies to get end-to-end visibility.

It is essential to focus on behaviour aspects of the driver while driving to ensure safety and zero accidents, so the logistics companies can protect their assets (e.g. the delivery van or truck) and the drivers' lives. Whether they're employees or contractors, the drivers expect some modicum of protection and safety standards as they buckle up and rush off to deliver packages.

In the face of increased e-pharma volumes and tight delivery windows, one might hire more drivers to solve the problem. Still, it would increase the logistics operations cost and the number of inexperienced drivers per route. The only solution to overcome these hurdles is to leverage technology for long-term sustainability. Figure 20.5 shows the importance of real-time visibility and how it can solve the three significant challenges—driver safety, vehicle safety, and environmental sustainability issues—faced due to an increase in e-pharma demand.

The end-to-end visibility in the last-mile supply chain through technology-powered is the need of the hour for the pharmaceutical industry. Whether it is temperature-sensitive or non-refrigerated pharmaceutical products, small issues like delivery delays can lead to the pharma supplies' discarding; hence, monitoring the product and delivery operator while in transit is extremely important.

Driver behaviour recognition is an integral part of safety. The logistics provider needs to underpin driver behaviour as the distance and scale of delivery operation increases. The logistics provider needs to prioritise the things that matter most in operation, which include the following:

- Driver safety: Delivery operator behavioural patterns should be the primary concern.
- Vehicle safety: Most often, the vehicle is owned by the logistics company, and if a delivery operator uses it, it could be one of the most significant expenses.
- Route safety: Optimise routes for safety and efficiency, minimise delays, prolonged idling, and unnecessary stops by the driver.

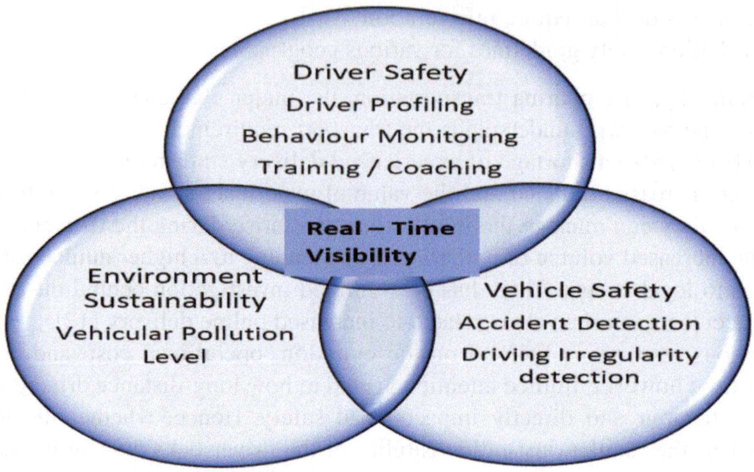

Fig. 20.5 Leveraging technology for real-time visibility in last-mile delivery

Many of the last-mile accidents are caused by the change in delivery operators' behaviour due to prolonged driving and distracted driving. Implementing a technology-driven driver profiling solution will provide an insight into this issue and provide real-time visibility and decision-making ability.

20.1.1 Key Psychological Factors of the Driver Leading to Accidents

While driving a vehicle for a more extended period, the driver is often multitasking. The driver often utilises all the cognitive resources for the completion of a safe journey to the destination. But distraction and attention-less driving mainly contribute to the majority of road accidents. Psychological factors like motivation, personality, fatigue, and stress level of the driver must also be considered.

Different surveys have shown that around 19% of all highway crashes involve fatigue, with some highways accounting for up to 48%. The primary reason for accidents is driver exhaustion. Due to the danger of sleepiness on the road, techniques to counteract its effects must be created. Driver care may be the consequence of the driving absence of alarm because of driver sleepiness and diversion.

Driver diversion happens when a person is drawn away from the driving job by an item or incident. Contrary to driver diversion, driver somnolence does not trigger an event but is marked instead by gradual removal of attention from street and traffic demand. However, both the rider's sleepiness and diversion could have the same impacts, i.e. reduced riding power, longer response time, and enhanced likelihood of a collision.

The lack of willingness to drive due to driver tiredness and distraction may be the result. Driver's distraction occurs when a person is far from the driving company by an object or opportunity.

In comparison with driver distraction, driver laziness does not involve a possible activating occasion but rather a vibrant departure from streets and congestion demands. Motorists' tranquillity and distraction can have comparable consequences, i.e. decreased driving performance, longer reaction times, and an increased risk of accidents. Currently, the problem of road accidents is severe, and their frequency increases annually. The critical problem behind the road malfunctions is the faintness of the driver and the driver's alcoholicity. Unprecedented progress is made to overcome this problem. These technologies are used to recognise laziness and to maintain road accidents. For laziness acceptance, the unique inventions are developed. Subsequent relies on the vehicle, where the guide wheel location, track location, and weight of the velocity pedal have always been noted. Furthermore, the behaviour relies on the eye's flashing recurrences, eye closure, yawning, and head current continuously noted.

The third is dependent on the physiological activity of ECG (electrocardiogram), EEG (electrooculography), and EMG (electromyogram) to control pulse and brain effects. Four key variables make the rider tired. There are rest, practice, daytime, and fitness.

This is about cultural dependence, in which a fluttering recurrence of the eye, nose, and head present is continuously noted. A steady measurement is suggested in a conventional camera video group to define the eye, bow, and head location. Ongoing milestone indices ready for wild datasets demonstrate superb power in head implementation, fluctuating illumination, and exterior looks.

This study aims to identify the driver locations by evaluating the closing and bowing dimensions of the eye. Further, we would suggest that calculation and milestone locations be successively assessed and lone scalar quantity eye viewpoint ratio (EAR) must be removed. Further, depicting the enlightenment in each case, the mouth aspect ratio (MAR) is also necessary. Finally, an SVM classification acknowledges glip and yawning in brief worldly windows as EAR and MAR esteem instances.

20.1.2 Prevailing System

The laws and criteria used to assess the driver's sharpness' prospective feasibility to observe developments and gadgets recognise the gadget's practical features and functional characteristics. In several instances, the speciality subtleties of this roundabout are not important to consider as helpful preconditions. However, it is essential to ensure that all gadgets or innovation are satisfied behind the checking motive, unpretentiously and constant, driver willingness, and, therefore, in essence, moderating engine accidents that are associated with driver exhaustion, to tend towards this overall customer recognition and consistent standards.

20.1.2.1 The Gap in the Prevailing System

To build an effective last-mile delivery process, the logistics provider needs the current systems to be integrated with artificial intelligence (AI) technology. The rapid pace of artificial intelligence (AI) developments provides unprecedented opportunities to enhance different industries and businesses' performance, including last-mile delivery. The technology-integrated solution will help to monitor the driver behaviour but at the same should have the following features:

1. Cost-effective: The hardware should be affordable with interoperability features.
2. Also as an easily downloadable mobile application.
3. Highly accurate: The technology should be able to provide driver profiling at any given time.
4. Scalable: Importantly, mobile-based solutions are far more scalable than hardware solutions, especially since last-mile delivery services often use contractors who may use their own vehicles.
5. Driver-centric: Mobile-based solutions are the only way to truly measure the *individual driver* instead of measuring the car or truck, which multiple drivers may use.

To address the poor driving behaviour, we need insight into various facial and psychological aspects so that the logistics provider can actively address high-risk behaviour and equally acknowledge and praise the low-risk drivers' behaviour for reinforcing their positive habits.

Recent advances in integrated vision technologies are briefed, and the literature on the identification of the face and eye in real time is reviewed. Real-time monitoring of drowsiness is carried out using multiple detection methods to analyse multiple input information kinds. First, the assessment of human physiological activity, such as brain wave (EEG), heart rate, or pulse frequency, is analysed [13] and presented with the hypothesis of proof, an ORD model for drowsiness detection scheme. ORD is a subjective evaluation of drowsiness, reflecting people's physical appearance and behaviour [14]. Driver sleepiness and diversion are detected using dynamic modelling based on HMM [15] in the latest publications. Fortunately, in distinct countries, the human face generates unique features. Many visual signs, such as blinding of your eye, yeast, and head motion, can be identified during sleepiness. A suggested scheme measures eye-blinding rates and eye shutter length. Hidden Markov model analyses the facial expressions of the rider to determine somnolence. The scheme comprises segmenting the skin, the face, and the iris's placement and detecting the blink [16]. A neural network estimate of the RGB skin colour histogram is used as part of the suggested skin segmentation process. This proposed a scheme centred on the "miscellaneous output-correction scheme" that used a proprietary driving simulator to conduct laboratory tests, causing drowsiness among the test riders. The scheme was suggested. These tests had the objective to acquire electrocardiogram and video sequences with eye blinks. A video camera has also tracked the riders and proposed a fresh technology for modelling driver somnolence using a multi-eyelid motion technology—partial least squares regression (PLSR)—to deal with the issue of powerful colinear relationships between eyelid motion characteristics. A proposal to evaluate the efficiency of the recent eye-tracking-based forecast procedures for vehicles' fatigue is oriented on a camera-based drowsiness identification. These works provide 3D data from a range camera alternative for driver surveillance and incident detection. The scheme incorporates 2D and 3D methods for assessing head positions and identifying areas of interest [17]. The points related to the top will be determined for further evaluation based on a recorded cloud of a 3D point from the sensor and an assessment of the 2-d projection.

20.2 Framework for the Efficient Delivery

The weakness of the driver leads to real harm to all other road accidents. Roughly 20% of fatal road problems include driver deficiency. This article describes a cutting-edge strategy that distinguishes driver fatigue from most weariness side impacts. The critical side effects of exhaust behaviour are eye assessment, yawning, and head tilting. The driver's weariness is also caused by a distracted road vehicle growth under exhaustion. The aim is to differentiate these side impacts for improved road conditions. Two cameras monitor these signs. This offers a strong structure that recognises external appearances, head tilting, and route for weariness. The results of the test of the method suggested and of the previous approach are compared. The results demonstrate high accuracy and reliable performance to avoid road malfunctions contrasting with the previous technology. The structure suggested is fundamental and retains a strategic distance from any complexity.

For a long time, an approach has been envisaged in a vehicle review sector to check and recognise a lazy or drunk driver. The past study uses detectors to detect exhaustion, for instance, an inferred camera for understudies. These methods can, in fact, recognise drivers' weariness, but they are not flexible nor intuitive to riders with external driving circumstances. In opposition to the previous methodology, we offer a weariness identification frame for the driver, which uses the driver's instance control button for the circumstances in front of the perspective. The frame uses a segregation sensor at the vehicle's front-end to capture an external event. The sensor data is ready using a mix of calculation and instructions based on decision tree learning. At every start-up of a car, the structure learns the method so that our structure is qualified to be adapted to every driver's driving style and behaviour. Similarly, depending on response models, we can acquire a driver fatigue rate.

Figure 20.6 is a logical representation of efficient delivery. This includes primarily the three main components, which includes detection of driver behaviour and drowsiness detection, and these two results are processed first, followed by GPS

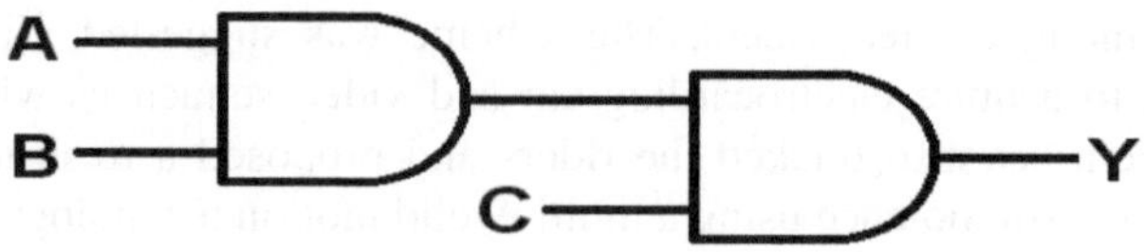

Fig. 20.6 Logical representation of an efficient delivery system. A: Detection of driver behaviour (fatigue and eye blink) | B: drowsiness alter system. C: GPS system | Y: Result

integrated with these results. The final alert is generated, which may be updated in the cloud for further analysis and understanding.

Over the last decades, *GPS (Global Positioning System)* has reshaped the logistics and transport sector. GPS is used to track and trace on the geographic position of the map and enables us to see the vehicle in motion and towards which direction. It also monitors the speed and provides routing direction, time management, and traffic status. Advancement in technology led to using GPS with Google Maps and cloud computing to collect and transfer the vehicle's information on a real-time basis. This intelligent monitoring system uses the various systems to transmit information like driver condition, tire condition and pressure, and fuel level. The GPS gathers all the essential information related to location, speed, and communication on a real-time basis via cellular or satellite to a centralised server in the cloud network [18]. The GPS's tracking systems enable a base control centre to keep updated information of the vehicles without the driver's intervention, whereas navigation system helps the driver reach the destination.

Now, GPS is one of the top navigation technologies which provide the driver with an increased variety of wayfinding information. The GPS antenna communicates with GPS satellite for transferring the geographic location details. The control centre servers are maintained in the cloud while the sensors are fitted with the vehicle [18].

Many research types have already explored strategy to minimise the driving distraction, but few research types focused on real-time monitoring and reducing distraction behaviours with system design.

The stand-alone GPS application provides information on the vehicle location (latitude and longitude), speed, and altitude. However, when integrated with advanced technologies like NB-IoT, the coverage area is enhanced many folds and low power consumption. According to [19], NB-IoT-based procedure can be broadly categorised into two phases: (1) random access and (2) transmission phase. Whenever a new alert is generated, the sensor attempts to detect the transmit signal from the location, and the tracking area code is decoded. We explore the conceptual framework based on GPS and NB-IoT integration to analyse the distraction behaviours and deliver the real-time status to the control centre server and alert to the drivers. Consequently, the drivers will either take a break or drive safely.

GPS (Fig. 20.7) will play a significant role in this framework. Any delivery from point A to point B needs real-time monitoring. Usually, all the routes between any two given points (source and destination) are almost fixed, and routing network is

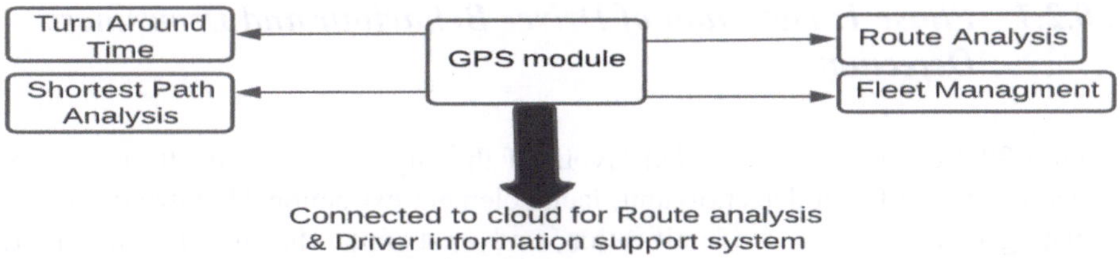

Fig. 20.7 Benefits of GPS in relation to the framework

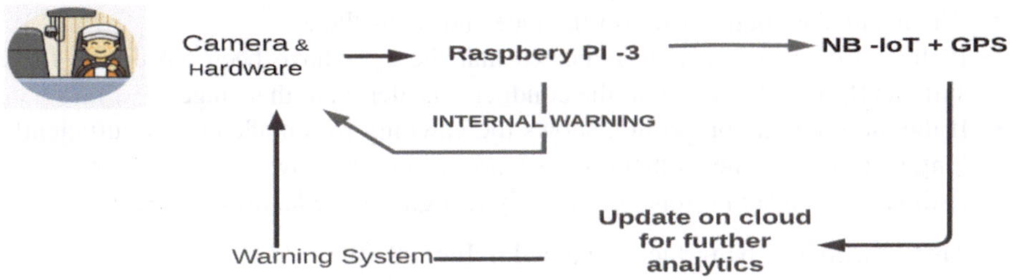

Fig. 20.8 Logical layout of adopted hardware system

standard. However, the number of alternate routes is more than one in between two points, but the numbers of route/city are almost fixed. With the NB-IoT and GPS system's help, continuous route information; average delivery time in a particular day, time, and month; and driver details can be recorded and transmitted to the centralised cloud server. This repository of information from all the routes can provide insight into the best possible delivery time at a destination from a given source.

This information can be used for fleet management, best route calculation at the given time in weekday/weekend accordingly. This will also help us if the time taken for delivery between point A and point B is deviating more than the average time required for delivery between those two points, which can be used for the route management.

Figure 20.8 represents the logical structure of adopted hardware system. Integrated camera at the primary phase will capture video of the driver, which will be further processed with the help of Raspberry Pi 3, and based on the internal processing and algorithm, internal warning will be issued. After certain warnings, this will be updated in the cloud with NB-IoT and GPS module help. From there, final warning can be issued to the driver, which can help avoid any dangerous situation. This entire layout is the combination of two different processes as following:

- Phase 1: Detection of driver behaviour and drowsiness detection.
- Phase 2: GPS module integration.

20.2.1 Phase 1: Detection of Driver Behaviour and Drowsiness Detection

Figure 20.9 discusses the detailed layout of the suggested system. It consists of video capture, a facial detection unit, facial element extraction, shut eye detection, yawning place, sleepiness identification, and alert unit. The overall flow of the calculation of languor identification is provided below:

- First, set up a camera that displays a flow for faces.
- When a face is found, discover the face and focus the eye.
- If the eye-view percentage indicates that the eyes have been closed off for a sufficiently lengthy moment, the conductor is alerted at that stage.
- If the mouth angle proportion shows the yawning for an adequately sufficiently long measure of time, at that point sounds a caution to awaken the driver.
- Estimation of head present additionally recognises the laziness of the driver.

This concept can be further explained in Fig. 20.10.

Video Capture First, install camera in the car to differentiate the driver's profile and impose a limitation on the milestone's face to display the nose and lips. The condition of the driver's head will also catch up. The collection of video from a web camera on a dashboard leading group of a car captures video securing photos of the driver and a language place noise warning system.

Face Detection The structure suggested will start one by one with the video descriptions. OpenCV offers wide assistance in the preparation of live recordings. The frame differentiates the shape of each case in the case image. This model uses an AI strategy for visual item identification, the Viola-Jones object locator. This is done using the hair calculation for the position of the face. Haar course provides an excellent computation based on the components, making a proficient distinction

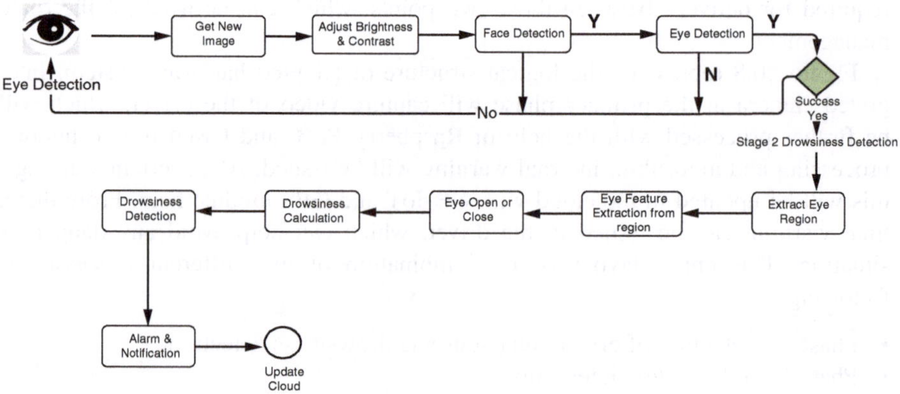

Fig. 20.9 Detailed process layout for detection of driver behaviour and drowsiness detection

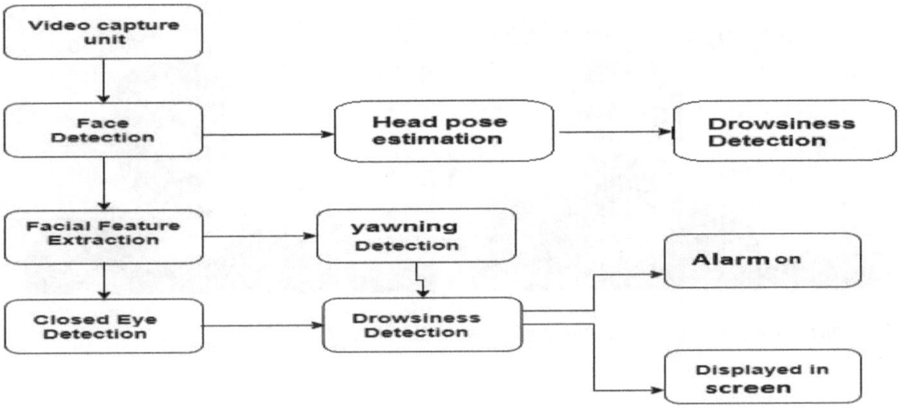

Fig. 20.10 The architecture of the proposed system

between the face images. With the use of jobs, Haar's calculation will naturally expel the non-face rivals. Moreover, the mixture of different hair highlights consists of each phase. Therefore, every component is marked by a hair classifier. The built-in OpenCV xml "haarcascade frontalface alt.xml" record is used to view and recognise the image in single borders. This paper includes multiple facial highlights and uses a number of beneficial and bad examples. At that stage, the course paper will first burden the purchased case with border identifying job identifying all imaginable items of different dimensions in the case. As the conductor's principle includes an enormous part of the image and not items of all conceivable dimensions distinguished, define the border index so that items of a given magnitude for a facial region can be identified. Next, the edge rates are removed, and the result is opposed to the course paper with the edge picture recognition. The output of this module is a face-known border.

The dlib library is used to track the eye and mouth's current milestone and to focus on the locals (Fig. 20.11). There is thus a two-stage method of recognising facial milestones:

- Localise the face in the picture.
- Detect the key facial structures on the face ROI.

Face discovery (step #1) can be accomplished in various ways. In Haar falls, we could use OpenCVs. We can explicitly apply the pre-prepared HOG + Linear SVM object locator for the assignment of face identification. Or we can even use in-depth learning calculations to limit our face. The true calculation used in the picture to recognise the face does not change in either case. Rather, it is important to achieve the face box (i.e. (x, y) direction in the image) by means of some approach.

Due to the face region, step #2 can be used to distinguish the eye district's main facial buildings. There is a range of facial landmarks, but basically, all methods try to limit and label the associated facial areas:

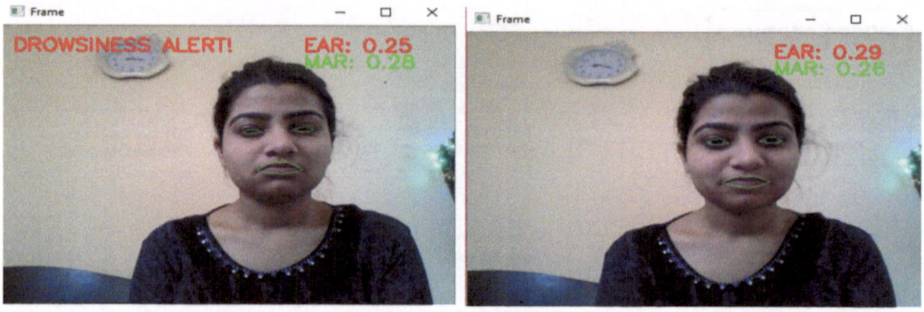

Fig. 20.11 Face detection (eye and mouth) using dlib library

- Mouth
- Right eyebrow
- Left eyebrow
- Right eye
- Left eye
- Nose
- Jaw

The facial milestone indicator incorporated into the dlib library is an execution of the One Millisecond Face Alignment with an Ensemble of Regression Trees paper. This strategy begins by utilising:

- A preparing set of named facial milestones on a picture. These pictures are physically named, determining explicit (*x*, *y*)-directions of areas encompassing every facial structure.
- Prior, of all the more explicitly, the likelihood of the separation between sets of information pixels.

Given this preparation information, a gathering of relapse trees is prepared to appraise the facial milestone positions straightforwardly from the pixel powers themselves (i.e. no "highlight extraction" is occurring).

The final product is a facial milestone indicator that can be utilised to recognise facial tourist spots progressively with great expectations. The pre-prepared facial milestone locator inside the dlib library is utilised to assess the area of 68 (*x*, *y*)-facilitates that guide to facial structures on the face. The records of the 68 directions can be imagined on the picture beneath:

These comments are a piece of the 68 point iBUG 300-W dataset which the dlib facial milestone indicator was prepared on. It's critical to note that different kinds of facial milestone indicators exist, including the 194 point display that can be prepared on the HELEN dataset. Notwithstanding which dataset is utilised, the equivalent dlib system can be utilised to prepare a shape indicator on the information preparing information—this is valuable because you might want to prepare facial milestone identifiers or custom shape indicators of your own. We can see that facial

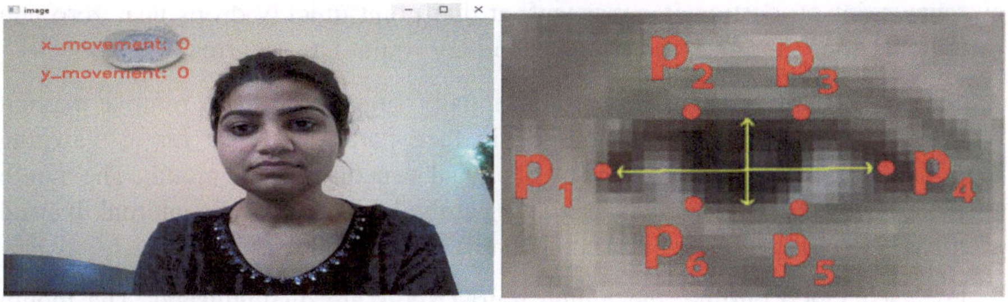

Fig. 20.12 Facial milestone identification

locales can be gotten to through basic Python ordering (expecting zero-ordering with Python since the picture above is one recorded):

1. The mouth can be gotten to through focuses [48, 68].
2. The right eyebrow through focuses [17, 22].
3. The left eyebrow through focuses [22, 27].
4. The right eye utilising [36, 42].
5. The left eye with [42, 48].
6. The nose utilising [27, 35].
7. And the jaw by means of [0, 17].

We can apply facial milestone identification to restrict critical areas of the face, including eyes, eyebrows, nose, ears, and mouth; it has appeared in Fig. 20.12.

Aspect Ratio of Eyes This additionally suggests that we can extricate explicit facial structures by knowing the specific face parts' records. Regarding flicker recognition, we are just intrigued by two arrangements of facial structures—eyes.

Each eye is spoken to by 6 (x, y)-arranges, beginning at the eye's left corner (as though you were taking a gander at the individual), after that working clockwise around the rest of the area. For each video outline, the eye milestones are distinguished. The eye viewpoint proportion (EAR) among tallness and the width of the eye are processed. Where p1, ..., p6 are the 2D milestone areas, delineated in Fig. 20.12.

For the most part, the EAR is consistent when an eye is open and is drawing near to zero while shutting an eye. It is halfway individual, and head presents uncaring. Angle proportion of the open eye has a little difference among people, and it is completely invariant to a uniform scaling of the picture and in-plane pivot of the face. Since eye squinting is performed synchronously by the two eyes, the two eyes' EAR arrives at the midpoint. The numerator of this condition registers the separation between the vertical eye tourist spots, while the denominator figures the separation between flat eye milestones. However weighting the denominator fittingly since there is just a single lot of even focuses two arrangements of vertical focuses. The eye viewpoint proportion is consistent, at that point quickly drops near zero and increments once more, demonstrating a solitary squint has occurred.

Aspect Ratio of the Mouth This additionally suggests we can remove explicit facial structures by knowing the specific face parts' lists. As far as yawning identification, we are just intrigued by the facial structures of the mouth. The mouth is spoken to by 8 (*x*, *y*)-arranges, beginning at the left corner of the internal lips and afterwards working clockwise around the rest of the locale:

For each video outline, the mouth tourist spots are distinguished. The mouth angle proportion (MAR) among tallness and the width of the mouth are figured.

Where p1, ..., p8 are the 2D milestone areas. The MAR is generally consistent when a mouth is open and is getting shifted during the opening of the mouth. It is incompletely individual, and head presents heartless. Viewpoint proportion of the shut mouth has a little difference among people, and it is completely invariant to a uniform scaling of the picture and in-plane turn of the face. This condition's numerator registers the separation between the vertical eye tourist spots, while the denominator figures the separation between even mouth milestones, weighting the denominator. It is consequently ascertaining mouth angle proportion.

Head Pose Estimation The following stage is to assess the driver's head present. Driver's face picture from head location and following has been balanced for head tilting. A strategy to evaluate the head present is following the head utilising the head's movement or the movement of highlights on the face. A famous strategy to obtain the movement is to utilise an optical stream calculation to follow an inflexible head-on video utilising optical stream. They utilised a method-assembled movement regularisation with an ellipsoid model as a base for the following procedure.

The fundamental thought is to locate the head that shows inflexible movement that accounts best for the optical stream. In the first place, the optical stream of each point is determined, and after that, they utilise an angled drop strategy to locate the head's best movement. Their test track is entirely steady over an extensive number of edges and even while utilising groupings with a low edge rate and uproarious pictures. The proposed optical stream based strategy to limit the movements of a deformable model is used to forestall floating brought by the optical stream, and used to join optical stream data and edge data.

Alert Unit The modelling of the alert unit is done when the driver is drowsy. The representation of the classification output is either 1 or 0, and the alert unit uses this number. Whenever the resultant value goes above a specified threshold, it implies that fatigue is detected and the alert system goes active and takes action according to the detected fatigue level.

Result and Analysis Eye viewpoint proportion is utilised as the marker of sleepiness in this eye shutting part, and mouth angle proportion is utilised as the pointer of tiredness in this yawning part. We extricate the video information to its casings. The edges contribute to the part eye and mouth district, figuring and looking at the eye viewpoint proportion and mouth perspective proportion with the limit esteem and distinguishing the sluggishness of the driver. On the off chance that the driver is tired, the caution will sound, and EAR and MAR esteem and the alarm will appear in a showcase. Additionally, investigating the head posture of the driver will recognise the driver's laziness.

20.3 Conclusion

Last-mile delivery is the most important part of e-pharmacy in a pandemic when the delivery of essential critical products is challenging. Most often, the customer growing demands next-day and same-day delivery, leading to a growing number of accidents, which is largely ignored. The factors influencing a driver's fatigue level due to long-distance driving and faster delivery stress are not monitored, mostly out of sight. For the last-mile delivery, the logistics provider is supposed to assume all the liability and legal cost for a vehicle accident and loss of life. Hence, monitoring of the movement, drivers tiredness level is essential. Driver fatigue and distraction levels need to be identified during the last-mile delivery to avoid fatal accidents. This fatigue technology monitors the necessary facial image, eyes and mouth, for instance. Recognition of the eye closure duration, head pose, and the nose is less precise than the scar's finding. Hence, we have used a mask to get detail features of the driver's eyes and mouths in this system. The assessment of its head situation will recognise the driver's tiredness. In terms of moment and accuracy, it improves the structure. The split into three units of the prepared frame is an efficient means of warning the delivery operator. It will alert the driver on a real-time basis, the fatigue level, and improve safety levels. The system seamlessly integrates with the logistics provider's system and continuously provides information and reports immediately if there is a minimal deviation from the specified levels. Real-time data analysis will also help the logistics provider improve driver performance and reach zero accident level.

References

1. Online Pharmacy Market (Global e-Pharma Market) 2020–2026 is Growing So Rapidly || Leading Players (n.d.), https://www.pharmiweb.com/press-release/2020-08-12/online-pharmacy-market-global-e-pharma-market-2020-2026-is-growing-so-rapidly-leading-players. Accessed 8 Sept 2020
2. J. Visser, T. Nemoto, M. Browne, Home delivery and the impacts on urban freight transport: A review. Procedia. Soc. Behav. Sci. **125**, 15–27 (2014). https://doi.org/10.1016/j.sbspro.2014.01.1452
3. R.D. Souza, M. Goh, H. Lau, W. Ng, P. Tan, Collaborative urban logistics – Synchronizing the last mile a Singapore research perspective. Procedia. Soc. Behav. Sci. **125**, 422–431 (2014). https://doi.org/10.1016/j.sbspro.2014.01.1485
4. R. Gevaers, E.V. Voorde, T. Vanelslander, Characteristics and typology of last-mile logistics from an innovation perspective in an urban context, in *City Distribution and Urban Freight*

Transport, (Edward Elgar Publishing, Cheltemham, UK, 2014). https://doi.org/10.4337/9780857932754.00009
5. R. Diebner, E. Silliman, K. Ungerman, M. Vancauwenberghe, Adapting customer experience in the time of coronavirus (2020), https://www.mckinsey.com/business-functions/marketing-and-sales/our-insights/adapting-customer-experience-in-the-time-of-coronavirus. Accessed 8 Sept 2020
6. J. Allen, M. Piecyk, M. Piotrowska, F. Mcleod, T. Cherrett, K. Ghali, et al., Understanding the impact of e-commerce on last-mile light goods vehicle activity in urban areas: The case of London. Transp. Res. Part D: Transp. Environ. **61**, 325–338 (2018). https://doi.org/10.1016/j.trd.2017.07.020
7. Y. Wang, D. Zhang, Q. Liu, F. Shen, L.H. Lee, Towards enhancing the last-mile delivery: An effective crowd-tasking model with scalable solutions. Transp. Res. Part E: Logistics Transp. Rev. **93**, 279–293 (2016). https://doi.org/10.1016/j.tre.2016.06.002
8. S. Digiesi, G. Mascolo, G. Mossa, G. Mummolo, *New Models for Sustainable Logistics. Internalization of External Costs in Inventory Management*, Springer Brief in Operations Management (Springer International Publishing, Cham, Switzerland, 2016) ISBN 978-3-319-19709-8
9. L. Ranieri, S. Digiesi, B. Silvestri, M. Roccotelli, A review of last mile logistics innovations in an externalities cost reduction vision. Sustainability **10**(3), 782 (2018). https://doi.org/10.3390/su10030782
10. X. Wang, L. Zhan, J. Ruan, J. Zhang, How to choose "last mile" delivery modes for E-fulfillment. Math. Probl. Eng. **2014**, 1–11 (2014). https://doi.org/10.1155/2014/417129
11. The last-mile delivery challenge - capgemini.com (n.d.), https://www.capgemini.com/wp-content/uploads/2019/01/Report-Digital-—Last-Mile-Delivery-Challenge1.pdf. Accessed 8 Sept 2020
12. N. Mcdonald, Q. Yuan, R. Naumann, Urban freight and road safety in the era of e-commerce. Traffic Inj. Prev. **20**(7), 764–770 (2019). https://doi.org/10.1080/15389588.2019.1651930
13. K.U. Anjali et al., Real-time nonintrusive monitoring and detection of eye blinking in view of accident prevention due to drowsiness, in *2016 International Conference on Circuit, Power and Computing Technologies (ICCPCT)*, (IEEE, New York, 2016)
14. O. Stan, L. Miclea, A. Centea, EyeGaze tracking method driven by Raspberry PI applicable in automotive traffic safety, in *2014 2nd International Conference on Artificial Intelligence, Modelling and Simulation (AIMS)*, (IEEE, New York, 2014)
15. G. Turan, S. Gupta, Road accidents prevention system using driver's drowsiness detection. Int. J. Adv. Res. Comput. Eng. Technol. **2** (2013)
16. R. Liu et al., Design of face detection and tracking system, in *2010 3rd International Congress on Image and Signal Processing (CISP)*, vol. 4, (2010), pp. 1840–1844
17. P. Goal et al., Hybrid approach of Haar cascade classifiers and geometrical properties of facial features applied to illumination invariant gender classification system, in *2012 International Conference on Computing Sciences (ICCS)*, (2012), pp. 132–136
18. D. Jose, S. Prasad, V. Sridhar, Intelligent vehicle monitoring using global positioning system and cloud computing. Procedia Comput. Sci. **50**, 440–446 (2015). https://doi.org/10.1016/j.procs.2015.04.012
19. S. Kavuri, D. Moltchanov, A. Ometov, S. Andreev, Y. Koucheryavy, Performance analysis of onshore NB-IoT for container tracking during near-the-shore vessel navigation. IEEE Internet Things J. 7(4), 2928–2943 (2020).

Chapter 21
Chest X-ray Images Analysis with Deep Convolutional Neural Networks (CNN) for COVID-19 Detection

Xavier Lessage, Saïd Mahmoudi, Sidi Ahmed Mahmoudi, Sohaib Laraba, Olivier Debauche, and Mohammed Amin Belarbi

21.1 Introduction

In a crisis context, health professionals need efficient tools allowing them to make the best decisions in an emergency. Following the example of meteorological modeling, artificial intelligence-based methods use epidemic modeling to propose an estimate of the number of caregivers that could be ill in the next few days at the scale of a hospital or a hospital department.

Since 2012, we have witnessed an increased use of artificial intelligence in various fields, particularly in computer vision and medical imaging. At the dawn of this fourth industrial revolution, we are witnessing the birth of new algorithms based mainly on deep learning. The enthusiasm is such that it is pushing the scientific community to apply these techniques in medical applications.

Over the last 10 years, deep learning has changed the IT landscape dramatically. In the 1980s and 1990s, a computer had to be programmed in order to enable it to learn. Today, by showing the algorithm annotated images, some containing cats and others with no cats for example, the computer learns to recognize cats from a library of images. After a certain number of images, the system starts to generalize and knows how to recognize the animal in pictures it has never seen. The data scientist no longer has to write the code to extract the desired characteristics from the image as he used to do with Machine Learning (ML) techniques. With Deep Learning, a convolutional neural network will learn them based on examples and thus identify the characteristics of the object. Indeed, Deep Learning is a sub-domain of Machine

X. Lessage · S. Mahmoudi (✉) · S. A. Mahmoudi · S. Laraba · O. Debauche · M. A. Belarbi
University of Mons, Mons, Belgium
e-mail: xavier.lessage@student.umons.ac.be; said.mahmoudi@umons.ac.be; sidi.mahmoudi@umons.ac.be; sohaib.laraba@umons.ac.be; olivier.debauche@umons.ac.be; mohammedamin.belarbi@umons.ac.be

L. Garg et al. (eds.), *Healthcare Informatics for Fighting COVID-19 and Future Epidemics*, EAI/Springer Innovations in Communication and Computing,
https://doi.org/10.1007/978-3-030-72752-9_21

Learning. It uses what is called deep neural networks, which are composed of a very high number of layers. It takes advantage of the increasing availability of large data volumes and the computing power of GPUs.

The latest advances in Convolutional Neural Networks (CNNs) have proven more than once their high accuracy in disease detection. They show great promise and may help to reduce the number of discrepancies and the recall rate without reducing the detection rate.

However, these technologies do not claim to replace the radiologist, but rather to increase his or her performance in detecting abnormalities by combining the two intelligences: the first, artificial, to make an initial analysis, and the second, human, to interpret the results and make the right diagnosis. The doctor's opinion remains essential before starting a complementary adjustment of the detected abnormalities (complementary radiographs, ultrasound, magnetic resonance, and/or biopsies).

This chapter proposes a new detection method based on deep learning-based algorithms for COVID-19 detection in chest X-rays images. The proposed approach applies, in an efficient way, the techniques of transfer learning and fine-tuning from pre-trained CNNs (InceptionV3 [1], VGG16 [2] and VGG11, MobileNet [3], Xception [4], DenseNet [5] and EfficientNet [6]).

21.2 Related Works

Medical imaging has been using machine learning algorithms for decades. In the mid-1960s, radiologists started using algorithms to help in analyzing radiographic images [7–9]. These algorithms made more progress in the 1980s and helped mainly in the detection and diagnosis of cancer from radiographs and mammograms [10, 11], and later on other modalities like computer tomography (CT) and ultrasound [12, 13].

Most of the proposed approaches since are based on classical ML methods which require the design of features manually [14–18]. Despite the effectiveness of these algorithms in terms of computation time and accuracy, hand-crafted features have a lot of drawbacks, like dataset-dependency. These features are designed on specific datasets and cannot be generalized on other datasets. Moreover, hand-crafted features require a lot of feature engineering and are time-consuming.

Currently, deep learning methods have been receiving a lot of attention due to the high performances they achieved in a variety of problems such as image classification, speech processing, object detection, and action recognition. Naturally, ML applications in a medical imaging context have increased significantly. Given the current COVID-19 context, we focus in this section on the last works proposed for the detection of pneumonia lesions.

Rajpukar et al. proposed in 2017 the **CheXNet** network for the classification of 14 different diseases from a dataset composed of chest X-ray images [19]. CheXNet architecture is a modified version of DenseNet [5] with 121 convolutional layers. The last fully-connected layer is replaced by a single output layer, after which a

Sigmoid non-linear function is applied. The model was trained on ChestX-ray14 dataset. [20] The network weights are initialized from a pre-trained model on the ImageNet dataset [21].

Recently, Mangal et al. [22] developed a COVID-19 detection system based on CheXNet, namely **CovidAID**. Their network contains 121 convolutional layers as in CheXNet, followed by a fully-connected layer. The network is trained on a dataset with four classes (COVID-19, normal, viral pneumonia, and bacterial pneumonia). The dataset is formed partially from ChestX-ray14, where a class corresponding to COVID-19 disease is added. In total, 6014 images are gathered in this dataset. The authors fine-tuned the ChexNet network and initialized their model with its weights. The training has been achieved in 2 steps: In the first step, the DenseNet backbone layers are frozen, and only the fully-connected layer is trained on 30 epochs. In the second step, all the layers have been re-trained on 10 epochs. The authors obtained an accuracy of 87.2%. They have also tested another configuration with three classes where they merged the images of viral and bacterial pneumonia and obtained an accuracy of 90.5%.

Hammoudi et al. [23] have shown that the DenseNet model with 169 layers [5] provides better results of classification on a 3-classes dataset (bacteria, normal, and virus) of 5232 chest X-rays images of children patients. They obtained a mean accuracy of 95.72% (97.97% for bacterial, 96.62% for virus, and 95.57% for normal cases).

Wang et al. presented **Covid-Net**[24], an architecture that exploits the residual architecture design principles for the detection of COVID-19 based on X-ray images. Their training dataset is composed of 5941 post-anterior chest X-rays across 2839 patients distributed in 1203 normal, 931 bacterial pneumonia, 660 non-COVID-19 viral pneumonia, and 45 COVID-19. The global accuracy obtained is 83.5%.

Kahn et al. proposed **CoroNet**[25], a deep CNNs model that uses Xception architecture [4] with a dropout layer and two fully-connected layers added at the end. The dataset used for the training is composed of 310 normal, 330 pneumonia bacterial, 327 pneumonia viral, and 284 COVID-19 images. They obtained an accuracy of 99% for two classes (COVID, non-COVID), 95% for three classes (COVID, pneumonia, normal), and 89.6% for four classes (COVID, pneumonia bacterial, pneumonia viral, normal).

Hemdan et al. [26] have proposed **COVIDX-NET**, a framework based on seven convolutional neural networks: VGG19 [2], DenseNet201 [5], InceptionV3 [1], ResNetV2 [27], InceptionRestNetV2 [28], Xception [4], and MobileNetV2 [29] to assist radiologists to detect COVID-19 from X-ray images. The models are trained on a dataset composed of 25 COVID-19 images, and 25 normal images. VGG-19 and DenseNet-201 have given the best value of accuracy (90%).

Apostolopoulos et al. [30] compared five different CNN architectures, VGG-19 [2], MobileNetV2, Inception, Xception, InceptionResNetV2 for COVID-19 classification. The results showed that VGG19 and MobilNetV2 provide the best accuracy results, respectively 98.75 and 97.40%, on two classes (COVID, normal), and 93.48 and 92.85% on three classes (COVID, pneumonia, normal). The dataset

Table 21.1 State-of-the-art results of COVID-19 classification from chest X-ray images

Model	Reference	# 2-classes	# 3-classes	# 4-classes	# Images
CovidAID	[22]	–	90.50%	87.20%	112,120
Covid-Net	[24]	–	–	83.00%	5941
COVIDX-Net	[26]	90.00%	–	–	50
CoroNet	[25]	99.00%	94.59%	89.60%	1211
DenseNet-169	[23]	–	–	95.72%	5941
VGG-19	[30]	98.75%	93.48%	–	1428
MobileNetV2	[30]	97.40%	92.85%	–	1428
MobileNetV2	[30]	96.78%	94.72%	–	1442
ResNet50	[31]	98.00%	–	–	100
COVID-CXNET	[34]	99.40%	–	–	3628
COVID-CXNET	[34]	–	87.21%	–	7700

is composed of 504 normal images, 224 COVID-19, and 700 bacterial pneumonia. On a second dataset composed of 224 COVID-19, 400 bacterial pneumonia, 314 viral pneumonia, and 504 normal cases images, MobileNetV2 provided an accuracy of 96.78% on using two classes and 94.72% using three classes.

Narin et al. [31] have also compared performances of three classical CNN architectures: ResNet50 [32], InceptionV3 [1], and InceptionResNetV2 [28]. They obtained the best accuracy with ResNet50 (98%). The training dataset is composed of 50 normal and 50 COVID-19 chest X-ray images. The models were trained using the transfer learning process by using the ImageNet database[21].

Wang et al. [33] have elaborated **ChestNet**, a deep neural network composed of two branches. The first is a classification step using a pre-trained ImageNet ResNet-152 model to label predictions. The second branch is composed of six convolutional layers: The first five layers use ReLU activation function while the last layer uses a Sigmoid one. The layers contain respectively 1×1, 3×3, 1×1, $14\ 1 \times 1$, $512\ 1 \times 1$, and 14×14 kernels. The model was trained on ChestX-ray14[20] and provided an average accuracy of 78.1% on a 14-classes dataset (Table 21.1).

Ahishali et al. [35] compared the performances of two sets of models for early detection of COVID-19. In the first set, they used classical machine learning algorithms (SRC, CRC, CSEN, MLP, SVM, and k-NN), while in the second set, they trained multiple CNN models (ChestXNet, DenseNet-121, ResNet-50, and InceptionV3). All models were tested over the Early-QaTa-COV19 dataset composed of 175 early-stage COVID-19 and 1579 normal images. Experimentation showed that CRC is the best compact model with an accuracy of 92.30% while the CNNs obtained better performances with an augmented dataset to 20,000 images. The obtained accuracy results for different CNN models are as follows: 99.26% for CheXNet, 99.49% for DenseNet-121, 99.37% for InceptionV3, and 99.43% for ResNet50.

Haghanifar et al. [34] have described **COVID-CXNET** based on DenseNet-121, followed by 10 fully-connected layers, a dropout layer of 0.2 dropping rate, and a

Sigmoid activation function. An accuracy of 99.04% is obtained on a two-classes dataset of 3628 images (428 COVID-19 and 3200 normal) and 81.04% for a three classes dataset with 7700 images (700 COVID-19, 3500 CAP, and 3500 normal).

In May 2020, El Asnaoui and Chawki [36] compared several recent deep learning models (VGG16[2], VGG19[2], DenseNet201[5], InceptionResNetV2[28], InceptionV3[1], Resnet50[32], and MobileNetV2[29]) for COVID-19 detection based on chest X-rays images classification. The dataset was formed by adding 231 COVID-19 X-ray images of chest to a second dataset of 5856 images constituted in 2018 by Kermany et al. [37]. This resulted in a dataset consisting of 6087 images with four classes (231 COVID-19 cases, 1583 normal, 2780 bacterial pneumonia, and 1493 viral pneumonia). Image pre-processing has also been performed to improve the contrast (CLAHE) [38]. In this work, the best results were achieved by InceptionResnetV2 which achieved 92.07% of F1-score and 92.18% of accuracy. The second model was DenseNet201 with an accuracy of 88.09%. On the contrary, VGG16 and VGG19 gave the lowest scores with 72.52% and 74.84% of accuracy, respectively.

21.3 Proposed Approach

Chest X-ray images analysis can be rethought as an image classification task, which represents a machine learning problem that can be effectively dealt with by employing Deep Learning Technology. In this chapter, we present a classification methodology that uses transfer learning (from pre-trained weights with ImageNet) and fine-tuning of several selected and most efficient recent convolutional neural network architectures.

21.3.1 Transfer Learning

The technique of transfer learning is highly used in the domain of deep learning. It takes advantage of previously acquired learning weights, and by analogy, it solves a related but different problem. The goal of the convolutional layers is feature extraction, and the fully-connected layers allow the classification task. The neural networks are stacked into multiple layers, and each one learns from the previous one. The first layers learn low-level features, like colors, edges, etc. The learned features are increasingly complex and abstract the deeper we go into the network. In the courses of the learning phase, the neural network adapts its weights. Indeed, it is effortless to take advantage of an existing neural network, without having to recalculate what has allowed it to reach its optimal configuration, calculated for the dataset and problem for which it was designed.

In this work, each Convolutional Neural Network (CNN) architecture is initialized with the pre-trained ImageNet[21] weights to benefit from a network that is already well trained. ImageNet is a freely accessible dataset containing 14 million images divided into 1000 categories [21].

21.3.2 Data Augmentation

The volume of the dataset available for our experimentation is reduced; that is why, we use the technique of data augmentation technique. To this aim we apply multiple transformations to input images. For this task, we apply classical transformations such as rotation, rescale, shear, and shift. This can be used, among other things, as a regularization technique to avoid overfitting due to the small size of the data. In our case, the dataset was increased with a ratio of 30% compared to the initial dataset.

21.3.3 The Proposed Method

The primary objective of the method described is the separation of X-ray images into two or three categories by selecting and adapting the best CNN architecture. The proposed method exploits a pre-trained architecture on ImageNet and applies different modifications:

1. From each pre-trained architecture, we removed the last layer of 1000 neurons, which was initially used for the classification of ImageNet images that represent 1000 classes;
2. Integration of 5 dense layers composed of 1024, 512, 256, 128, and 64 layers that allow to fine-tune the weights in a progressive way since our problem tends to classify 3 classes only;
3. Definition of the size of the last layer (output): 3 classes (normal, COVID-19, other pathology) or 2 classes (normal, COVID-19).

In order to avoid oscillations of accuracy and loss values between epochs during the training process, we suggest to use the rate decay method that allows to optimize the learning rate value and thus accelerate the convergence and ensure accurate results. To improve the performance of the classifier in terms of sensitivity and specificity, an additional test based on the probability of classification has been added. The COVID-19 lesions will only be classified if the probability is at least 85%. Otherwise, the detected lesion will be classified as other pathologies.

21.4 Evaluation Dataset

We use a recent chest X-ray anonymized dataset from an Italian hospital thanks to a retrospective study. It is composed of three classes (normal, COVID-19, other

Table 21.2 Content of the used dataset

	# Normal	# COVID-19	# Other pathologies
Training	938	153	948
Validation	268	44	270
Testing	135	22	127

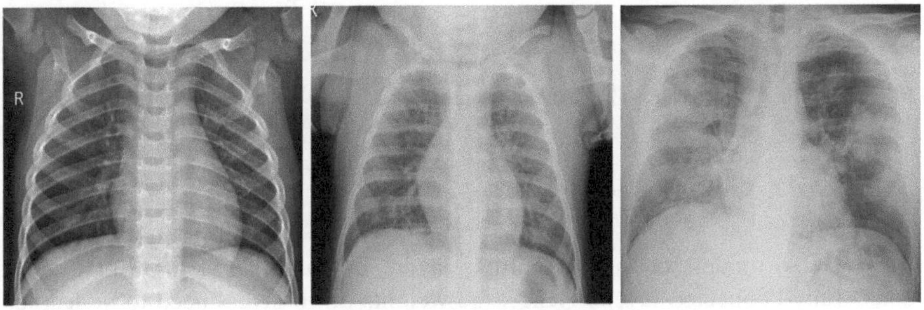

(a) "Normal" (b) "Other pathology" (c) "COVID-19"

Fig. 21.1 Example of chest X-ray images. Respectively, from left to right, a normal chest image (**a**), another pulmonary pathology (**b**), an image showing traces of COVID-19 (**c**)

pathologies) with a total number of 2905 images. This dataset was randomly splitted into three parts (70% for training, 20% for validation, and 10% for test) as shown in Table 21.2 to obtain an efficient evaluation of the proposed models.

Figure 21.1 presents some examples of its content. As can be in this figure, the image showing traces of COVID-19 is very characteristic by the presence of spots in the lower part of the lung.

Note that this dataset contains only X-rays of children's chests.

21.5 Experimental Results

The dataset of X-rays images is represented by three separate class folders: normal (1341 images), COVID-19 (219 images), and other pathologies (1345 images). For our experiments, we divided the dataset into three parts: training 70%, validation 20%, and test 10%. The training and validation datasets are used during the training process, while the test dataset is used to obtain an independent test composed of unknown images by the neural network. As described above, we benchmark the performance of the proposed method and compared it within several CNNs architectures. We will first briefly illustrate the VGG16 architecture, as it is simple, yet explanatory of CNNs.

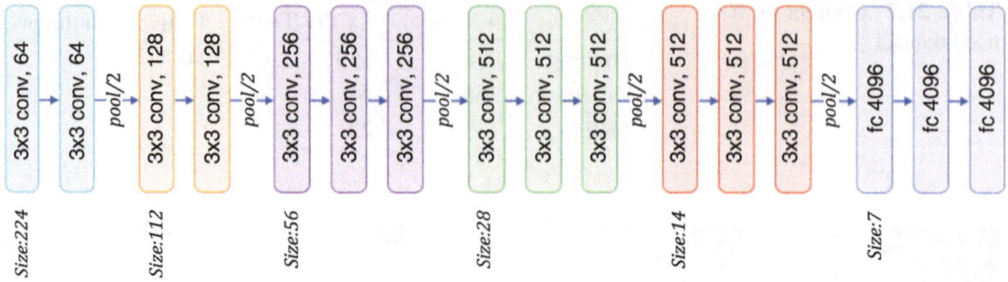

Fig. 21.2 Illustration of the VGG16 architecture

21.5.1 VGG16

The VGG16 model consists of multiple layers, containing 13 convolution layers and 3 fully-connected layers. Hence, the weights of 16 layers need to be learned. VGG 16 architecture takes a 224 × 224 pixels color image as input, after that it is classified into one of the *n* classes. Finally, a vector of size *n* is returned. This vector represents the probabilities related to each class. The architecture of VGG16 is illustrated in Fig. 21.2.

21.5.1.1 Training and Validation

With this model, a classifier of 3 classes is trained on 50 epochs and stopped by Early Stopping at 48 epochs, we obtain the best result as shown above. Figures 21.3, 21.4, and 21.5 show successively the progression of the training accuracy, the training loss, and the validation accuracy. Figure 21.3 shows an evolution of the accuracy from 94.3% at the first epoch to 97.8% at epoch 48. We can also notice that the loss evolves from 0.25 to 0.11 when the training is finished. Finally, the validation rate of accuracy evolves from 88.6% at the beginning and finishes with a value of 94.1% at the end of the training.

The best results were obtained by calibrating the CNNs with the following hyperparameters: an image size of 224 × 224 pixels, a number of epochs equal to 50 with batch size of 10 images. The FC_size (fully-connected layer size) is equal to three, and all the layers are trained in two steps. During the first step namely transfer learning, the RMSprop optimizer is used with a learning rate (lr) of 1e–04, a ρ parameter of 0.9, an ϵ parameter of 1e–08, and a decay of 1e–04. The second step namely fine-tuning used the optimizer SGD with a learning rate of 1e–04, and a momentum of 0.9.

The analysis of these results shows that the accuracy tends towards 98% and the loss towards 11%. Although the results are very encouraging, we have taken care to test this classifier with a set of test images that the model has never seen. We also added a threshold of 85% based on the detected lesion probability in order to classify the image as COVID-19. Otherwise, it will be classified as other

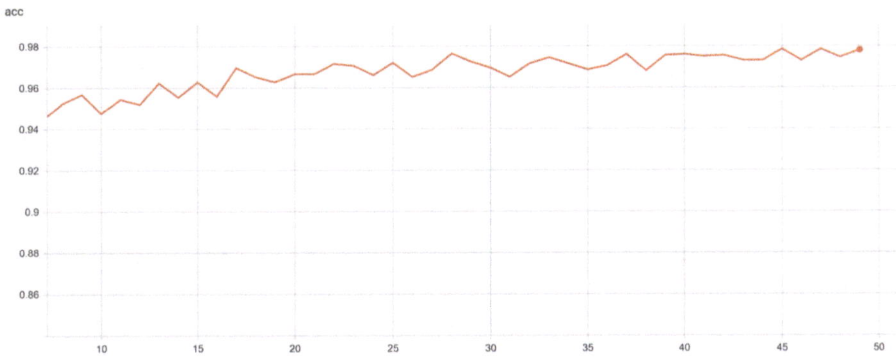

Fig. 21.3 Progression of the training accuracy using VGG16 model

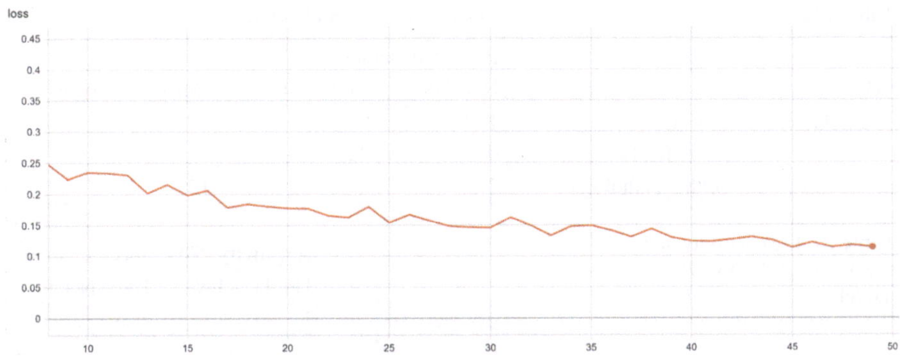

Fig. 21.4 Progression of the training loss using VGG16 model

pathologies. Thanks to this threshold, we were able to reduce the number of false negatives in the classifier.

21.5.1.2 Confusion Matrix

The confusion matrix expresses the number of true positive (the number of examples that are correctly classified as infected), false positives (the number of examples classified as infected, while they are normal), true negatives (the number of examples that are correctly classified as normal), and false negatives (the number of examples classified as normal, while they are infected). By infected, we mean that the corresponding patients have either signs of COVID-19 or other pathologies. We note these values TP, FP, TN, and FN respectively. The confusion matrix in Table 21.3 presents the results obtained with the threshold enabled.

The number of false positives (FP) and false negatives (FN) are only 5 and 2 respectively. If we disable the threshold, FP is slightly higher (8 instead of 5). The number of FN remains unchanged.

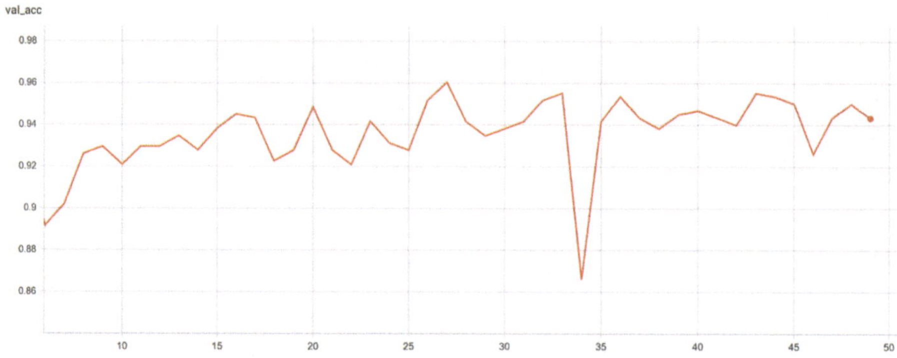

Fig. 21.5 Progression of the validation accuracy using VGG16 model

Table 21.3 Confusion matrix of test results using VGG16 architecture

VGG16		Predicted classes		
		Normal	COVID-19	Other pathologies
True classes	Normal	130	0	5
	COVID-19	0	22	0
	Other pathologies	2	0	125

Table 21.4 Sensitivity and specificity of the VGG16 model

Sensitivity (%)	Specificity (%)
TP/(TP + FN)	TN/(TN + FP)
98.7	98.5

21.5.1.3 Sensitivity and Specificity

The sensitivity of a model reflects its ability to provide the highest FN (i.e., its ability to not missing any infected person). The specificity, on the other hand, is the ability of the model to provide the minimum FP (i.e., its ability to detect only the infected persons). The sensitivity is very important from the medical point of view, where a reliable system should be able to spot all the infected patients. The specificity is less important, as a patient who is healthy and classified as sick will not cause a lot of damages to other people.

Our results with the VGG16 architecture show excellent scores, as shown in Table 21.4.

21.5.1.4 Impact of Regularization on Model Training

In order to avoid overfitting, i.e., prevent that the model adjusts too much to the dataset during the learning phase, without being able to generalize correctly, various techniques are recommended. Regularization is one of them and consists of acting at the level of the cost function by making the model less flexible through additional constraints.

We have tested the regularization techniques with a view to further improving the results and control overfitting. But, against all expectations, despite a learning curve that reached 98% and an even smaller loss of around 6%, the test with the same dataset (284 images) was not as good as with the model without regularization.

Figures 21.6, 21.7, and 21.8 show respectively the progression of the training accuracy, the training loss, and the validation accuracy obtained.

Table 21.5 compares the confusion matrix and results obtained for different combinations of threshold and regularization.

The analysis of Table 21.5 shows that regularization increased the number of false negatives from 2 to 9 with the same threshold, while the number of false positives remained the same, at 5.

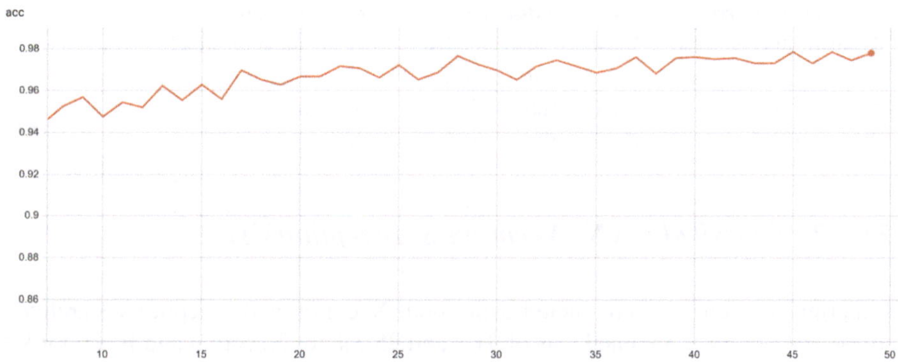

Fig. 21.6 Progression of the VGG16 training accuracy after regularization

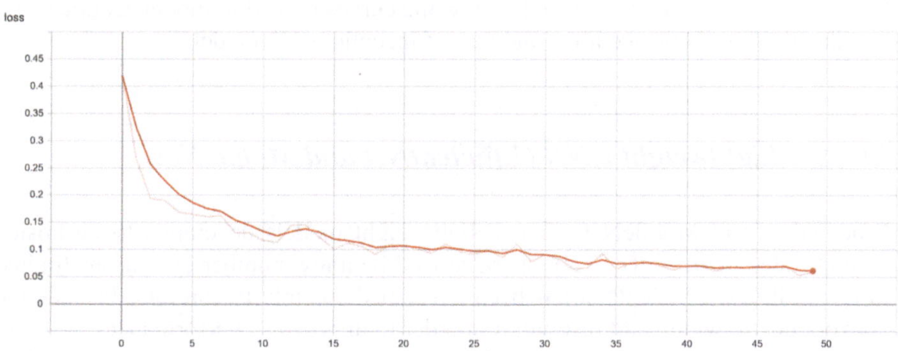

Fig. 21.7 Progression of the VGG16 training loss after regularization

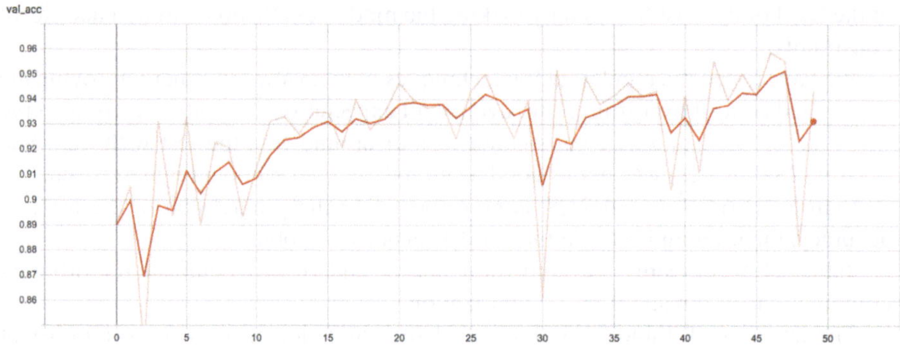

Fig. 21.8 Progression of the VGG16 validation accuracy after regularization

Table 21.5 Comparison of confusion matrix

Threshold **enabled**			Threshold **disabled**			Threshold **enabled**		
Regularization **enabled**			Regularization **enabled**			Regularization **disabled**		
	True	False		True	False		True	False
True	139	5	True	160	2	True	147	5
False	9	131	False	18	104	False	2	130

21.5.2 Classical CNN (Xception & InceptionV3)

Experiments were also conducted using both Xception and InceptionV3 architectures. The accuracy obtained was of 91.2 and 95.7% for Xception and InceptionV3.

Figures 21.9, 21.10, 21.11, and 21.12 show the curves related to model accuracy and loss and the validation accuracy and loss of Xception model. On the other hand, Figs. 21.13, 21.14, 21.15, and 21.16 show the curves related to model accuracy and loss and the validation accuracy and loss of Inceptions V3 model.

21.5.3 Lightweight CNN (EfficientNet and MobileNet)

EfficientNet and MobileNet are two lightweight models developed to be hosted on embedded devices. They are characterized by a low number of neurons limited to few millions. EfficientNet has been developed recently to carefully balance the network depth, width, and resolution in order to improve its performance.

The results obtained by MobileNet model are very promising. Indeed, we obtained 99.3% of accuracy, 98.7% of specificity, and 98.7% of sensitivity. This model has a tiny size (24.8 MB), which allows it to be exploitable on mobile devices without the need for cloud hosting.

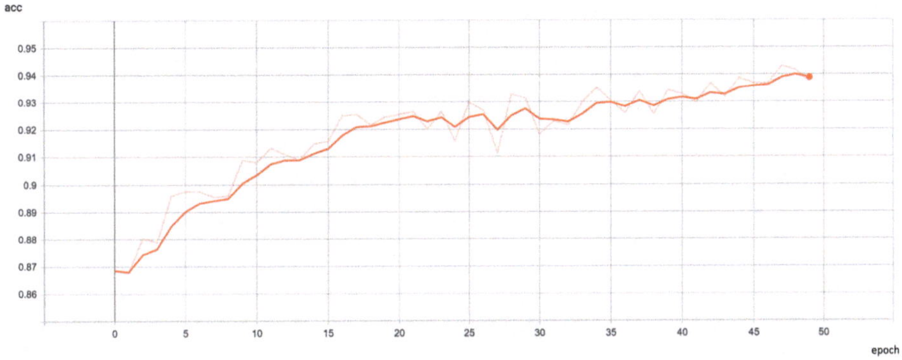

Fig. 21.9 Progression of the training accuracy of Xception

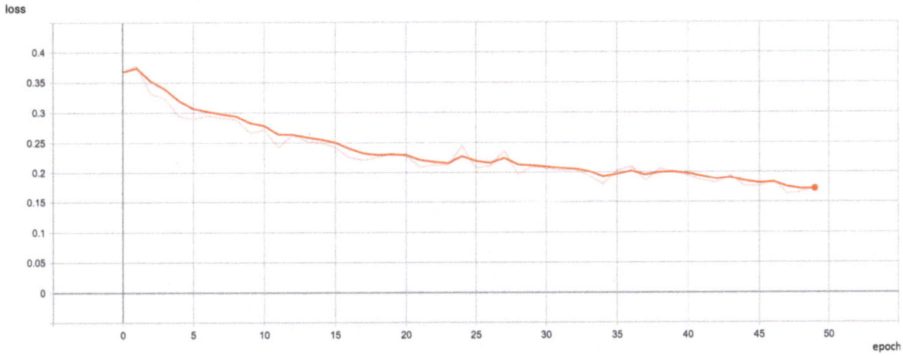

Fig. 21.10 Progression of the training loss of Xception

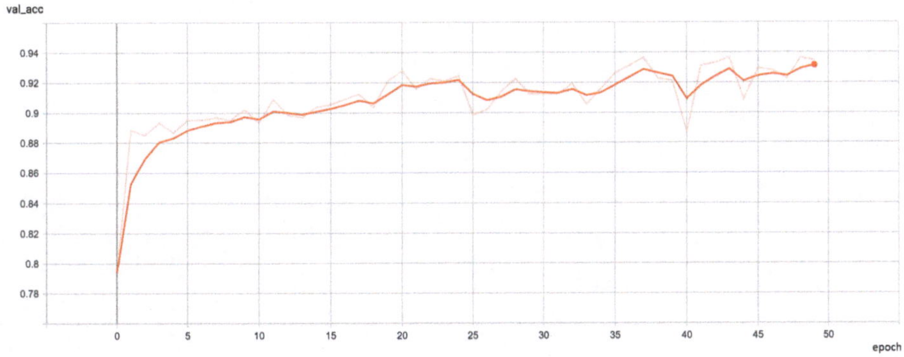

Fig. 21.11 Progression of the validation accuracy of Xception

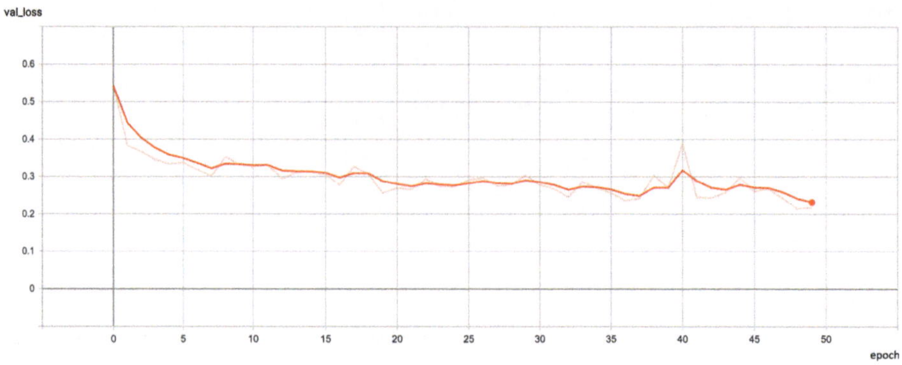

Fig. 21.12 Progression of the validation loss of Xception

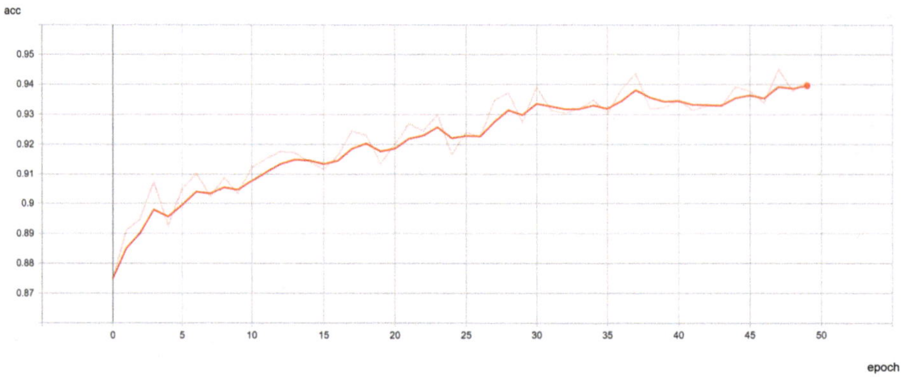

Fig. 21.13 Progression of the training accuracy of InceptionV3

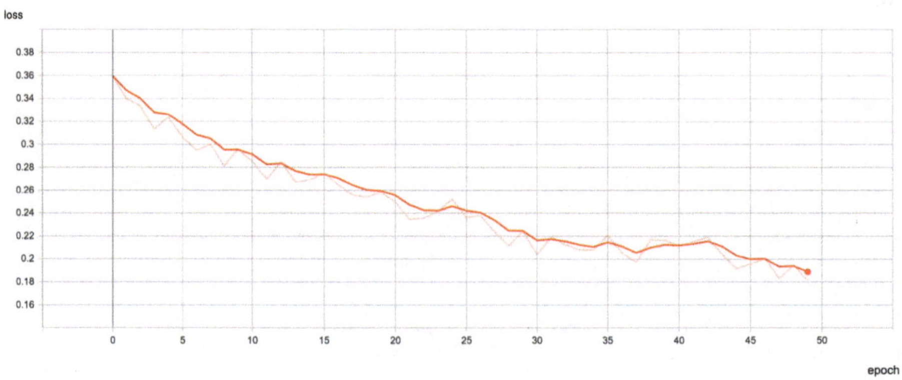

Fig. 21.14 Progression of the training loss of InceptionV3

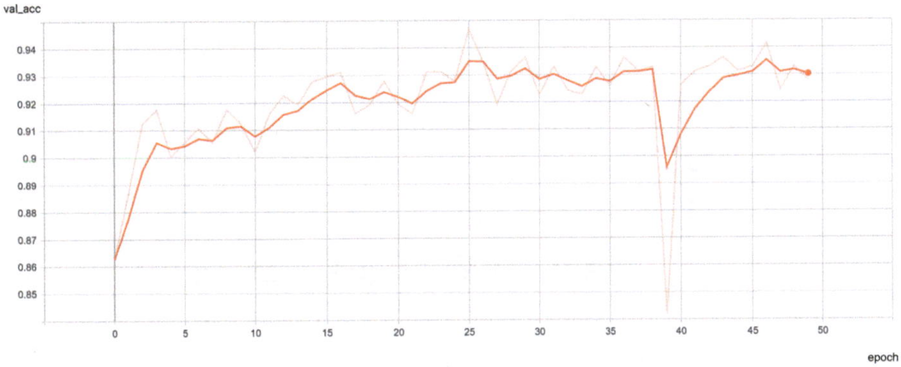

Fig. 21.15 Progression of the validation accuracy of InceptionV3

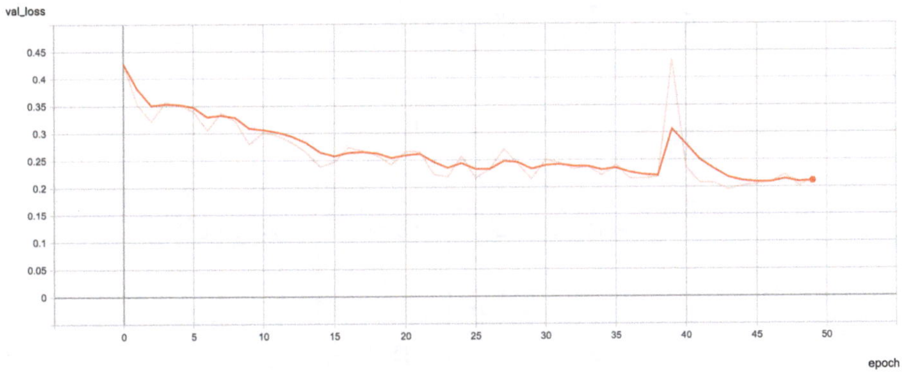

Fig. 21.16 Progression of the validation loss of InceptionV3

21.6 Benchmark Results

In this chapter, we have compared well-known state-of-the-art CNNs: VGG16, MobileNet, InceptionV3, Xception, DenseNet-169, and a recent model Efficient-NetB0, in order to evaluate their performance to identify COVID-19 on X-rays of children chests. We use the VGG16 as a baseline for our comparison with other models. The analysis of Table 21.6 shows that MobileNet and VGG16 are the best models in terms of accuracy. Indeed, the performances comparison of the different architectures shows that MobileNet and VGG16 provide the highest scores: 99.3% and 98.7% of accuracy respectively, 98.7% and 96.3% of sensitivity respectively, and 98.7% of specificity for both models.

We can notice that MobileNet presents only one false negative detection, and VGG16 two false negative detection. This fact is also confirmed by the high sensitivity value of both models (99.3% and 98.7% for MobileNet and VGG16

Table 21.6 Performance comparison of different algorithms

Features	VGG16	MobileNet	Xception	InceptionV3	EfficientNetB0	DenseNet169
Training						
Epochs	48	48	48	48	48	48
# Training images	2039	2039	2039	2039	2039	2039
# Validation images	588	588	588	588	588	588
Test						
Test accuracy	97.5%	99.3%	91.2%	95.7%	85.5%	90.1%
# Images	284	284	284	284	284	284
Model						
Sensitivity	98.7%	99.3%	91.3%	95.9%	96.6%	85.9%
Specificity	96.3%	99.2%	91.1%	95.6%	73.3%	94.8%
F1-score	97.5%	99.3%	91.2%	95.7%	83.4%	90.1%
Details of true/false positive/negative						
True positives (TP)	147	152	136	139	143	128
False positives (FP)	5	1	12	6	36	7
False negatives (FN)	2	1	13	6	5	21
True negatives (TN)	130	130	123	129	99	128

respectively). These results are very promising because they prove the capacity of these two models to identify all possible COVID-19 cases.

On the other hand, the accuracies obtained with Xception and InceptionV3 architectures were 91.2% and 95.7% respectively, which are acceptable scores. However, the number of false negatives (respectively 12 and 6) is more important for both models. The sensitivity ratio of 91.3% and 95.9% respectively for Xception and InceptionV3 confirms that fact.

EfficientNet presents a lower accuracy of 85.5%, meanwhile, this architecture shows an acceptable false negative ratio (only five false negative detection). However, the specificity of this architecture is not good (73.3%) which means that this model provides a high number of false positives detection (36) and tends to assert that non-infected patients are positive COVID-19 cases.

The last model DenseNet presents also a low-test accuracy of 90.1%. This model shows also a bad sensitivity ratio of 85.9% with 21 false negative detection.

We can conclude that MobileNet and VGG16 models provide the best results. MobileNet architecture presents the additional advantage to be lightweight and suitable for mobile devices.

21.7 Web Application

Figure 21.17 shows the graphical user interface of our web application. This web portal allows users to upload their X-ray images for analysis. This approach has the advantage of not requiring the installation or configuration of libraries. The user can upload an X-ray image which is used by the proposed pre-trained Artificial Intelligence algorithm to detect the presence or the absence of COVID-19. Three examples are also proposed to the user for demonstration purpose. The algorithm tags the image with the result of the diagnostic and gives the probability for each of the three categories and also the execution time.

After the analysis, the image is erased by the server. We plan to add a box that allows the user to keep the uploaded image on our server in order to extend our dataset. Another option that will be added to the interface is to get the feedback of the doctors who use the platform to confirm the model decisions and provide more improvements.

21.8 Conclusions and Future Work

In this chapter, we described a deep learning-based approach that exploits the transfer learning technique in an efficient way for the detection of COVID-19, or other pathologies, from chest X-ray images. Our approach allowed us to solve the problems of underfitting and overfitting during the training process, with the use of data augmentation and regularization techniques.

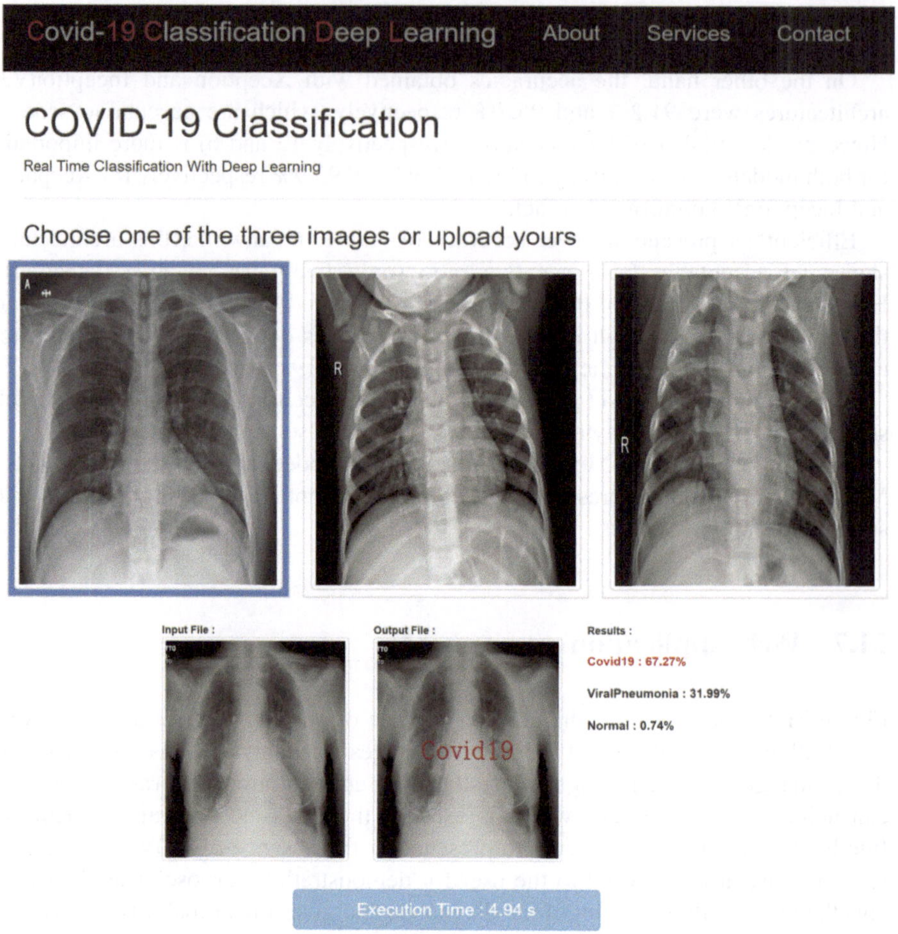

Fig. 21.17 Real-time classification with deep learning

Our results show that the best classification results for the three classes (COVID-19, others pathologies, normal) are obtained with the MobileNet and VGG16 architectures. MobileNet architecture presents an accuracy of 99.3%. On the other hand, VGG16 architecture allows to predict the presence of COVID-19 with an accuracy of 97.5%.

In our future work, we will continue to extend our approach to CT images and to use a larger dataset.

References

1. C. Szegedy, V. Vanhoucke, S. Ioffe, J. Shlens, Z. Wojna, Rethinking the inception architecture for computer vision, in *Proceedings of the IEEE Conference on Computer Vision and Pattern Recognition* (2016), pp. 2818–2826. https://arxiv.org/abs/1512.00567. Cited 6 Aug 2020
2. K. Simonyan, A. Zisserman, Very deep convolutional networks for large-scale image recognition (2014). https://arxiv.org/abs/1409.1556. Cited 12 Aug 2020
3. A.G. Howard, M. Zhu, B. Chen, D. Kalenichenko, W. Wang, T. Weyand, M. Andreetto, H. Adam, Mobilenets: Efficient convolutional neural networks for mobile vision applications (2017). https://arxiv.org/abs/1704.04861. Cited 9 Aug 2020
4. F. Chollet, Xception: Deep learning with depthwise separable convolutions, in *Proceedings of the IEEE Conference on Computer Vision and Pattern Recognition* (2017). https://arxiv.org/abs/1610.02357. Cited 8 Aug 2020
5. G. Huang, Z. Liu, L. Van Der Maaten, K.Q. Weinberger, Densely connected convolutional networks, in *Proceedings of the IEEE Conference on Computer Vision and Pattern Recognition* (2017), pp. 4700–4708. https://arxiv.org/abs/1608.06993. Cited 2 Aug 2020
6. M. Tan, Q.V. Le, EfficientNet: Rethinking model scaling for convolutional neural networks (2019). https://arxiv.org/abs/1905.11946. Cited 5 Aug 2020
7. P.H. Meyers, C.M. Nice Jr, H.C. Becker, W.J. Nettleton Jr, J.W. Sweeney, G.R. Meckstroth, Automated computer analysis of radiographic images. Radiology **83**(6), 1029–1034 (1964). https://doi.org/10.1148/83.6.1029
8. H.C. Becker, W.J. Nettleton, P.H. Meyers, J.W. Sweeney, C.M. Nice, Digital computer determination of a medical diagnostic index directly from chest X-ray images. IEEE Trans. Biomed. Eng. **11(3)**, 67–72 (1964). https://doi.org/10.1109/TBME.1964.4502309
9. G.S. Lodwick, T.E. Keats, J.P. Dorst, The coding of roentgen images for computer analysis as applied to lung cancer. Radiology **81**(2), 185–200 (1963) . https://doi.org/10.1148/81.2.185
10. H.P. Chan, K. Doi, S. Galhotra, C.J. Vyborny, H. MacMahon, P.M. Jokich, Image feature analysis and computer-aided diagnosis in digital radiography. I. Automated detection of microcalcifications in mammography. Med. Phy. **14**(4), 538–548 (1987) . https://doi.org/10.1118/1.596065
11. M.L. Giger, K. Doi, H. MacMahon, Image feature analysis and computer-aided diagnosis in digital radiography. 3. Automated detection of nodules in peripheral lung fields. Med. Phys. **15**(2), 158–166 (1988) . https://doi.org/10.1118/1.596247
12. K. Kanazawa, Y. Kawata, N. Niki, et al., Computer-aided diagnosis for pulmonary nodules based on helical CT images. Comput. Med. Imaging Graph. **22** 157–167 (1998). https://doi.org/10.1016/S0895-6111(98)00017-2
13. C. Abe, C.E. Kahn, K. Doi, S. Katsuragawa, Computer-aided detection of diffuse liver-disease in ultrasound images. Invest Radiol. **27**, 71–77 (1992). https://doi.org/10.1097/00004424-199201000-00015
14. K. Kourou, T.P. Exarchos, K.P. Exarchos, M.V. Karamouzis, D.I. Fotiadis, Machine learning applications in cancer prognosis and prediction. Comput. Struct. Biotechnol. J. **13**, 8–17 (2015). https://doi.org/10.1016/j.csbj.2014.11.005
15. G.F. Cooper, C.F. Aliferis, R. Ambrosino, J. Aronis, B.G. Buchanan, R. Caruana, et al., An evaluation of machine-learning methods for predicting pneumonia mortality. Artif. Intell. Med. **9**(2), 107–138 (1997). https://doi.org/10.1016/S0933-3657(96)00367-3
16. S.Y. Kim, J. Diggans, D. Pankratz, J. Huang, M. Pagan, N. Sindy, et al., Classification of usual interstitial pneumonia in patients with interstitial lung disease: assessment of a machine learning approach using high-dimensional transcriptional data. Lancet Respir. Med. **3**(6), 473–482 (2015). https://doi.org/10.1016/S2213-2600(15)00140-X
17. R.T. Sousa, O. Marques, F.A.A. Soares, I.I. Sene Jr, L.L. de Oliveira, E.S. Spoto, Comparative performance analysis of machine learning classifiers in detection of childhood pneumonia

using chest radiographs. Procedia Comput. Sci. **18**, 2579–2582 (2013). https://doi.org/10.1016/j.procs.2013.05.444

18. O. Salem, A. Guerassimov, A. Mehaoua, A. Marcus, B. Furht, Anomaly detection in medical wireless sensor networks using SVM and linear regression models. Int. J. E-Health Med. Commun. **5**(1), 20–45 (2014). https://doi.org/10.4018/ijehmc.2014010102
19. P. Rajpurkar, J. Irvin, K. Zhu, B. Yang, H. Mehta, T. Duan, D. Ding, A.B. Curtis, C. Langlotz, K. Shpanskaya, M.P. Lungren, A.Y. Ng, CheXNet: Radiologist-Level Pneumonia Detection on Chest X-Rays with Deep Learning (2017). https://arxiv.org/abs/1711.05225. Cited 12 Aug 2020
20. X. Wang, Y. Peng, L. Lu, Z. Lu, M. Bagheri, R. Summers, ChestX-ray8: hospital-scale chest X-ray database and benchmarks on weakly-supervised classification and localization of common thorax diseases, in *Proceedings of CVPR* (2017), pp. 3462–3471
21. J. Deng, W. Dong, R. Socher, L.J. Li, K. Li, L. Fei-Fei, Imagenet: A large-scale hierarchical image database, in *2009 IEEE Conference on Computer Vision and Pattern Recognition* (2009), pp. 248–255. https://doi.org/10.1109/CVPR.2009.5206848
22. A. Mangal, S. Kalia, H. Rajgopal, K. Rangarajan, V. Namboodiri, S. Banerjee, C. Arora, CovidAID: COVID-19 Detection Using Chest X-Ray (2020). https://arxiv.org/abs/2004.09803. Cited 11 Aug 2020
23. K. Hammoudi, H. Benhabiles, M. Melkemi, F. Dornaika, I. Arganda-Carreras, D. Collard, A. Scherpereel, Deep Learning on Chest X-ray images to Detect and Evaluate Pneumonia Cases at the Era of COVID-19 (2020). https://hal.archives-ouvertes.fr/hal-025533605. Cited 11 Aug 2020
24. L. Wang, A. Wong, COVID-Net: A Tailored Deep Convolutional Neural Network Design for Detection of COVID-19 Cases from Chest X-Ray Images (2020). https://arxiv.org/abs/2003.09871. Cited 12 Aug 2020
25. A.I. Khan, J.L. Shah, M.M. Bhat, Coronet: A deep neural network for detection and diagnosis of COVID-19 from chest X-ray images. Comput. Methods Programs Biomed. **196**, 105581 (2020) . https://doi.org/10.1016/j.cmpb.2020.105581
26. E.E.D. Hemdan, M.A. Shouman, M.E. Karar, COVIDX-Net: A framework of deep learning classifiers to diagnose COVID-19 in X-ray images (2020). https://arxiv.org/abs/2003.11055. Cited 12 Aug 2020
27. K. He, X. Zhang, S. Ren, J. Sun, Identity mappings in deep residual networks, in *European Conference on Computer Vision* (Springer, Cham, 2020), pp. 630–645. https://arxiv.org/abs/1603.05027. Cited 10 Aug 2020
28. C. Szegedy, S. Ioffe, V. Vanhoucke, A.A. Alemi, Inception-v4, inception-resnet and the impact of residual connections on learning, in *Thirty-First AAAI Conference on Artificial Intelligence* (2017). https://arxiv.org/abs/1602.07261. Cited 10 Aug 2020
29. M. Sandler, A. Howard, M. Zhu, A. Zhmoginov, L.C. Chen, Mobilenetv2: Inverted residuals and linear bottlenecks, in *Proceedings of the IEEE Conference on Computer Vision and Pattern Recognition* (2018), pp. 4510–4520. https://arxiv.org/abs/1801.04381. Cited 10 Aug 2020
30. I.D. Apostolopoulos, T.A. Mpesiana, Covid-19: automatic detection from X-ray images utilizing transfer learning with convolutional neural networks. Physic. Eng. Sci. Med. **43** 635–640 (2020) . https://doi.org/10.1007/s13246-020-00865-4
31. A. Narin, C. Kaya, Z. Pamuk, Automatic detection of coronavirus disease (COVID-19) using X-ray images and deep convolutional neural networks (2020). https://arxiv.org/abs/2003.10849. Cited 12 Aug 2020
32. K. He, X. Zhang, S. Ren, J. Sun, Deep residual learning for image recognition, in *Proceedings of the IEEE Conference on Computer Vision and Pattern Recognition* (2016), pp. 770–778. https://arxiv.org/abs/1512.03385. Cited 10 Aug 2020
33. H. Wang, Y. Xia, Chestnet: A deep neural network for classification of thoracic diseases on chest radiography (2018). https://arxiv.org/abs/1807.03058. Cited 13 Aug 2020
34. A. Haghanifar, M.M. Majdabadi, S. Ko, COVID-CXNet: Detecting COVID-19 in Frontal Chest X-ray Images using Deep Learning (2020). https://arxiv.org/abs/2006.13807. Cited 13 Aug 2020

35. M. Ahishali, A. Degerli, M. Yamac, S. Kiranyaz, M.E. Chowdhury, K. Hameed, T. Hamid, R. Mazhar, M. Gabbouj, A Comparative Study on Early Detection of COVID-19 from Chest X-Ray Images (2020). https://arxiv.org/abs/2006.05332. Cited 7 Aug 2020
36. K. Elasnaoui, Y. Chawki, Using X-ray images and deep learning for automated detection of coronavirus disease. J. Biomol. Struct. Dyn. 1–22 (2020) . https://doi.org/10.1080/07391102.2020.1767212
37. D.S. Kermany, K. Zhang, M. Goldbaum, Labeled optical coherence tomography (Oct) and chest X-ray images for classification. Mendeley Data (2018) . https://doi.org/10.17632/rscbjbr9sj.2
38. K. El Asnaoui, Y. Chawki, A. Idri, Automated methods for detection and classification pneumonia based on X-ray images using deep learning (2020). https://arxiv.org/abs/2003.14363. Cited 13 Aug 2020

Index

L. Garg et al. (eds.), *Healthcare Informatics for Fighting COVID-19 and Future Epidemics*, EAI/Springer Innovations in Communication and Computing,
https://doi.org/10.1007/978-3-030-72752-9

D

E